CBT FOR CHILDREN AND ADOLESCENTS WITH HIGH-FUNCTIONING AUTISM SPECTRUM DISORDERS

CBT for Children and Adolescents with High-Functioning Autism Spectrum Disorders

edited by
ANGELA SCARPA
SUSAN WILLIAMS WHITE
TONY ATTWOOD

THE GUILFORD PRESS
New York   London

© 2013 The Guilford Press
A Division of Guilford Publications, Inc.
370 Seventh Avenue, Suite 1200, New York, NY 10001
www.guilford.com

Paperback edition 2016

Printed in the United States of America

This book is printed on acid-free paper.

Last digit is print number: 9 8 7 6 5

The authors have checked with sources believed to be reliable in their efforts to provide information that is complete and generally in accord with the standards of practice that are accepted at the time of publication. However, in view of the possibility of human error or changes in behavioral, mental health, or medical sciences, neither the author, nor the editors and publisher, nor any other party who has been involved in the preparation or publication of this work warrants that the information contained herein is in every respect accurate or complete, and they are not responsible for any errors or omissions or the results obtained from the use of such information. Readers are encouraged to confirm the information contained in this book with other sources.

Library of Congress Cataloging-in-Publication Data

CBT for children and adolescents with high-functioning autism spectrum disorders /
edited by Angela Scarpa, Susan Williams White, Tony Attwood.
    pages cm
Includes bibliographical references and index.
ISBN 978-1-4625-1048-1 (hardcover : alk. paper)
ISBN 978-1-4625-2700-7 (paperback : alk. paper)
1. Children with autism spectrum disorders—Rehabilitation.   2. Autistic children—
Rehabilitation.   3. Cognitive therapy for children.   4. Cognitive therapy for
teenagers.   I. Scarpa, Angela, editor of compilation.   II. White, Susan Williams,
editor of compilation.   III. Attwood, Tony, editor of compilation.   IV. Title:
Cognitive-behavioral therapy for children and adolescents with high-functioning
autism spectrum disorders.
RJ506.A9C397 2013
618.92′85882—dc23
                                                                        2013017187

To my son Hugh, who is my inspiration
for this volume,
and to my other children,
Emilia, Sal, and Dan, and my husband, Bruce,
for their unending support and love

To my clients, for the privilege of knowing you
—A. S.

To the clients who've taught me so much
—S. W. W.

To my inspiring clients, colleagues,
and family members
—T. A.

About the Editors

Angela Scarpa, PhD, is Associate Professor of Psychology at Virginia Polytechnic Institute and State University (Virginia Tech), founder and codirector of the Virginia Tech Autism Clinic, and director of the Virginia Tech Center for Autism Research. She is a clinical psychologist whose research and practice focus on the mental health of children, adolescents, and young adults with autism spectrum disorders (ASD). Dr. Scarpa is coauthor (with Anthony Wells and Tony Attwood) of *Exploring Feelings for Young Children with High-Functioning Autism or Asperger's Disorder: The STAMP Treatment Manual.*

Susan Williams White, PhD, is Assistant Professor of Psychology at Virginia Tech and codirector of the Virginia Tech Autism Clinic. She is a clinical psychologist specializing in the treatment of people affected by neurodevelopmental disorders such as ASD. Dr. White has a special interest in interventions for social deficits and co-occurring psychiatric problems, such as anxiety in individuals with ASD, and exploration of transdiagnostic processes such as emotional and behavioral self-regulation. She is the author of *Social Skills Training for Children with Asperger Syndrome and High-Functioning Autism.*

Tony Attwood, PhD, is a clinical psychologist and Chairperson of the Minds and Hearts Clinic in Brisbane, Australia, and Adjunct Professor at Griffith University in Queensland. With over 35 years of clinical experience, he is considered a leading international expert in the field. His publications include *The Complete Guide to Asperger's Syndrome* and *Asperger's Syndrome: A Guide for Parents and Professionals.*

Contributors

Tony Attwood, PhD, Minds and Hearts Clinic, Brisbane, Queensland, Australia

Nirit Bauminger-Zviely, PhD, Graduate Program in Special Education, School of Education, Bar-Ilan University, Ramat-Gan, Israel

Renae Beaumont, PhD, Social Skills Training Institute, Queensland, Australia

Audrey Blakeley-Smith, PhD, JFK Partners, Anschutz Medical Campus, School of Medicine, University of Colorado, Aurora, Colorado

Shulamite A. Green, MA, Department of Psychology, University of California at Los Angeles, Los Angeles, California

Isabelle Hénault, PhD, Department of Psychology, University of Québec, Montréal, Québec, Canada

Gloria K. Lee, PhD, Department of Counseling, School of Educational Psychology, University at Buffalo, The State University of New York, Buffalo, New York

Christopher Lopata, PsyD, Institute for Autism Research, Canisius College, Buffalo, New York

Jill Lorenzi, MS, Department of Psychology, Virginia Polytechnic Institute and State University, Blacksburg, Virginia

Carla A. Mazefsky, PhD, Department of Psychiatry, University of Pittsburgh School of Medicine, Pittsburgh, Pennsylvania

Thomas H. Ollendick, PhD, Department of Psychology, Virginia Polytechnic Institute and State University, Blacksburg, Virginia

Judy Reaven, PhD, JFK Partners, Anschutz Medical Campus, School of Medicine, University of Colorado, Aurora, Colorado

Nuri Reyes, MS, Department of Psychology, Virginia Polytechnic Institute and State University, Blacksburg, Virginia

Lawrence Scahill, MSN, PhD, Marcus Autism Center, Emory University, Atlanta, Georgia

Angela Scarpa, PhD, Department of Psychology, Virginia Polytechnic Institute and State University, Blacksburg, Virginia

Kate Sofronoff, PhD, School of Psychology, University of Queensland, St. Lucia, Brisbane, Australia

Marcus L. Thomeer, PhD, Institute for Autism Research, Canisius College, Buffalo, New York

Martin A. Volker, PhD, Department of Counseling, School of Educational Psychology, University at Buffalo, The State University of New York, Buffalo, New York

Susan Williams White, PhD, Department of Psychology, Virginia Polytechnic Institute and State University, Blacksburg, Virginia

Jeffrey J. Wood, PhD, Division of Human Development and Psychology, University of California at Los Angeles, Los Angeles, California

Preface and Acknowledgments

The goal of this book is to provide scientists, practitioners, and students with a single-source overview of promising interventions that use a psychosocial approach to teach cognitive and behavioral skills to children and adolescents with high-functioning autism spectrum disorders (HFASD), including disorders formerly referred to as autistic disorder, Asperger syndrome, and pervasive developmental disorder not otherwise specified. The growing body of research on the effective application of cognitive-behavioral therapy (CBT) to treat children and adolescents with HFASD prompted our conceptualization of this resource. While behavioral therapies for HFASD have been used and recommended for decades, the addition of cognitive components has only recently come to this stage. The inclusion of both cognitive and behavioral strategies seems especially helpful for youth with HFASD who have no concurrent cognitive or intellectual impairment. Often, these individuals can use their tendency toward logical thinking to evaluate biases or assumptions that also affect their feelings and behaviors, and they can learn new ways to understand and monitor these thoughts, feelings, and actions.

The timing of this book coincides with the publication of the DSM-5 (American Psychiatric Association, 2013), thus necessitating some change in diagnostic labels. In this book, we aim to be consistent with the current nosology provided in the DSM-5. In the DSM-5 former labels of autistic disorder, Asperger's disorder, and pervasive developmental disorder are subsumed under the overall label of Autism Spectrum Disorder (ASD), and the presence of co-occurring intellectual impairment is listed as a specifier. In the extant research, individuals with ASD and no co-occurring intellectual impairment are often referred to as having HFASD. To be consistent with this research and the DSM-5, we will use the following terminology:

HFASD (to refer to ASD with no intellectual disability), ASD with intellectual impairment (to refer to ASD in the presence of intellectual impairment), and ASD (to refer to the broad spectrum, regardless of intellectual ability). However, there may be times when chapter authors refer to published work on samples with former diagnostic labels (e.g., autistic disorder, Asperger's disorder), and we may use those labels as needed in order to accurately represent the research.

For lack of better terminology, in this book we aim to address interventions for the population of children and adolescents with HFASD, meaning that they have a diagnostic label of ASD and are not globally intellectually impaired. Nonetheless, it is clear that these youth are not "high-functioning" in every domain, and indeed are often exceedingly poor in adaptive functioning. In other words, these children and adolescents may do well in terms of assessed intellectual ability, and can sometimes function quite well academically or in terms of their knowledge base, but they still may not maintain friendships or meaningful age-appropriate relationships; they may be removed from school or may get in legal troubles; and later in life, they may not be able to get or keep a job. Common difficulties in living and behavioral problems frequently seen in this population that get in the way of their adaptive functioning and quality of life include mood/anxiety and behavior problems, social skills deficits, and concerns about intimacy and sexuality. As such, these specific areas of concern are targeted in this book.

Despite the prevalence of these specific problems in people with HFASD, to date, no treatments for them are designated as "well established," or even "probably efficacious" according to the standards put forward by the 1995 American Psychological Association (APA) Task Force on Promotion and Dissemination of Psychological Procedures. Therefore, this book is the first to specify in one volume currently available treatments that are likely to achieve such status in the future. A treatment is considered "promising" if there is at least one empirical study supporting its efficacy, based on 1995 APA Task Force criteria. More specifically, to be included in this book, there needs to be at least one study showing efficacy of the treatment in either a randomized clinical trial (RCT; with at least a wait-list or no-treatment control condition) or in a small series ($n > 3$) of well-controlled (i.e., through using multiple-baseline, reversal, or alternating-treatment designs) single-case experiments. Pilot or preliminary studies with less stringent criteria were also considered for some understudied areas (e.g., affection, sexuality). Chambless and Hollon (1998) have suggested that findings from such studies are promising and would receive a label of "possibly efficacious" pending replication. In other words, although these interventions show some initial evidence of efficacy, they require additional objective verification. The chapters of this volume demonstrate a broad range of treatment intensity (e.g., from weekly outpatient therapy to intensive, all-day programs) as well as research design (e.g., preliminary open trials to RCTs with active comparators). Our hope is that this compilation of CBT interventions will spur additional work and research in this exciting and encouraging field.

To this end, the psychosocial treatments that were chosen are manualized, brief, and easily transported to practice. The treatments address difficulties related to anxiety, aggression/behavior problems, and social competence in youth with HFASD. A section addressing sexuality/affection in young people with high-functioning ASD is included, because this area is being recognized as an increasingly important and unaddressed need. The psychosocial interventions in this book draw heavily on the cognitive-behavioral approach to therapy, which emphasizes the identification and modification of thought patterns/processes and teaches concrete behavioral skills that can improve functioning. While relying heavily on CBT, however, other modalities are sometimes included as supplements to the treatment (e.g., ecological models described by Bauminger-Zviely in Chapter 10) or may involve a very specific tool (e.g., computer-based instruction described by Beaumont & Sofronoff in Chapter 8) to teach new thoughts or skills.

Part I of the book addresses theoretical issues related to the use of cognitive-behavioral interventions in the HFASD population, including the general principles of CBT (Chapter 1, by Scarpa & Lorenzi), how CBT may need to be modified to take into account the special needs of children with HFASD (Chapter 2, by Attwood & Scarpa), and the roles of assessment and conceptualization in guiding treatment for this population (Chapter 3, by Mazefsky & White). Part II then focuses on CBT to address anxiety and behavior problems in HFASD (Chapters 4–7). Chapter 4, by Wood and Green, focuses on individual treatment of anxiety in school-age children with HFASD that includes a parent training component and additional school involvement. Chapter 5, by Reaven and Blakely-Smith, further discusses the importance of including parents as part and parcel of the treatment program for anxiety in youth with HFASD. In Chapter 6, by White, Scahill, and Ollendick, the bidirectional relationship between social skills and anxiety is expanded upon, and its treatment in adolescents with HFASD is reviewed using an integrated individual and group therapy format. Anxiety and behavior problems as a result of skills deficits and cognitive biases in stressful situations are both targeted in the treatment described in Chapter 7, by Scarpa, Reyes, and Attwood, using a group format that is developmentally adapted for younger children with HFASD.

Part III emphasizes CBT for improving social competence (Chapters 8–10), a core impairment of ASD. Chapter 8, by Beaumont and Sofronoff, describes a novel computer-assisted intervention for school-age children with high-functioning ASD that is supplemented with groups and school involvement to address issues of social understanding. Chapter 9, by Lopata, Thomeer, Volker, and Lee, reviews the development of an intensive manualized summer group treatment program for improving specific social skill deficits in 7- to 12-year-old children with ASD. Chapter 10, by Bauminger-Zviely, expands on the combination of social understanding and social performance deficits and discusses a treatment that addresses both components in an ecological model.

Part IV of this volume is devoted to the emerging area of affection and sexuality in youth with ASD. While Chapter 11, by Attwood, focuses on affection more broadly as it applies to family, friends, and romantic partners, Chapter 12, by Hénault, targets issues directly related to sexuality and sex education in adolescents with high-functioning ASD.

Part V concludes the book with a chapter by the editors that synthesizes the knowledge to date and suggests areas of future direction.

All chapters follow a similar format in order to simplify comparison across programs. Specifically, chapter contributors were asked to provide historical background and significance of the treatment, practical considerations, an overview of the sessions, research to date on the treatment, and future directions. It is our hope that this format will make the information accessible to all readers, including scientists, professionals, and students. We also hope this format will provide the reader with enough information to understand the basic premise and practicalities of each program as a point of reference, while not overwhelming with too much detail.

It has been truly a pleasure to prepare this edited volume and to sense the passion of clinical scientists and practicing clinicians alike for using CBT in a steadily growing portion of the youth with ASD in need of novel treatments to address a specific combination of abilities and deficits. The number of CBT treatments for people with ASD has risen, even since we began to compile this volume, and the research support continues to develop. In addition to medical and pharmacological treatments for ASD, psychosocial treatments are critical to addressing difficulties that impair adaptive functioning in daily life. We believe that CBT, especially when provided early in childhood and adolescence, can halt a cycle of escalating difficulties and distress that could otherwise impair the quality of life of individuals with ASD and their families. We hope our optimism is passed on to all of our readers.

*   *   *

Before ending, we would like to acknowledge and thank the many people who contributed to this volume. We thank all the chapter authors for so graciously describing their programs, and for all the time and energy they put into their research programs to better the lives of affected individuals with ASD. We acknowledge the support of our respective universities and workplaces for permitting us the time and resources to complete this work. We thank our families for supporting us through our editing, despite having to give up some nights and weekends, and for being such a source of happiness. We thank Tom Ollendick for his mentoring and guidance. At The Guilford Press, we thank Kitty Moore for encouraging the development of this volume and for her helpful suggestions to improve the quality of topics and contributors, Sawitree Somburanakul for seeing this book through its preproduction stages, and all the Guilford staff members who saw this book through to completion. We could not have completed this effort without all of you. Most importantly, we thank all of the families and youth with ASD who have allowed us the opportunity and the genuine privilege to work with them and get to know them. This book is dedicated to all of you!

ANGELA SCARPA
SUSAN WILLIAMS WHITE
TONY ATTWOOD

REFERENCE

Chambless, D. L., & Hollon, S. D. (1998). Defining empirically supported therapies. *Journal of Consulting and Clinical Psychology, 66,* 7–18.

Contents

PART I. THEORETICAL BACKGROUND

1. **Cognitive-Behavioral Therapy with Children
   and Adolescents: History and Principles**   3
   Angela Scarpa and Jill Lorenzi

   Definition and Guiding Principles of CBT 4
   Philosophical Roots of CBT 5
   Historical Bases of CBT 7
   Strategies Used in CBT 10
   CBT with Children and Adolescents 12
   Developmental Modifications Needed in CBT 13

2. **Modifications of Cognitive-Behavioral Therapy
   for Children and Adolescents with High-Functioning
   ASD and Their Common Difficulties**   27
   Tony Attwood and Angela Scarpa

   Learning Profile Associated with ASD 29
   Language Profile Associated with ASD 36
   Interpersonal and Social Abilities Associated with ASD 37
   Sensory Profile Associated with ASD 38
   Additional Aspects That May Be Helpful in a CBT Program 39
   Concluding Comments 41

3. **The Role of Assessment in Guiding Treatment
   Planning for Youth with ASD**   45
   Carla A. Mazefsky and Susan Williams White

   Choosing and Administering Measures 46
   Assessment Purpose 47
   Case Example: Assessment and Conceptualization
   for CBT 60
   Summary 63

PART II. ANXIETY AND BEHAVIOR PROBLEMS

4. Cognitive-Behavioral Therapy for Anxiety Disorders   73
in Youth with ASD: Emotional, Adaptive,
and Social Outcomes
Shulamite A. Green and Jeffrey J. Wood

     Historical Background and Significance of the Treatment   73
     Practical Considerations in Implementing CBT with
     Children with ASD   76
     BIACA: Overview of Sessions   79
     Research to Date on the Treatment   86
     Future Directions   91

5. Parental Involvement in Treating Anxiety in Youth   97
with High-Functioning ASD
Judy Reaven and Audrey Blakeley-Smith

     Historical Background and Significance of the Treatment   97
     Practical Considerations   107
     FYF: Session by Session   112
     Research to Date on the Treatment   115
     Conclusions and Future Directions   116

6. Multimodal Treatment for Anxiety and Social Skills   123
Difficulties in Adolescents on the Autism Spectrum
Susan Williams White, Lawrence Scahill,
and Thomas H. Ollendick

     Historical Background and Significance of the Treatment   124
     Practical Considerations: Background and Theoretical
     Basis for MASSI   128
     Overview of Sessions   131
     Research to Date on the Treatment   136
     Future Directions   137
     Case Example   138
     Conclusion   140

7. Cognitive-Behavioral Therapy for Stress and Anger   147
Management in Young Children with ASD:
The Exploring Feelings Program
Angela Scarpa, Nuri Reyes, and Tony Attwood

     Historical Background and Significance of the Treatment   148
     The Exploring Feelings Intervention for Emotion Regulation
     in Children with High-Functioning ASD   151

Practical Considerations for Exploring Feelings as Adapted
in STAMP   154
Overview of STAMP Sessions   158
Research Support for the Treatment   163
Future Directions   164

PART III. SOCIAL COMPETENCE

8. Multimodal Intervention for Social Skills Training   173
in Students with High-Functioning ASD:
The Secret Agent Society
Renae Beaumont and Kate Sofronoff

Historical Background and Significance of the Treatment   173
Overview of Sessions   177
Practical Considerations   186
Research to Date on the Treatment   195
Future Directions   196

9. A Manualized Summer Program for Social Skills   199
in Children with High-Functioning ASD
Christopher Lopata, Marcus L. Thomeer,
Martin A. Volker, and Gloria K. Lee

Historical Background and Significance of the Treatment   199
Practical Considerations   204
Overview of the Manualized Summer Program for Children
with HFASD   206
Research to Date on the Manualized Summer Program
for Children with HFASD   213
Future Directions   220

10. Cognitive-Behavioral-Ecological Intervention   226
to Facilitate Social-Emotional Understanding
and Social Interaction in Youth
with High-Functioning ASD
Nirit Bauminger-Zviely

Historical Background and Significance of the Treatment   226
The Multidimensional Social Deficit in HFASD:
Social Cognition and Social Interaction   227
Multifaceted Social Interventions for HFASD   230
Cognitive-Behavioral-Ecological Intervention:
Practical Considerations and Overview of Sessions   241
Research to Date on the Treatment   245

Summary, Conclusions, and Future Directions
for School-Based Social CBT for HFASD 250

PART IV. SEXUALITY AND AFFECTION

11. Expressing and Enjoying Love and Affection: 259
A Cognitive-Behavioral Program for Children
and Adolescents with High-Functioning ASD
Tony Attwood

Historical Background and Significance of the Treatment 260
A Cognitive-Behavioral Therapy Program for Affection 267
Future Directions and Conclusions 275

12. Understanding Relationships and Sexuality   278
in Individuals with High-Functioning ASD
Isabelle Hénault

Historical Background and Significance for the Treatment 278
Practical Considerations 286
Overview of Sessions from the Sociosexual Skills
Educational Program 289
Research to Date on the Treatment 291
Future Directions 295

PART V. CONCLUDING REMARKS

13. What Do We Know about Psychosocial Interventions   303
for Youth with High-Functioning ASD,
and Where Do We Go from Here?
Susan Williams White, Angela Scarpa,
and Tony Attwood

Theoretical Grounding and Conceptualization 304
CBT for Anxiety and Behavioral Problems in ASD 306
Social Competence 308
Sexuality/Affection 311
Where Are We and Where Do We Go from Here? 312

Index   317

CBT FOR CHILDREN AND ADOLESCENTS WITH HIGH-FUNCTIONING AUTISM SPECTRUM DISORDERS

PART I

THEORETICAL BACKGROUND

1

Cognitive-Behavioral Therapy with Children and Adolescents

History and Principles

ANGELA SCARPA AND JILL LORENZI

Psychological theories are important because they offer explanations for normal and abnormal behavior that inform our understanding of the etiology and maintenance of disorders, as well as suggest possible targets of intervention. Cognitive-behavioral theory of psychopathology and its treatment form the common bases of the clinical approaches described in this book. Cognitive-behavioral therapy (CBT) is an approach that merges behavior therapy with cognitive therapy, using short-term, problem-focused cognitive and behavioral strategies based on empirical data and theory from learning and cognition. The cognitive components of CBT primarily focus on helping clients identify and change maladaptive attitudes and beliefs that subsequently change cognitive processing, emotional experiences, and problem behaviors, but CBT can also include techniques to change behavior through modifying associated responses and/or antecedents and consequences in the situation (Craske, 2010). The therapeutic process generally involves teaching and guiding the client toward more adaptive ways to think and behave, making use of both cognitive and behavioral strategies to varying degrees. While this approach historically was developed for and is traditionally used to treat adults, there is a general consensus that CBT approaches have empirical support for treating psychological disorders of childhood (e.g., Weisz & Kazdin, 2010); however, a simple downward extension from adults to children is insufficient; that is, CBT approaches for children must consider developmental issues (Ollendick, Grills, & King, 2001). The history and guiding principles for using CBT, and its application with children and adolescents, are reviewed in this chapter.

DEFINITION AND GUIDING PRINCIPLES OF CBT

According to the Association for Behavioral and Cognitive Therapies (ABCT; 2012), CBT is a class of interventions and techniques based on cognitive and behavioral theories and supported by scientific evidence (see Craske, 2010; Dobson & Dobson, 2009; Dobson, 2010, for reviews). Behavioral perspectives within CBT consider how behaviors are learned through paired associations, and cognitive perspectives within CBT emphasize the role of thinking in how we act and feel. As such, CBT is partly based on the notion that cognitions or thoughts mediate our emotional and behavioral responses, implying that it is not external events (i.e., people, situations) that cause our responses but rather our thoughts about those events. Therefore, if we change our thoughts, we can change our behaviors and feelings. In addition to assuming cognitive mediation, CBT is rooted in principles of learning theory that grew out of the experimental analysis of behavior and has applications in behavior therapy. According to this view, it is believed that all behavioral and emotional responses are learned and can therefore be "unlearned" by replacing unwanted responses with new ways of reacting. While it does not specify particular techniques, CBT does classify an array of therapies that have common principles. Five common guiding principles in CBT outlined by the ABCT include the following:

1. *Collaborative effort between client and therapist.* CBT involves collaboration between the client and the therapist, whereby the client elaborates on goals and the therapist helps the client achieve those goals. While the therapist is viewed as having the theoretical and technical expertise, the client is viewed as an expert about him- or herself who actively participates in the treatment. Clients are taught the process of therapy so that they become self-sufficient and do not need to rely on the relationship with the therapist for change to occur.

2. *Promotes self-efficacy to tolerate emotions and change behavior.* Some approaches to CBT are based on the philosophy of Stoicism (see section below on CBT's philosophical roots), which suggests that destructive emotions are often caused by errors in judgment. Stoics suggested that we can calmly accept difficult situations in our lives, since undesirable events

occur whether we are upset about them or not. In this vein, CBT encourages clients to use scientific or inductive reasoning via logic and Socratic questioning to evaluate their unwanted or upsetting thoughts, rather than basing their emotional reactions and behaviors on perceptions that may be inaccurate. Moreover, clients are taught that they can tolerate negative emotions and choose new ways to behave.

3. *Short-term and directive.* CBT is intended to be time-limited and based on achieving goals that are initially set by the client and the therapist. It is structured and directive, with an agenda of skills to be taught by the therapist that focus on helping the client to achieve his or her goals. Typically, therapists provides instruction and homework assignments (e.g., reading, journal recording, and practice) to complement what is taught in the session.

4. *Present-focused and goal-oriented.* While recognizing that current problems may have arisen from early experiences, the CBT therapist does not focus on developmental origins of behavior. Instead, CBT emphasizes things that can be done now to resolve current difficulties and achieve goals in a step-by-step fashion.

5. *Monitors progress toward goals.* Throughout CBT, progress toward goals is tracked and monitored via objective behavior as well as self-report. Consistent with the empirical approach, therapy is modified as needed if progress is not being made.

PHILOSOPHICAL ROOTS OF CBT

Aspects of CBT can be found in various philosophical schools, including Stoicism, the Socratic method, and constructivist epistemology (i.e., the philosophy of what can be known), among others. Although CBT theorists do not adhere to all the components of these philosophies, some conceptual and methodological themes are shared with today's CBT.

Stoicism is a school of Hellenistic philosophy that was founded by Zeno of Citium in the third century B.C.E.. CBT has some commonalities with the ethical and epistemological considerations noted in Stoicism concerning virtue, destructive emotions, and reason. Specifically, Stoics believed that knowledge could only be obtained through the use of reason. While they believed in a true external reality that stimulated the senses and left an impression (or copy) on the mind, they stated that the mind then has the ability to judge the impression, thereby approving or rejecting it. It is through this process that a person achieves comprehension of reality.

According to Stoic philosophers, destructive emotions resulted from errors in judgment, whereas a person who retained the use of reason and clear unbiased thinking could be free from negative emotions. This notion is exemplified in a quote credited to Marcus Aurelius, a philosopher in the late Stoic phase: "If thou are pained by an external thing, it is not this thing that disturbs thee, but thine own judgment about it" (as cited in Ingram & Siegle, 2010, p. 79). In this way, emotions could be transformed through clear judgment and inner calm. The notion of a "Stoic calm" suggests that one can remain calm in the face of positive or negative external events and maintain emotional detachment from reality, over which one has no direct control. Healthy methods used to achieve this state of calmness include logic, self-dialogue, reflection on current problems and possible solutions, and training attention and concentration to stay in the present moment. These methods have direct parallels to strategies used in modern-day CBT (Robertson, 2010), which also include recent conceptualizations of mindfulness (i.e., nonjudgmental awareness) and acceptance (i.e., being open to subjective experiences, including emotions) of negative emotions (Fruzzetti & Erikson, 2010). These ideas suggest that we can objectively acknowledge and accept distressing situations without added suffering over and above the objective reality.

Zeno's Stoic ideas developed from those of the Cynics, an ancient school of Greek philosophers who rejected conventional desires for wealth, power, health, and fame by living simple lives, free from all possessions. They, too, emphasized self-discipline through reasoning and believed that suffering results from false judgments of what is truly valuable in this world by succumbing to societal conventions and customs. The Cynics' founder, who had been a student of Socrates, thus may be the link through which the Stoics adopted logic as a method to achieve knowledge. Credited as one of the founding fathers of Western philosophy, Socrates is probably best known for his legacy of the Socratic method of questioning, which is a form of debate in which viewpoints are expressed and elaborated through asking and answering a series of questions. It involves a negative form of hypothesis testing (i.e., disproving the null, or default, hypothesis or supposition). By identifying and eliminating hypotheses that lead to contradictions of the original belief, beliefs become clearer and can lead to better hypotheses. Based on his own belief that he had no true wisdom, Socrates used this technique as a method to confirm his ignorance and the ignorance of others. As with most hypothesis testing in the scientific method, this form of logic is thought to promote critical thinking and to clarify ideas that encourage more insight into the current issue of debate. The Socratic method of questioning has been adopted in many forms of CBT as a way to challenge potentially inaccurate belief systems by helping clients to examine their own beliefs and the validity of those beliefs rather than automatically accepting their beliefs as fact.

Finally, Mahoney (1988) suggests that most of the philosophical foundations of CBT can be found in *constructivist epistemology*, which maintains that reality is simply a social construction that exists only as a function of the observer who constructs it. Note that this view is in contrast, however, to Stoic epistemology, which maintains that knowledge is based in actual sense experiences from which we then make a judgment. Nonetheless, constructivism holds the view that the only reality we can know is that which is represented in our own minds; therefore, knowledge is always a human construction. This notion, developed in reaction to associationist principles suggesting that humans passively gather information from the environment, instead maintains that humans actively construct and give meaning to their own experiences. While this view is extreme, it is consistent with cognitive therapies that focus exclusively on challenging the way clients make sense out of the events that occur in their lives.

HISTORICAL BASES OF CBT

The historical roots of CBT grew out of behavior therapy that developed in the early 20th century and cognitive therapy in the 1950s and 1960s, which later merged. Therefore, whereas some CBT clinicians and researchers are more behaviorally oriented, others are more cognitively oriented, and still others try to achieve a more balanced integration (Harwood, Beutler, & Charvat, 2010).

Behavior therapy grew out of dissatisfaction with the psychoanalytic approaches to psychotherapy at that time, which were viewed as nonscientific, in that many of the concepts were not clearly observable or measurable. In contrast, principles of learning theory, through the experimental analysis of behavior, suggested new scientifically grounded approaches that could be applied to change behavior. This new, empirically guided approach led to behavior therapy (or applied behavior analysis).

Especially influential were the works of Ivan Pavlov on classical (respondent) conditioning, and B. F. Skinner on operant (instrumental) conditioning (see Craske, 2010, for a review). *Classical conditioning* refers to the paired association between a previously neutral stimulus and an evocative (or unconditioned) stimulus, so that the neutral stimulus comes to evoke the same response as the unconditioned stimulus. For example, a person may come to fear and avoid driving a car after an automobile accident, because the car (i.e., previously neutral, but now a conditioned stimulus) has become associated with trauma (i.e., unconditioned response) and now automatically evokes a fear response (i.e., conditioned response). Based on this experimental work on classical conditioning in animals, Watson and Rayner (1920), through their famous case study of "Little Albert," showed that a phobia can be classically conditioned in humans. Jones (1924) was possibly the first to use the behavioral approach to eliminate fears in children. Later, Wolpe (1958) was able to demonstrate that human anxiety can be reduced through repeatedly pairing graduated exposure to the feared image and a relaxation response (using progressive muscle relaxation developed by Jacobson, 1938). This counterconditioning technique became known as *systematic desensitization* and was the initial basis for many of the exposure-based therapies we use today in the treatment of anxiety disorders, although cognitive exposure-based therapies question the need for relaxation during the exposure and instead emphasize mastery of the distress and use of coping skills (e.g., Francis & Beidel, 1995; Marks, 1975, as cited in Kendall, 2012).

Instrumental conditioning (Thorndike, 1898; Skinner, 1938) refers to the modification of behavior based upon its consequences. In this model, behavior is thought to operate on its environment based on the likelihood of receiving certain consequences, and is therefore also referred to as *operant conditioning*. *Reinforcers* are consequences that increase the likelihood of a response, while *punishers* are consequences that decrease the likelihood of a response. For example, if a compulsive behavior, such as hand washing, is followed by anxiety reduction, the hand-washing behavior is likely to increase in frequency. On the other hand, if oppositional behavior from a child is followed by the removal of a privilege, that behavior is less likely to occur again. Skinner (1953) directly translated principles of instrumental conditioning into behavior modification techniques for humans, suggesting that undesirable behaviors could be extinguished and desirable behaviors could be taught and shaped via varying schedules of reinforcement.

Both classical and instrumental approaches to behavior therapy assumed that abnormal behaviors result from faulty learning, which can be modified with behavioral procedures. The growth and popularity of behavior modification techniques was strengthened via the influential work of Hans Eysenck (1952, 1960), who challenged traditional psychoanalytic therapy and argued that the only effective therapies to date were based on learning theory (e.g., systematic desensitization and instrumental procedures).

Later, during the later 1960s, it was becoming more apparent that the radical behaviorist approach was not comprehensive enough to explain behavior fully. Bandura's (1965, 1969) work on vicarious learning suggested that behavior could be learned without direct experience, and the "cognitive revolution" movement in psychology established information processing as a mediating factor in behavior (Dobson & Dozois, 2010). In general, research was pointing to the role of cognitive variables as important influences on human behavior, and it became clear that cognitive phenomena needed to be incorporated into behavioral theory. In his social learning theory, Bandura (1973) proposed that motivation was influenced by cognitive factors, including thinking about future consequences, setting goals, and engaging in self-monitoring and self-evaluation. One specific cognitive mediator that he proposed was *self-efficacy*, the confidence that one's ability to execute a behavior would achieve certain outcomes (Bandura, 1977). In Bandura's model of *reciprocal determinism*, self-efficacy expectations determine the choice of, and persistence in, certain behaviors.

As the notion of cognitive mediation became more popular, and the work of researchers such as Lazarus and colleagues identified the importance of cognitive appraisal in outcomes such as anxiety (Lazarus, 1966; Lazarus & Averill, 1972; Lazarus & Folkman, 1984), cognitive therapy approaches emerged. The primary assumption of cognitive therapy is that thoughts determine mood and behavior; therefore, changing dysfunctional thoughts can lead to behavior change. Two influential leaders in the cognitive therapy movement were Albert Ellis and Aaron Beck. Ellis's (1962) rational-emotive behavior therapy proposed that the impact of events on people is determined by their interpretations of those events. In his ABC model, *activating events* (A) trigger certain *beliefs* (B) that lead to the emotional or behavioral *consequences* (C) in reaction to the event. Specifically, ideas that were "irrational," or unlikely to be supported or confirmed, would lead to negative emotional reactions to adverse events. These irrational beliefs become automatic through repeated use and need to be challenged.

Similarly, Beck (1972) proposed that faulty thinking leads to emotional distress. He initially applied his theory to the conceptualization and treatment of depression. Specifically, he suggested that cognitive biases (e.g., minimizing the positive) can prevent individuals from benefiting emotionally from reinforcement. In addition, negative beliefs about the self (e.g., personalizing or catastrophizing) can interfere with the performance of social skills needed to obtain reinforcement from others. In both cases, the lack of perceived reinforcement exacerbates depressive thoughts and feelings. One assumption of Beck's model is that the negative beliefs reflect underlying schemas, or belief systems, that color the way people perceive themselves, others, and the future, and thereby influence their reactions to negative events. His model of cognitive therapy therefore seeks to clarify information that competes with the dysfunctional schema and provides new, adaptive, compensatory schema.

Overall, behavioral and cognitive therapies share an emphasis on empirical science, an assumption that behavior is learned, and a present-oriented focus on behavior change. Modern CBT merges these two approaches to provide efficient, time-limited therapy that targets specific, typically circumscribed problems. Therefore, depending on the problem being addressed and the expertise of the clinician, some CBTs may emphasize behavioral strategies, others may emphasize cognitive strategies, while still others may represent a blend or combination of both.

STRATEGIES USED IN CBT

In this new era of empirically informed practice, CBT has become widely adopted as the treatment of choice by clinicians. Stewart and Chambless (2007) report, for example, that 45.4% of randomly surveyed American Psychological Association (APA) members labeled themselves as holding a CBT orientation, compared to 21.9% endorsing psychodynamic, 19.8% eclectic, 4.4% humanistic, 3.9% family systems, and 4.6% other orientations. The widespread use of CBT is due in part to its evidence base. Indeed, the majority of empirically supported treatments cited by Division 12 of the APA Task Force on Promotion and Dissemination of Psychological Procedures (1995), updated by Chambless and Ollendick (2001), includes cognitive, behavioral, and cognitive-behavioral therapies. As noted earlier, cognitive therapy was initially developed in the treatment of depressed adults (Beck, 1967), but CBT is currently used to treat a wide array of additional disorders and problems in adults, such as anxiety disorders, eating disorders, schizophrenia, somatoform disorders, substance use disorders, personality disorders, sexual offending, marital difficulties, and chronic pain, to name a few. CBT has also been extended for use in children and adolescents (as reported in the APA Division 53 listing for Evidence-Based Mental Health Treatment for Children and Adolescents, 2012), with appropriate developmental modifications, as described in a separate section below.

Multiple strategies may be used in CBT. Mahoney and Arnkoff (1978) divided the major CBTs into three categories: (1) cognitive restructuring, (2) coping skills therapies, and (3) problem-solving therapies. More recently, Craske (2010) also identified three categories of CBT strategies: cognitively based, skills and reinforcement based, and exposure based. In this conceptualization, while cognitive restructuring remains in its own category, coping skills and problem-solving therapies are combined into the "skills and reinforcement based" category, and exposure-based strategies are included as an additional category.

Cognitively based therapies in the cognitive restructuring category assume that maladaptive thoughts lead to negative reactions; therefore, these thought patterns are challenged, and the goal is to replace them with more appropriate and adaptive beliefs. Beck's cognitive therapy of depression and Ellis's rational-emotive behavior therapy, described earlier, are prime examples of cognitively based therapies. Craske (2010) also considers self-instruction training (SIT) to be cognitively based, in that Meichenbaum (1977) combined Ellis's model of irrational self-talk with the knowledge of typical development of internal speech and its control over behavior in children. In SIT, these internal verbalizations are viewed as a cognitive mediator of behavior, so clients are taught to use inner speech as a way to bring their behavior under their own control. In this approach, modeling, behavioral rehearsal, and cognitive rehearsal of appropriate strategies are used as primary teaching methods (Meichenbaum & Goodman, 1971).

Skills and reinforcement based CBT strategies are largely based on behavioral principles, and include teaching coping skills and problem-solving skills as general strategies to help clients cope or solve problems in a variety of situations, consistent with the idea of teaching process-oriented skills that generalize to a wide variety of problems that clients might encounter. As such, they are not specific to a particular disorder but instead target a core deficit that is believed to cut across various disorders or distress reactions. Examples of these include self-control treatment (e.g., Goldfried & Davison, 1976), stress inoculation training (Meichenbaum & Cameron, 1973), and problem-solving therapy (D'Zurilla & Nezu, 2010; Kazdin, 2010).

Systematic rational restructuring, for example, is a form of self-control treatment whereby clients are taught the process of exposing themselves to anxiety-provoking images or situations, monitoring cognitions, developing rational reevaluations, and measuring subsequent changes in anxiety levels (Goldfried & Davison, 1976). In behavioral monitoring, a strategy used in this treatment, clients are taught to observe and record their own feelings, thoughts, and behaviors as they occur, so that they can become aware of the relationships between these variables, then institute cognitive and behavioral changes. Similarly, stress inoculation training involves educating clients about the nature of stress, teaching coping skills (e.g., relaxation exercises, appropriate self-statements), and ultimately rehearsing these new skills during exposures to stressors (Meichenbaum & Cameron, 1973). In this treatment, *relaxation training* (e.g., progressive muscle relaxation or diaphragmatic breathing) and *behavioral rehearsal* (i.e., teaching skills through instruction, modeling, role play, and feedback) are two further examples of skills-based strategies. Finally, problem-solving therapy stresses the importance of learning the process of problem solving, which includes identifying problems, clarifying goals, generating possible solutions, evaluating the possible outcomes, then implementing and evaluating the solution (e.g., D'Zurilla & Nezu, 2010; Kazdin, 2010). These skills-based strategies equip clients with the tools they need to deal effectively with future stressors or difficulties. Much of the recent work in evidence-based practices is disorder- rather than treatment-based (e.g., Barlow, 2008; Weisz & Kazdin, 2010), but it is important to note that these techniques can still be incorporated throughout CBTs.

Finally, exposure-based CBT strategies are based on principles of extinction of classically conditioned responses and are mostly used to treat anxiety, although they are also sometimes used to treat substance use or eating disorders. In exposure-based therapies, clients are exposed to the feared object/situation (or object that causes cravings) repeatedly without reinforcement or avoidance, until the object/situation loses its association with the fear or craving (Francis & Beidel, 1995). *Systematic desensitization*, in which the feared object is gradually and progressively paired with a relaxation response (described earlier), is one example of an exposure-based therapy. Another example includes the technique of response prevention, often used to treat obsessive–compulsive disorder (OCD), in which the client is progressively presented with situations that evoke obsessive thoughts, but then blocked from engaging in the corresponding compulsive, avoidant behaviors (e.g., Pediatric OCD Treatment Study Team, 2004). In this manner, it is believed that the client is prevented from experiencing the compulsion's negative reinforcement, which is maintaining the anxious response. Exposure based therapies are also thought to promote change by challenging anxiety-promoting beliefs about the consequences of encountering the feared object or situation. For example, a client who fears all dogs because of the belief that any dog will bite him or her may learn through exposure to a number of friendly dogs that this belief is inaccurate.

CBT WITH CHILDREN AND ADOLESCENTS

CBT has been used to treat a number of psychological disorders or other problems, such as anxiety disorders, depression, substance abuse, anger–aggression, and eating disorders with general success (see Epp & Dobson, 2010, for a review of the evidence). Most of this work has been conducted with adult populations, but researchers using downward extensions have attempted to apply CBT to children and adolescents.

DEVELOPMENTAL MODIFICATIONS NEEDED IN CBT

Even though some have questioned the appropriateness of CBT at young ages given children's immature level of cognitive understanding, there is growing empirical support for the benefits of CBT in treating young children if developmental issues are carefully considered (Choate-Summers et al., 2008; Grave & Blissett, 2004; Ollendick et al., 2001; Southam-Gerow & Kendall, 2000). Consideration needs to be given to developmental issues related to the fact that children are dependent upon larger systems within which they are embedded and display a wide range of cognitive maturation or ability. To be sensitive to these issues, the CBT approach can be modified, for example, to include parents or other key caregivers in the treatment process, to incorporate concrete and tangible examples, to use methods that match the child's cognitive abilities, and to incorporate lessons into developmentally appropriate play routines.

Since children and adolescents are arguably more dependent upon larger systems than adults (or less self-sufficient), it is common that they are referred to treatment by adults (e.g., parents, teachers) rather than self-referred. Therefore, motivation to attend therapy is a critical component that needs to be considered in CBT with youth. For this reason, it is critical that therapists assess the child's motivation and use methods that make the treatment a generally enjoyable experience, so that the child will want to attend. In addition, it may be important to include parents in the treatment process, especially with children of younger ages or developmental levels, when parental involvement is ecologically appropriate. In adolescence, a decision needs to be made about whether it is appropriate to include parents. However, further research is needed to determine whether parental involvement is beneficial at all ages and for all disorders. Finally, parents or other caregivers may need to be included in treatment if their behavior is assessed as directly impacting the child's referral problem (e.g., harsh or ineffective parental discipline, ineffective parent–child communication, impact of parental anxiety on child). In these cases, parental behaviors may be considered targets of treatment. Child sessions that involve parents or other family members also carry the benefit of temporarily shifting the focus away from the child in order to determine how other important people in the child's life may best be able to help.

When involving families in treatment of a children, parents may consider discussing upcoming events and challenges with their children to help prepare them for difficult situations (Pahl & Barrett, 2010). Children may be better prepared for difficult situations if they can anticipate the event and have thought about what coping skills might be helpful. Parents are encouraged to focus on the positive aspects of the anticipated event and to remind children of their repertoires of coping skills.

Besides considering the optimal level of parent involvement, other social contexts must also be considered. For the most optimal benefits, children should be able to generalize acquired skills to domains beyond the therapy setting, such as at home, at school, and with friends. As the role of the peer group becomes more prominent in late childhood and early adolescence, it may become worthwhile to incorporate role plays based on typical or challenging social situations in order for children to practice some of the encounters they are likely to face in real-life situations. Themes of interpersonal relations taking on additional importance and the need for greater autonomy from parents can also be woven into therapy (Crawley, Podell, Beidas, Braswell, & Kendall, 2010).

As mentioned earlier, lack of motivation to attend therapy may often present a challenge when working with child clients. A complicating factor involved in potential lack of motivation is that children may neither see their behavior as problematic nor view their behaviors as excessive or their expectations unrealistic. They may be more likely to deny their symptoms and less likely to desire help as the potential for self-reflection continues to develop over the elementary school years. Therefore, an emphasis on psychoeducation may be more critical in the case of a child, than in the case of an adult who recognizes his or her own symptoms and desires to overcome them. This may come in the form of providing information to the child and family about the purpose for engaging in certain exercises, and by having the child summarize frequently during sessions to gauge his or her level of understanding. It may also be important to help children understand why therapy is relevant, or what about it might be motivating from the child's point of view. Child-specific motivators for attending therapy might include finding it easier to make friends following successful treatment, or experiencing less "nagging" about problem behaviors from one's parents.

Some researchers suggest that meeting more frequently than once a week is beneficial for young CBT clients. Stark, Streusand, Arora, and Patel (2012) suggest that meeting more frequently may improve the efficacy of CBT, because it helps children retain what is discussed in each session and decreases the amount of time between assigning homework and evaluating how the assignment went. Additional advantages relate to greater efficiency, in that less time is needed for review from one session to the next, rapport and cohesion can be developed more quickly, and the impact of distractions between sessions can be minimized. Therefore, semiweekly meetings may be considered an adaptation to CBT that increases accessibility for children and adolescents, although more research is needed to confirm whether this modification is essential.

Other modifications of CBT relate more to the actual developmentally appropriate method of delivery. These methods include making examples more concrete and tangible, using methods that are appropriate to the child's cognitive abilities, and incorporating lessons into play routines. Each of these strategies may help to increase the probability of successful treatment.

Using more concrete and behaviorally based examples to illustrate the benefits of therapy helps to facilitate therapeutic progress in young children, because cognitive sophistication and abstract thinking may be lacking in early elementary school children. Children and adolescents may truly need to "see it before they believe it"—whereby learning comes easier once benefits of the skills training are actually experienced. Therefore, children may benefit from more behavioral interventions (e.g., deep breathing) earlier in treatment to demonstrate the effectiveness of coping skills (e.g., Stark et al., 2012). Therapists working with a group of children with depression might initiate a fun and energizing activity, meant to create intense positive emotional engagement, to allow children to experience a boost in mood during session. Experiential learning serves as a powerful tool in proving to youngsters the effectiveness of coping skills and strategies, and demonstrating cognitive constructs in a more concrete way.

Examples from a child's own life can also help to make learning cognitive constructs more concrete. The link between thoughts and emotions can be solidified by using examples that are real-to-life and therefore easier to understand. Depending on the target of intervention, stories and videotaped vignettes may help to make abstract ideas more concrete. Particularly if the characters are easy to relate to (e.g., similar in age, same gender), child clients are more likely to imitate their appropriate behavior. For example, a videotaped vignette may show a child using appropriate anger management skills in order to demonstrate that there are alternatives other than reacting explosively in challenging situations.

Visual aids can help to make examples more concrete. For example, children may benefit from labeling a cutout of a child's body with the locations in which they feel the physical sensations of an emotional experience. Additionally, cartoons with blank thought bubbles can help to promote thinking about what another individual may be experiencing. A visual thermometer can be used to label and monitor the child's intensity of emotion. Finally, visuals can be used to document treatment progress, both within single sessions and over the course of treatment. For example, visually charting the frequency of a target behavior on a daily basis helps to make treatment progress more understandable and accessible. This modification is helpful both to remind a client what has been learned and what still remains, and to boost confidence by documenting how far a client has come.

Another important modification to the delivery of CBT involves matching delivery methods to the child or adolescent's cognitive abilities. Cognitive constructs should be labeled with more understandable terms. In many CBT programs for treating OCD in children and adolescents, it is typical for youth to be asked to give OCD a "nasty nickname" to which they can then "talk back" (March & Benton, 2006). When metaphors are used, they should be age-appropriate and simple to understand. Metaphors involving popular television characters, scenes from video games, or sports references might be applicable. For example, a child who likes Toy Story might imagine that he and his therapist are "Woody" and "Buzz," working together to defeat his OCD, which they might call "Sid" (the boy next door in the story, who set out to torture Woody, Buzz, and the other toys).

Relaxation strategies, which are common to many CBT programs, should also be taught at a developmentally appropriate level. Scripts that incorporate the notion of a "tin soldier" (tensing) and "rag doll" (relaxed) can be simpler for children and adolescents to follow than standard relaxation training language (Deblinger, Behl, & Glickman, 2012). In the initial stages of relaxation training, children and adolescents may also benefit from pictures that demonstrate the specific muscles that are to be tensed and relaxed as the sequence progresses. With practice, the need for visual aids will likely decrease. Relaxation for children should also be shorter in duration, with fewer distinctions between different muscle groups than is typical for training relaxation skills in adults (Kendall, 2012).

There are many different ways in which lessons can be incorporated into play routines. In some treatment programs, activities can even be tailored to the specific interests of the child or group of children, in order to maximize interest and engagement. As a general recommendation, creative expressions such as drawing, writing stories, dancing, and singing can be used to reinforce key concepts. For example, putting a list of coping skills to music and singing together as a group can be a fun way to help children to remember the skills at their disposal. Puppet shows can demonstrate examples of successful cognitive restructuring. Other games, such as musical chairs, "hot potato," duck–duck–goose, and board or card games (e.g., checkers, Go Fish) can be modified to include an educational component. Ideally, the educational component could, in later sessions, transition into a practical component, whereby children have the opportunity to practice skills that they have learned. For example, a game of "hot potato" in the first half of treatment could require a child to identify an emotional expression, while a similar game in the second half of treatment could require a child to find a way to turn a negative thought into a positive one. When selecting techniques, therapists may need to be sensitive to the needs and abilities of older children who may resent games or activities that they view as immature. For older children and adolescents, games such as Pictionary or Hangman can be used to reinforce key concepts. In later sessions, older children and adolescents might practice learned skills by demonstrating how they would teach the skills to a younger child.

Affective education can be enhanced in the form of games or other child-friendly activities. The ACTION program for depression recommends teaching children a simplified model of depression before encouraging them to work as "emotion detectives" to investigate the experience of the "three B's: brain, body, and behavior" (Stark, Schnoebelen, et al., 2005; Stark, Simpson, et al., 2005). Sessions may also include a soft, spongy ball that children can pass around to signal turn taking during group discussions. Analogous modifications may both better match a child's level of cognitive ability and become integrated into play-based activities.

Other forms of creative play include end-of-treatment activities whereby children can demonstrate and show pride in what they have learned. Examples include creating a television commercial or "talk show," art project, or puppet show. In teaching others what they have learned, children can become more confident in their own skills.

Research Support for CBT in Young Children

In a meta-analysis of 64 studies that used CBT to modify children's behavioral or social functioning and specifically *excluded* CBT programs that involved parents, Durlak, Fuhrman, and Lampman (1991) concluded that CBT without parental involvement was more effective for older children (i.e., 11–13 years old; effect size [ES] = 0.92) than younger children (i.e., 5–7 years old; ES = 0.57). Although this meta-analysis may seem to suggest that CBT is not effective for young children, it is important to note that the ES of 0.57 was sizable in its own right, and it was significant for younger children. Furthermore, the inclusion of parents is a critical modification needed in therapies with young children, and it is quite likely that the effects for younger children found by Durlak et al. would have been enhanced if studies involving parents had been included in the analysis. This meta-analysis, however, did not report an ES for treatment as usual (TAU) or a non-CBT treatment. However, a similar meta-analysis of CBT for anxiety disorders in children and adolescents that did not exclude studies involving parents reported an overall ES of 0.68 for CBT compared to a no-treatment group, and a small yet still significant ES of 0.27 for a CBT group versus other treatment (e.g., TAU) (Ishikawa, Okajima, Matsuoka, & Sakano, 2007).

In recent years, several studies with appropriate developmental modifications have supported the use of CBT in children as young as 3 years old. In the pediatric psychology literature, for example, Powers (1999) reviewed 13 CBT studies that included children as young as 3 years old and concluded that CBT is a well-established treatment (using Chambless et al. [1996] criteria) for coping with procedure-related pain in pediatric samples of children and adolescents. In another randomized controlled trial (RCT), Zelikovsky, Rodrique, Gidycz, and Davis (2000) found developmentally modified CBT techniques useful in teaching coping strategies and lowering distress in 3- to 7-year-old children undergoing a stressful medical procedure. Similarly, in a study of trauma-focused CBT, children ages 3–7 made improvements in posttraumatic symptoms compared to children in a wait-list control group (Scheeringa, Weems, Cohen, Amaya-Jackson, & Guthrie, 2011). Two studies targeting anxiety disorders found that 4- to 7-year-old children (Hirshfeld-Becker, Micco, Mazursky, Bruett, & Henin, 2011) and 5- to 7-year-old children (Monga, Young, & Owens, 2009) showed decreased rates of anxiety disorders after treatment compared to children in a wait-list condition. Likewise, an open pilot trial found that a modified form of CBT including parent involvement led to significant improvement on multiple rating scales in children between the ages of 3 and 7 with anxiety (Minde, Roy, Bezonsky, & Hashemi, 2010). Despite the many findings supporting CBT, research directly comparing CBT to behavioral therapy (BT) alone in young children is largely absent from the literature and would be a valuable contribution. As such, both in adults and children, the relative contribution of cognitive and behavioral components in CBT is still an open question.

Several case studies have used CBT approaches successfully to treat encopresis and night terrors in 5- to 8-year-old children (Ronen, 1993a, 1993b; Knell & Moore, 1991). These studies each accounted for developmental issues and recommended modifications that may help to make CBT more accessible when working with young children.

With regard to specific support for the likelihood of young children possessing the ability to engage in cognitive therapy, Doherr, Reynolds,

Wetherly, and Evans (2005) examined the performance of 5- to 7-year-old children on tasks typically required for participation in CBT. These tasks included generating alternative explanations, identifying emotions, and connecting thoughts and feelings. Results of this study indicated that most participants were able to engage in all three tasks, suggesting that young children may be appropriate candidates for CBT provided that developmentally appropriate modifications are made. The authors noted that children who are thought to be deficient in any one meta-cognitive area may need additional assistance in developing particular skills prior to engaging in standard CBT. A similar study of 4- to 7-year-old children also found that many participants were able to differentiate among thoughts, feelings, and behaviors. Participants also benefited from the use of cues such as puppets, suggesting that comparable accommodations may serve as useful therapeutic tools to aid in this differentiation (Quakley, Reynolds, & Coker, 2004).

Specific CBT programs for children and adolescents have been recognized for their effectiveness. Kendall's (2000) Coping Cat program (known as the C.A.T. Project for adolescents) targets anxiety disorders in children and incorporates standard CBT components such as psychoeducation, relaxation, problem solving, contingent reinforcement, modeling, exposure, and coping skills in a developmentally modified format. The typical duration of the treatment is 16 sessions, with the first half comprising skills training and the second half comprising skills practice in anxiety-provoking situations. This program concludes with the production of a "commercial" (in the form of a video, book, or other creative project) in order for the young client to teach others what he or she has learned. Recent research has shown that individual and family formats of this program were superior to a family-based education–support–attention service (active control) in reducing the presence of the primary anxiety disorder in children, and gains were maintained 1 year later (Kendall, Hudson, Gosch, Flannery-Schroeder, & Suveg, 2008).

Another program with empirical support is the ACTION program for depression, a manualized group treatment that was evaluated in a 5-year study by the National Institutes of Mental Health (Stark, Schnoebelen, et al., 2005; Stark, Simpson, et al., 2005). The manuals and workbooks were designed for groups of girls between ages 9 and 13 but can be modified to apply to boys and to individual clients as well. This particular program, conducted in small groups during the school day, comprised 20 group and two individual sessions over the course of 11 weeks. Some participants were also assigned to receive parent training, which occurred outside of the school day and involved the child client in a portion of the parent sessions. The program is meant to be "fun and engaging" as it teaches skills to apply to depressive symptoms, interpersonal challenges, and other life difficulties (Stark et al., 2012). The focus of the sessions begins with affective education, coping, and problem-solving skills before shifting into learning and applying cognitive restructuring, and finally improving sense of self. CBT for depression has been identified as a "well-established" treatment for depressed children and adolescents (David-Ferdon & Kaslow, 2008).

Meta-analyses have also supported the effectiveness of CBT for problems related to anger and aggression in children and adults (Beck & Fernandez, 1998; Fossum, Handegard, Martinussen, & Morch, 2008). One cognitive-behavioral intervention that can be used to address anger and aggression in children is known as Keeping Your Cool (Nelson & Finch, 2008). This program makes use of verbal self-talk, relaxation training, problem solving, assertion training, and humor to manage anger. The program uses illustrations, diagrams, video lessons, and child-friendly "antecedent–behavior–consequence" handouts to convey important concepts. Also included in the workbook are suggestions for prompts or other external cues that may be useful for children with newly acquired anger management skills in challenging situations. From a cognitive-behavioral perspective, the goal of this program is to provide youth with the necessary skills to manage anger, subsequently resulting in more appropriate behavioral responses to stressful situations. Other empirically supported techniques that are present in Keeping Your Cool include perspective taking, goal setting, and changing irrational beliefs.

One final example is the multimodality trauma treatment (MMTT; March, Amaya-Jackson, Murray, & Schulte, 1998) for youth who have experienced symptoms of trauma as a result of terrorism or natural disaster. In youth between ages 10–15, this 18-session group CBT program led to significant improvements in levels of posttraumatic stress disorder (PTSD) that were maintained 6 months later (March et al., 1998). The treatment included standard components of CBT, such as habituating anxiety and teaching coping strategies, and also practice of imaginal exposures during sessions.

Research regarding CBT in young children (i.e., age 7 or younger) is mounting and typically suggests that CBT may be an appropriate intervention for this age range. Additionally, specific cognitive-behavioral interventions such as the Coping Cat program for anxiety, the ACTION program for depression, and many others, have been recognized for their success in producing desired outcomes. Future research may guide the essential modifications that should accompany traditional CBT programs when working with children and adolescents.

Conclusions

Overall, CBT with children and adolescents involves the same theoretical principles as do standard forms of CBT with adults. CBT for children and adolescents typically includes both performance-based and cognitive strategies to produce change in thoughts, feelings, and behavior. CBT seeks to provide clients with a wider range of coping skills, so as to promote adaptive behavior. There is empirical support for CBT in treating a wide range of disorders, from anxiety to substance use to eating disorders. Like CBT for adults, child-directed CBT can be delivered in either individual or group settings, with manualized treatment plans available for many different psychological disorders. Key components of CBT include self-monitoring, role playing, exposure to avoided stimuli, relaxation training, and homework assignments.

CBT interventions for children must consider developmental issues in order to be successful. First, it is important to recognize that because children typically do not refer themselves to treatment, their motivation to attend may differ from that of adults. Level of family involvement, incorporation of the peer group context, and frequency of sessions are all issues that require attention when enacting a CBT intervention for youth. In treatment delivery, the therapist should consider inclusion of concrete examples, matching of the treatment to the child's cognitive abilities, and using play and other creative strategies to teach CBT skills. Failure to attend to these details and to make necessary developmental modifications may jeopardize the success of any program. However, more research must inform current treatments as to the optimal level of certain developmental modifications (e.g., how much family involvement is ideal, how frequently sessions should occur).

The body of research related to CBT interventions in children and adolescents is growing and provides some initial support for using CBT with children as young as 3 years of age. CBT has been defined as a "well-established" treatment for children with certain psychological disorders, but research should continue to evaluate its effectiveness. Given its success when used with adults, there is hope that children may be able to experience similar benefits of CBT given consideration of appropriate developmental issues and modifications.

REFERENCES

Association for Behavioral and Cognitive Therapies. (2012). *What is cognitive behavior therapy (CBT)?* Retrieved June 6, 2012, from *http://abct.org/Public /?m=mPublic&fa=WhatIsCBTpublic#aTop*.

Bandura, A. (1965). Influence of models' reinforcement contingencies on the acquisition of imitative responses. *Journal of Abnormal and Social Psychology, 66,* 575–582.

Bandura, A. (1969). *Principles of behavior modification.* New York: Holt, Rinehart & Winston.

Bandura, A. (1973). *Aggression: A social learning analysis.* Englewood Cliffs, NJ: Prentice Hall.

Bandura, A. (1977). Self-efficacy: Toward a unifying theory of behavioral change. *Psychological Review, 84,* 191–215.

Barlow, D. H. (Ed.). (2008). *Clinical handbook of psychological disorders: A step-by-step treatment manual* (4th ed.). New York: Guilford Press.

Beck, A. T. (1967). *Depression: Clinical, experimental, and theoretical aspects.* New York: Harper.

Beck, A. T. (1972). *Depression: Causes and treatment.* Philadelphia: University of Pennsylvania Press.

Beck, R., & Fernandez, E. (1998). Cognitive behavioral therapy in the treatment of anger: A review analysis. *Cognitive Therapy and Research, 22,* 63–74.

Chambless, D. L., & Ollendick, T. H. (2001). Empirically supported psychological interventions: Controversies and evidence. *Annual Review of Psychology, 52,* 685–716.

Chambless, D. L., Sanderson, W. C., Shoham, V., Bennett Johnson, S., Pope, K. S., Crits-Christoph, P., et al. (1996). An update on empirically validated therapies. *Clinical Psychologist, 49,* 5–18.

Choate-Summers, M. L., Freeman, J. B., Garcia, A. M., Coyne, L., Przeworski, A., & Leonard, H. L. (2008). Clinical considerations when tailoring cognitive behavioral treatment for young children with obsessive–compulsive disorder. *Education and Treatment of Children, 31*(3), 395–416.

Craske, M. G. (2010). *Cognitive-behavioral therapy.* Washington, DC: American Psychological Association.

Crawley, S. A., Podell, J. L., Beidas, R. S., Braswell, L., & Kendall, P. C. (2010). Cognitive behavioral therapy with youth. In K. Dobson (Ed.), *Handbook of cognitive behavioral therapies* (3rd ed., pp. 375–410). New York: Guilford Press.

David-Ferdon, C., & Kaslow, N. (2008). Evidence-based psychosocial treatments for child and adolescent depression. *Journal of Clinical Child and Adolescent Psychiatry, 37*(1), 62–104.

Deblinger, E., Behl, L. E., & Glickman, A. R. (2012). Trauma-focused cognitive behavioral therapy for children who have experienced sexual abuse. In P. C. Kendall (Ed.), *Child and adolescent therapy: Cognitive-behavioral procedures* (4th ed., pp. 345–375). New York: Guilford Press.

Dobson, D., & Dobson, K. S. (2009). *Evidence-based practice of cognitive-behavioral therapy.* New York: Guilford Press.

Dobson, K. S. (Ed.). (2010). *Handbook of cognitive-behavioral therapies* (3rd ed.). New York: Guilford Press.

Dobson, K. S., & Dozois, D. J. A. (2010). Historical and philosophical bases of the cognitive-behavioral therapies. In K. S. Dobson (Ed.), *Handbook of cognitive-behavioral therapies* (3rd ed., pp. 3–38). New York: Guilford Press.

Doherr, L., Reynolds, S., Wetherly, J., & Evans, E. H. (2005). Young children's ability to engage in cognitive therapy tasks: Associations with age and educational experience. *Behavioural and Cognitive Psychotherapy, 33*(2), 201–215.

Durlak, J. A., Fuhrman, T., & Lampman, C. (1991). Effectiveness of cognitive-behavior therapy for maladapting children: A meta-analysis. *Psychological Bulletin, 110*(2), 204–214.

D'Zurilla, T. J., & Nezu, A. M. (2010). Problem-solving therapy. In K. S. Dobson (Ed.), *Handbook of cognitive-behavioral therapies* (3rd ed., pp. 197–225). New York: Guilford Press.

Ellis, A. (1962). *Reason and emotion in psychotherapy.* Secaucus, NJ: Lyle Stuart.

Epp, A., & Dobson, K. S. (2010). The evidence base for cognitive-behavioral therapy. In K. S. Dobson (Ed.), *Handbook of cognitive-behavioral therapies* (3rd ed., pp. 39–73). New York: Guilford Press.

Evidence-based Mental Health Treatment for Children and Adolescents. (2012). In APA Division 53 (SCCAP), retrieved June 6, 2012, from *www.effectivechild-therapy.com.*

Eysenck, H. J. (1952). The effects of psychotherapy: An evaluation. *Journal of Consulting Psychology, 16,* 319–324.

Eysenck, H. J. (Ed.). (1960). *Behavior therapy and the neuroses.* Oxford, UK: Pergamon.

Fossum, S., Handegard, B. H., Martinussen, M., & Morch, W. M. (2008). Treatment of oppositional defiant and conduct problems in young Norwegian children. *European Child and Adolescent Psychiatry, 17,* 438–451.

Francis, G., & Beidel, D. (1995). Cognitive-behavioral psychotherapy. In J. S. March (Ed.), *Anxiety disorders in children and adolescents* (pp. 321–340). New York: Guilford Press.

Fruzzetti, A. E., & Erikson, K. R. (2010). Mindfulness and acceptance interventions in cognitive-behavioral therapy. In K. S. Dobson (Ed.), *Handbook of cognitive-behavioral therapies* (3rd ed., pp. 347–372). New York: Guilford Press.

Goldfried, M. R., & Davison, G. L. (1976). *Clinical behavior therapy.* New York: Holt, Rinehart & Winston.

Grave, J., & Blissett, J. (2004). Is cognitive behavior therapy developmentally appropriate for young children?: A critical review of the evidence. *Clinical Psychology Review, 5*(3), 161–172.

Harwood, T. M., Beutler, L. E., & Charvat, M. (2010). Cognitive-behavioral therapy and psychotherapy integration. In K. S. Dobson (Ed.), *Handbook of cognitive-behavioral therapies* (3rd ed., pp. 94–130). New York: Guilford Press.

Hirshfeld-Becker, D. R., Micco, J. A., Mazursky, H., Bruett, L., & Henin, A. (2011). Applying cognitive-behavioral therapy for anxiety to the younger child. *Child and Adolescent Psychiatric Clinics of North America, 20*(2), 349–368.

Ingram, R. E., & Siegle, G. J. (2010). Cognitive science and the conceptual foundations of cognitive-behavioral therapy: Viva la evolution! In K. S. Dobson (Ed.), *Handbook of cognitive-behavioral therapies* (3rd ed., pp. 74–93). New York: Guilford Press.

Ishikawa, S., Okajima, I., Matsuoka, H., & Sakano, Y. (2007). Cognitive behavioural therapy for anxiety disorders in children and adolescents: A meta-analysis. *Child and Adolescent Mental Health, 12*(4), 164–172.

Jacobson, E. (1938). *Progressive relaxation.* Chicago: University of Chicago Press.

Jones, M. C. (1924). A laboratory study of fear: The case of Peter. *Pedagogical Seminar, 31,* 308–315.

Kazdin, A. (2010). Problem-solving skills training and parent management training for oppositional defiant disorder and conduct disorder. In J. R. Weisz & A. E. Kazdin (Eds.), *Evidence-based psychotherapies for children and adolescents* (2nd ed., pp. 211–226). New York: Guilford Press.

Kendall, P. C. (2012). Anxiety disorders in youth. In P. C. Kendall (Ed.), *Child and adolescent therapy: Cognitive-behavioral procedures* (4th ed., pp. 143–189). New York: Guilford Press.

Kendall, P. C., Hudson, J., Gosch, E., Flannery-Schroeder, E., & Suveg, C. (2008). Cognitive behavioral therapy for anxiety disordered youth: A randomized clinical trial evaluating child and family modalities. *Journal of Consulting and Clinical Psychology, 76*(2), 282–297.

Knell, S. M., & Moore, D. J. (1991). Cognitive-behavioral play therapy in the treatment of encopresis. *Journal of Clinical Child Psychology, 19,* 55–60.

Lazarus, R. S. (1966). *Psychological stress and the coping process.* New York: McGraw-Hill.

Lazarus R. A., & Averill, J. (1972). Emotion and cognition with special reference to anxiety. In C. D. Spielberger (Ed.), *Anxiety: Current trends in theory and research* (Vol. 2, pp. 242–283). New York: Academic Press.

Lazarus, R. S., & Folkman, S. (1984). *Stress, appraisal, and coping.* New York: Springer.

Mahoney, M. J. (1988). The cognitive sciences and psychotherapy: Patterns in a developing relationship. In K. S. Dobson (Ed.), *The handbook of cognitive behavioral therapies* (pp. 357–386). New York: Guilford Press.

Mahoney, M. J., & Arnkoff, D. B. (1978). Cognitive and self-control therapies. In S. L. Garfield & A. E. Bergin (Eds.), *Handbook of psychotherapy and behavior change: An empirical analysis* (pp. 689–722). New York: Wiley.

March, J. S., Amaya-Jackson, L., Murray, M. C., & Schulte, A. (1998). Cognitive-behavioral psychotherapy for children and adolescents with posttraumatic stress disorder after a single incident stressor. *Journal of the American Academy of Child and Adolescent Psychiatry, 37,* 585–593.

March, J. S., & Benton, C. M. (2006). *Talking back to OCD: The program that helps kids and teens say "no way"—and parents say "way to go."* New York: Guilford Press.

Marks, I. M. (1975). Behavioral treatments of phobic and obsessive-compulsive disorders: A critical appraisal. In M. Hersen, R. M. Eisler, & P. M. Miller (Eds.), *Progress in behavior modification* (pp. 65–158). New York: Academic Press.

Meichenbaum, D. (1977). *Cognitive-behavior modification: An integrative approach.* New York: Plenum.

Meichenbaum, D. H., & Cameron, R. (1973). Training schizophrenics to talk to themselves. *Behavior Therapy, 4,* 515–535.

Meichenbaum, D., & Goodman, J. (1971). Training impulsive children to talk to themselves: A means of developing self-control. *Journal of Abnormal Psychology*, 77, 115–126.

Minde, K., Roy, J., Bezonsky, R., & Hashemi, A. (2010). The effectiveness of CBT in 3–7 year old anxious children: Preliminary data. *Journal of the Canadian Academy of Child and Adolescent Psychiatry*, 19(2), 109–115.

Monga, S., Young, A., & Owens, M. (2009). Evaluating a cognitive behavioral therapy group program for anxious five to seven year old children: A pilot study. *Depression and Anxiety*, 26(3), 243–250.

Nelson, W. M., III, & Finch, A. J., Jr. (2008). *Keeping Your Cool: The anger management workbook* (2nd ed., Parts 1 & 2) Ardmore, PA: Workbook Publishing.

Ollendick, T. H., Grills, A. E., & King, N. (2001). Applying developmental theory to the assessment and treatment of childhood disorders: Does it make a difference? *Clinical Psychology and Psychotherapy*, 8, 304–314.

Pahl, K. M., & Barrett, P. M. (2010). Interventions for anxiety disorders in children using group CBT with family involvement. In J. Weisz & A. Kazdin (Eds.), *Evidence-based psychotherapies for children and adolescents* (2nd ed., pp. 61–79). New York: Guilford Press.

Pediatric OCD Treatment Study Team (2004). Cognitive-behavioral therapy, sertraline, and their combination for children and adolescents with obsessive–compulsive disorder: The Pediatrics OCD Treatment Study (POTS) randomized controlled trial. *Journal of the American Medical Association*, 292, 1969–1976.

Powers, S. W. (1999). Empirically supported treatments in pediatric psychology: Procedure related pain. *Journal of Pediatric Psychology*, 24, 131–145.

Quakley, S., Reynolds, S., & Coker, S. (2004). The effect of cues on young children's abilities to discriminate among thoughts, feelings, and behaviours. *Behaviour Research and Therapy*, 42(3), 343–356.

Robertson, D. (2010). *The philosophy of cognitive-behavioural therapy: Stoicism as rational and cognitive psychotherapy*. London: Karnac.

Ronen, T. (1993a). Intervention package for treating encopresis in a 6 year old boy: A case study. *Behavioural Psychotherapy*, 21, 127–135.

Ronen, T. (1993b). Self-control training in the treatment of sleep terror disorder: A case study. *Child and Family Behavior Therapy*, 15, 53–63.

Scheeringa, M. S., Weems, C. F., Cohen, J., Amaya-Jackson, L., & Guthrie, D. (2011). Trauma focused cognitive-behavioral therapy for posttraumatic stress disorder in three through six year-old children: A randomized clinical trial. *Journal of Child Psychology and Psychiatry*, 52, 853–860.

Skinner, B. F. (1938). *The behavior of organisms*. New York: Appleton–Century–Crofts.

Skinner, B. F. (1953). *Science and human behavior*. New York: Macmillan.

Southam-Gerow, M. A., & Kendall, P. C. (2000). A preliminary study of the emotion understanding of youth referred for treatment of anxiety disorders. *Journal of Clinical Child Psychology*, 29, 319–327.

Stark, K. D., Schnoebelen, S., Simpson, J., Hargrave, J., Molnar, J., & Glenn, R. (2005). *Treating depressed children: Therapist manual for ACTION*. Ardmore, PA: Workbook Publishing.

Stark, K. D., Simpson, J., Schnoebelen, S., Glenn, R., Hargrave, J., & Molnar, J. (2005). *ACTION workbook*. Ardmore, PA: Workbook Publishing.

Stark, K. D., Streusand, W., Arora, P., & Patel, P. (2012). Childhood depression: The ACTION treatment program. In P. C. Kendall (Ed.), *Child and adolescent therapy: Cognitive-behavioral procedures* (4th ed., pp. 190–233). New York: Guilford Press.

Stewart, R. E., & Chambless, D. L. (2007). Does psychotherapy research inform treatment decisions in private practice? *Journal of Clinical Psychology, 63*, 267–281.

Task Force on Promotion and Dissemination of Psychological Procedures, Division of Clinical Psychology, American Psychological Association. (1995). Training in and dissemination of empirically validated psychological treatments: Report and recommendations. *Clinical Psychologist, 48*, 3–23.

Thorndike, E. L. (1898). Animal intelligence: An experimental study of the associative processes in animals. *Psychological Review Monograph Supplement 2*(4, Whole No. 8).

Watson, J. B., & Rayner, R. (1920). Conditioned emotional reactions. *Journal of Experimental Psychology, 3*(1), 1–14.

Weisz, J. R., & Kazdin, A. E. (Eds.). (2010). *Evidence-based psychotherapies for children and adolescents* (2nd ed.) New York: Guilford Press.

Wolpe, J. (1958). *Psychotherapy by reciprocal inhibition*. Stanford, CA: Stanford University Press.

Zelikovsky, N., Rodrique, J. R., Gidycz, C. A., & Davis, M. A. (2000). Cognitive behavioral interventions help young children cope during a voiding cystourethrogram. *Journal of Pediatric Psychology, 25*, 535–543.

2

Modifications of Cognitive-Behavioral Therapy for Children and Adolescents with High-Functioning ASD and Their Common Difficulties

Tony Attwood and Angela Scarpa

Cognitive-behavioral therapy (CBT) can be broadly conceived as the integration of cognitive and behavioral approaches for making specific targeted changes in thoughts, feelings, or behaviors (Craske, 2010; see also Scarpa & Lorenzi, Chapter 1, this volume, for a description of CBT history, principles, and its application to children and adolescents). The therapeutic approach of CBT is to encourage the person to be more consciously aware of his or her emotional state, to learn to respond more appropriately and effectively to the situation or emotion, and to become more sensitive to how others are feeling. Much of the early work in cognitive therapy focused primarily on adults with depression (e.g., Beck, Rush, Shaw, & Emery, 1979; Ellis, 1962). Since then, however, the incorporation of cognitive with behavioral techniques has been extended to numerous problems, such as anxiety, marital difficulties, substance abuse, eating disorders, attention-deficit/hyperactivity disorder (ADHD), and many others. Morover CBT has been extended downward to work with children and adolescents and is generally thought to be effective if appropriate developmental considerations and modifications are put into place (e.g., parent involvement, use of visuals, incorporation of play; Grave & Blissett, 2004; Ollendick, Grills, & King, 2001).

Typically, because of the focus on measurable change, CBT programs begin with an assessment of the nature and degree of problems associated with specific emotions or behaviors, using self-report scales and a clinical interview. After an adequate assessment of the problem, multiple strategies may be implemented to promote change, including psychoeducation, somatic management via relaxation, cognitive restructuring, problem solving, exposure therapy, and relapse prevention (Velting, Setzer, & Albano, 2004). For example, affective education may be used to increase the person's knowledge of emotions within him- or herself and others. Discussion and activities explore the connection among thoughts, emotions, and behavior, and identify the ways in which the person conceptualizes emotions and perceives various situations. For anxiety-related problems, some clinicians may incorporate behavioral exposures to the feared situation, while also challenging distorted cognitions. If a problem seems related to a behavioral skills deficit (e.g., social skills), education and behavioral rehearsal or role plays may be implemented in order to teach and practice the skill. Finally, to address cognitive biases, cognitive restructuring may be used to correct distorted conceptualizations and dysfunctional beliefs, and to constructively manage emotions. Then, therapist and client may plan a schedule of activities for practicing these new cognitive skills to comprehend and express emotions in real-life situations.

Linking thoughts with feelings and behaviors is often an integral part of CBT, and is often encouraged via Socratic questioning and verbal psychoeducation. Thus, CBT provides an opportunity to learn self-awareness, self-control, and more constructive strategies to repair emotions, as well as to improve social cognition and social competence. Yet self-reflection and reflection on the thoughts and feelings of others is particularly difficult for those with autism spectrum disorders (ASD; Frith & Happe, 1999; Hobson, 2010). They also have limited repertoires of behavioral responses to emotional arousal (Attwood, 2007), and may have language impairments that affect comprehension and self-assessment (American Psychiatric Association, 2013). Based upon the knowledge of some of these deficits in ASD, this chapter focuses on modifications of CBT to improve its accessibility for children and adolescents with ASD. Since the evidence for CBT in the ASD population, especially youngsters, is still emerging and mechanisms are as yet unclear (see, e.g., Lang, Regester, Lauderdale, Ashbaugh, & Haring, 2010; Rotheram-Fuller & MacMullen, 2011), this chapter relies heavily on clinical experiences and observations, while noting appropriate supporting research when applicable.

Multiple cognitive, language, and emotional skills need to be considered when adapting a CBT program for children and adolescents with ASD

(Rotheram-Fuller & MacMullen, 2011). The distinctive learning profile (as described below) associated with ASD, for example, needs to be recognized by the clinician, especially during the affective education and cognitive restructuring components. The therapy session is also affected by the profile of language abilities associated with ASD, especially impaired pragmatic and semantic language abilities. In line with the focus of this book, this chapter refers primarily to working with children and adolescents with ASD who are verbal and cognitively higher functioning. It seems plausible, however, that CBT can also be used with nonverbal people with ASD who have the cognitive capability and a functional communication system that the therapist can use (however, we are aware of no research on this issue). CBT can be implemented in a one-on-one (therapist and child) or group format. Whether the CBT is conducted on an individual or a group basis, there need to be adjustments to the therapy to accommodate the interpersonal and social abilities of the person(s) with ASD, including the explanation of the social conventions and protocol expected in the individual or group social situation. Finally, there needs to be consideration of the sensory profile of the person with an ASD in terms of sensory sensitivity (auditory, olfactory and tactile) to aspects of the therapy environment. Some of the issues to consider in adapting a CBT program are specific to ASD, whereas others may be more generally applicable but especially pertinent to working with someone with ASD. This chapter explores each of these modifications to a conventional CBT program and provides practical advice on other characteristics associated with ASD that can inhibit or enhance the effectiveness of CBT for such children and adolescents.

LEARNING PROFILE ASSOCIATED WITH ASD

Children and adolescents with an ASD have a different and clinically distinctive way of perceiving, thinking, and learning, and tend to perform at the extremes of cognitive ability (Attwood, 2007). Despite having IQs in the normal range, they usually have very uneven cognitive profiles on IQ tests. For the clinician designing a CBT program, information from an evaluation, which may include an assessment of the child's cognitive and processing abilities, can be invaluable in determining learning strengths and weaknesses. For example, if the child or adolescent has relatively advanced verbal reasoning skills and reading comprehension abilities, understanding of the concepts and strategies used in CBT may be improved by the inclusion of relevant literature in the program. When reading a text, there are no interpersonal or conversational skills required, and the child or adolescent with an ASD may be able to give full cognitive attention to the text. If the child or adolescent has relatively advanced visual reasoning abilities, learning may be facilitated by computer programs, demonstration, observation, and visual imagery, placing less emphasis on conversation. The phrase "a picture is worth a thousand words" may be particularly relevant to such children.

Children or adolescents with ASD can also be very logical in their thinking, and CBT programs help explain to them why we have emotions, how to identify and measure emotions, and how to explore new strategies to communicate and manage emotions. In a review of CBT programs for children with ASD, Rotheram-Fuller and MacMullen (2011), for example, have noted that some programs focus on teaching the child with ASD about the physical symptoms associated with anxiety rather than simply relying on the subjective emotional feeling, in order to help the child concretely identify when he or she is feeling anxious. As noted earlier, using visual aids or hands-on activities can also make discussions more concrete and improve comprehension of the abstract concept of emotions. This approach appeals to the logical, scientific thinking of children and adolescents with ASD (Anderson & Morris, 2006). We now have resources specifically designed to help children and adolescents with ASD learn about emotions in a concrete and logical way to complement the affective educational component of CBT (Attwood, Callesen, & Nielsen, 2008).

It is also important to be aware that children and adolescents with ASD may have difficulty with socioemotional processing, memory for sequential information, and processing information in novel contexts (Baron-Cohen, 2001; Boucher & Lewis, 1989; Hill, 2004). Therefore, the clinician conducting the CBT program should be aware of the time it may take for children with ASD cognitively, rather than intuitively, to process and respond to socioemotional information. It is thus very important that the clinician remain patient, and it may be helpful to supplement verbal with written instructions to aid processing and minimize the need for the child to rely on memory.

ADHD and Executive Function

Extensive research has confirmed that children and adolescents with ASD are at risk of difficulties associated with ADHD (Fein, Dixon, Paul, & Levin, 2005; Goldstein, Johnson, & Minshew, 2001; Sturm, Fernell, & Gillberg, 2004), although by convention the current diagnostic guidelines state that ADHD cannot be diagnosed in the presence of ASD, because the symptoms are assumed to be secondary to the underlying ASD syndrome.

Nonetheless, inattention and hyperactivity–impulsivity may still be present and can cause significant functional impairment in children and adolescents with ASD. Attention difficulties in ASD can include problems with sustaining attention that are similar to those in ADHD; however, children with ASD more often have difficulties with shifting attention. As such, they may be distracted by inner imagination (i.e., daydreaming) or may restrict the focus of their attention. If present, these attentional characteristics obviously affect the content and duration of many of the components of a CBT program. If the child or adolescent shows impulsivity or hyperactivity, these characteristics would also need to be accommodated and can require that the clinician provides more vigilant supervision, especially if the CBT is being conducted in a group format. A targeted behavioral intervention within the therapy session may be helpful, since it has been shown that children with ADHD tend to respond better to frequent schedules of reinforcement (Carlson & Tamm, 2000). For example, the clinician may use within the session a token economy whereby the client can earn tokens (or points, stars, coins, etc.) for following rules and completing activities. Also, stimulant medication is widely used, and often (though not always) is effective in the management of ADHD symptoms (Spencer, Biederman, & Wilens, 2000). A review of the literature for drug therapy in children with ASD recently concluded that atypical antipsychotics may provide substantial benefits, and the stimulant methylphenidate, as well as some other medications, may provide moderate benefits in reducing inattention and hyperactivity (Hazell, 2006). However, this review emphasized that many studies are still equivocal and limited to uncontrolled designs. Therefore, if stimulant medication is helpful for the client being seen, clinical experience has indicated that administering the medication prior to the CBT session can facilitate concentration and cooperation. Any change in medication use, however, should be carefully monitored and discussed with the child's prescribing physician.

Executive functioning deficits that are core to both ASD and ADHD may impact a CBT program. Problems with organizational and planning abilities, working memory, and time management indicate that others, such as the clinician and a parent supervising the between-sessions projects and practice in real-life situations, may have to become "executive secretaries" to minimize impaired executive function (Attwood, 2007). Consistent with educational modifications that have been found to be helpful for children with ADHD (DuPaul & Stoner, 2003), children and adolescents with ASD are more responsive to programs that are highly structured, with short discrete activities and assignments broken down into smaller units, in keeping with the children's attention spans. Other helpful educational modifications that can be adapted for use in CBT include highlighting relevant information, using graphics or visual aids, clearly posting rules, repeating instructions, and providing a visual schedule. The clinician should regularly monitor and give feedback to maintain attention, and the amount of environmental distractions should be reduced.

One-Track Mind

Another executive deficit that is characteristic of ASD involves a lack of flexibility in thinking and problem solving (Hill, 2008). A metaphor for this learning characteristic is a train on a singular track, representing a "one-track mind." Unfortunately, clinical and teaching experience has indicated that those with ASD are often the last to know and seek help if they are on the "wrong track" and cannot solve a problem. Sometimes referred to as having a problem in set shifting (Ozonoff et al., 2004), they tend to continue using incorrect strategies, not learning from mistakes—that is, they fail to "switch tracks" to get to the destination (i.e., find a solution). The inability to conceptualize an alternative response or strategy clearly influences the progress of a CBT program. It is therefore important that to encourage flexible thinking, the clinician ask, "What else could you do?" and provide multiple-choice options rather than anticipate the generation of spontaneous alternatives. Because cognitive inflexibility may increase with anxiety, clinical experience has suggested that strategies to improve relaxation (e.g., deep breathing, muscle relaxation, positive self-talk) can also be used to facilitate flexible thinking within the CBT session and in real-life practice situations, although research to test this possibility is needed.

Problems with set shifting may also contribute to the often-noted difficulties with generalization of skills learned in therapy to the child's natural settings in daily life (National Research Council, 2001). As such, role plays, behavioral rehearsal, and practice in real-life situations need to be included in the program to a greater extent than might occur with a typical child. In some cases, it might be helpful to begin with a cognitive picture rehearsal (e.g., Groden & LeVasseur, 1995) or social story (e.g., Gray, 1995) to help the child mentally clarify, illustrate, and rehearse the skills in a new situation before practicing *in vivo*.

Fear of Making a Mistake

Attwood (2007) has suggested that the rigidity in children with ASD can be associated with fear of making a mistake. When unsure what to do or say, the situation may become a trigger for flight, fight or freeze responses. Research on the cognitive abilities of children and adults with ASD has identified a tendency to notice more detail and errors than do typical children (Frith & Happé, 1994). When combined with a fear of appearing stupid and being ridiculed by peers, this can have a significant effect on the ability to learn. We have observed clinically that some children and adolescents with ASD may refuse to attempt a new activity that could result in failure, with the attitude "If you don't try, you don't make a mistake." Another reaction we have observed is to become extremely anxious, which can disintegrate into a feeling of panic or extreme frustration, possibly leading to explosive and agitated behavior. This observation is partially supported by research showing that social anxiety mediates the relationship between ASD features and hostile attitudes in a nonclinical sample of young adults (White, Kreiser, Pugliese, & Scarpa, 2012). Attwood speculates that over the long term, the pervasive fear of failure can lead to a need to be right and a tendency to criticize others in order to feel good about one's own abilities. This is a form of compensation, whereby criticism may be a way of demonstrating intellectual prowess to others as a counterbalance to feeling incompetent and stupid when making a mistake. The sometimes pathological fear of making mistakes (yet avidly pointing out others' mistakes) can affect cooperation and cohesion within the CBT sessions, especially when using a group format. Future research may help to clarify how cognitive biases such as the ones mentioned here can influence self-efficacy, behavior, and social competence in youth with ASD.

It is important that the clinician encourage any suggestion without criticism and adopt a positive approach, implying that a mistake is not a tragedy or sign of mental deficiency. The clinician can model how to handle mistakes by not catastrophizing when a mistake is made, and by reframing how making a mistake provides information that is useful in discovering the elusive solution. In other words, "We learn more from our mistakes than our successes." As noted earlier, people with ASD can be very sensitive to any indication of intellectual impairment and some develop a form of intellectual arrogance as a compensation mechanism. A valuable motivation in a learning situation can be to appeal to intellectual vanity by remarking on the ASD child's or adolescent's intellectual abilities. This verbal encouragement can be a more effective reinforcement than any altruistic desire to please the clinician. Thus, a comment such as "That suggestion demonstrates your amazing intellectual ability" can be a more powerful motivator than "You have just made my day," though the clinician should monitor how the child or adolescent responds to such remarks and only use this strategy if it is helpful in boosting the client's self-concept. Another useful strategy when encouraging self-control can be to use the self-talk comment, "If I stay calm, I'll find the solution more quickly" or "If I stay calm, I will be smarter."

Consistency and Certainty

Children and adolescents with ASD seem to have a strong desire to seek consistency and certainty in their daily lives; they thrive on routine and predictability. Such insistence on sameness was first described by Kanner (1943). Because of this desire to maintain sameness, they often need careful preparation for unexpected change. Thus, it is very helpful for the child or adolescent to have a schedule of activities for the session, with clear information on the objectives and the duration of each activity (Dalrymple, 1995). There can also be a compulsion for closure (i.e., not being able to change activities or "switch tracks" until the activity is complete to the satisfaction of the child or adolescent). Unfortunately, such children can also be very pedantic, overfocus on detail, and be perfectionistic, thereby resisting a clinician's attempts to hurry up.

Special Interests and Talents

One of the central characteristics of ASD is the development of restricted interests (American Psychiatric Association, 2013). With children and adolescents who have an IQ in the normal range, this can include collecting objects such as rocks or spark plugs; amassing information on topics, such as the life cycle of a butterfly; or having an encyclopedic knowledge of presidents of the United States or television programs, such as *Star Trek* or *The Power Rangers*. This special interest's many functions include feelings of enjoyment or euphoria in acquiring new items or knowledge of a specific theme; intense mental focus acting as a thought blocker for feelings of anxiety, sadness or anger; and acting as a means to demonstrate an admired talent to parents and peers. The interest can be incorporated into a CBT program, for example, as an antidote to feeling sad and as a thought blocker for anxiety. A special interest in a character such as Harry Potter can provide an illustration of how a perceived hero copes with adversity, becoming a model of how to cope with feelings, such as anger, when being bullied and tormented by peers.

The interests and talents associated with ASD can also be used to improve motivation, attention, and conceptualization (Koegel & Koegel, 2006). For example, if the special interest of a child with ASD is weather systems, his or her emotions may be expressed as a weather report. The special interest can also be used in the affective education component of CBT. A project or field study for an adolescent whose special interest is trains can be to visit a station to observe the emotions of passengers saying farewell, greeting friends and relatives, and waiting for a ticket.

Alexithymia

Research on theory of mind abilities has identified the problems children and adolescents with ASD have in "reading"ional states in themselves and others, which also may be related to the separate skill of facial emotion recognition (Berthoz & Hill, 2005; Tani et al., 2004). Deficits in facial emotion recognition have been found in individuals with ASD, possibly due to decreased functional connectivity among multiple brain regions in response to emotional faces (Harms, Martin, & Wallace, 2010). These authors posit, however, that higher functioning individuals with ASD may use other mechanisms to compensate for their lack of automatic ability to recognize facial emotions. CBT therapists might be able capitalize on this ability by encouraging and teaching children with ASD more cognitive–analytic processing of faces and social situations.

In addition to deficits in the fundamental processing of emotions, some individuals with ASD may experience characteristics of *alexithymia,* a diminished vocabulary to describe the different levels of emotional experience, especially the more subtle or complex emotions. Affective education within CBT aims to improve the vocabulary of the child or adolescent with ASD to describe emotions, thereby diminishing the effects of alexithymia. One approach is to quantify the degree of expression, such that if the precise word is elusive, the child or adolescent can calibrate and express his or her degree of emotion using a thermometer or numerical rating, thus indicating the intensity of emotional experience.

Converting Thoughts and Emotions to Speech

Clinical experience indicates that some children and adolescents with ASD may have considerable difficulty describing their thoughts and emotions in a face-to-face conversation. Although the person may have acquired, through the affective education component of CBT, a reasonable and precise vocabulary to describe a particular depth of emotion, there can still be considerable difficulty answering questions such as "What were you thinking and feeling?" or providing a coherent and cogent answer to the question "Why did you do that?" This is consistent with reports of poor pragmatics in people with ASD (see below). However, there can be greater communication of inner thoughts and feelings using communication systems other than a face-to-face conversation. If the explanation is incoherent or elusive, a child can often achieve greater clarity and insight by typing rather than talking. The clinician can request that the explanation be included in an e-mail or text message. Greater insight into inner thoughts and feelings can also be achieved using music; for example, an adolescent may choose a CD track that, through the music or lyrics, explains his or her inner thoughts and emotions. Sometimes, creating a drawing, cartoon, or collage may help to express the inner workings of the mind of the person with ASD.

LANGUAGE PROFILE ASSOCIATED WITH ASD

Although children and adolescents with high-functioning ASD do not necessarily experience a language delay or deficits in verbal speech, they often have difficulties with the pragmatics of language (Twachtman-Cullen, 2000). *Pragmatics* refers to the use of language in social contexts and the ways people produce and comprehend meanings through language (Bishop, 1997). Problems with pragmatics can occur in multiple areas of communication, such as inappropriate initiation (e.g., talking to anyone; talking repetitively about things that others may not be interested in), lack of coherence (e.g., difficulty describing a sequence of events or providing a clear account of an event), stereotyped language (e.g., including overprecise information in the conversation; turning the conversation to a favorite theme), poor use of context (e.g., being overliteral; misinterpreting situations), and difficulty with rapport (e.g., ignoring conversational initiations by others; not using gestures or facial expressions to convey a meaning or to interpret others' feelings) (Bishop & Baird, 2001).

The mere syntax or literal interpretation of language can be confusing or ambiguous, unless one takes the context into account. For example, to say "Flying planes can be dangerous," can mean two different things, depending on the context to which the speaker is referring. By the same token, intonation of voice or emphases on certain words can change the meaning of a sentence. For example, "I never said I liked *him*" means something completely different than "I never said I *liked* him." The main point here is that youth with ASD often do not perceive, appreciate, or accurately interpret how intonation and emphasis affect meaning. They also struggle with literal interpretation, which affects their use and comprehension of idioms, metaphor, and sarcasm. Therefore, it is important that the CBT clinician provide very concrete examples of constructs and double-check to be sure that the child with ASD has understood the information correctly. This can be done using visual aides to supplement verbal instruction, and hands-on learning such as role plays or real-life practice assignments. Simple metaphors can also be used to make ideas more concrete, as in the metaphor of a toolbox full of tools to "repair" feelings.

In addition, children and adolescents with ASD can vary widely in the amount of language they produce, from being pedantic and providing too much information to the opposite—being overly quiet and not elaborating. They can also display problems with narrative in terms of being able to provide a coherent, sequential, and logical description of events. These styles can make it difficult for them to "get to the point," so that the clinician may find that they go off-topic or on tangents. As such, the CBT therapist may need to remind the client with ASD about the initial topic or question and provide cues to either cut off tangents or help the client expand upon a specific point.

Finally, a key difficulty in ASD involves rapport or social reciprocity, which can impair the "art" of conversation. The child or adolescent with ASD may not engage in social chitchat or the give-and-take of conversation, making it harder for the CBT therapist to sustain the interaction. Shorter sessions or training in conversational skills may be helpful. The clinician also needs to appreciate how direct or "blunt" and honest the child can be, due to difficulties with theory of mind and the social conventions of conversation, and not to be offended by hearing the truth from the ASD client's perspective.

INTERPERSONAL AND SOCIAL ABILITIES ASSOCIATED WITH ASD

Children with ASD display deficits in social skills. Indeed, a core feature described in the current diagnostic criteria (American Psychiatric Association, 2013) is persistent deficits in social communication and social interaction across contexts including deficits in social–emotional reciprocity, nonverbal communicative behaviors used for social interaction and developing and maintaining relationships appropriate to developmental level. As noted earlier, nonverbal behaviors are often needed to clarify meaning in conversation and to understand the emotions of others. CBT clinicians may need to teach children with ASD "mind reading," that is, the ability to read the nonverbal cues that indicate the emotions or intentions of others, and how to use facial expressions or nonverbal communication to convey emotions. Several computer-assisted programs are now available to help children learn to read facial expressions in others (e.g., Beaumont & Sofronoff, Chapter 8, this volume; Golan et al., 2010; Hopkins, 2011; LaCava, Golan, Baron-Cohen, & Smith-Myles, 2007; Silver & Oakes, 2001; Tanaka, 2010). However, it should be noted that no study has yet demonstrated that improvement in facial emotion recognition directly affects social competence.

Because of the difficulty with social reciprocity, children and adolescents with ASD may not appear to develop relationships or attachments as easily as other clients; however, it would be wrong to conclude that they are not feeling emotions. Indeed, it is often the case that they feel emotions quite strongly but do not know how to express themselves, or they simply have a limited range of affective display (Ben Shalom et al., 2006). This seemingly aloof attitude can interfere with the therapist–client alliance if the clinician is not aware of this tendency in advance. Many individuals with ASD express their connection with someone through actions rather than words or facial expression. Therefore, the CBT clinician is advised to be mindful of actions that reflect alliance with the the therapist, as well as others, and to teach the client words and expressions (via affective education) that might be more accepted/recognized in the social world.

SENSORY PROFILE ASSOCIATED WITH ASD

Sensory issues in some children with ASD can contribute to emotional dyscontrol. In a recent study of 170 toddlers with ASD, for example, those with high frequencies of sensory symptoms or a mixture of both over- and underresponsivity but low sensory-seeking behavior were rated by parents as having more negative emotionality, anxiety, and depression (Ben-Sasson et al., 2008). Interestingly, Liss, Mailloux, and Erehull (2008) found that overresponsivity to sensory stimulation was related to autistic characteristics in a nonclinical sample of college students and was particularly related to anxiety in individuals who also experienced symptoms of alexithymia (i.e., being unable to identify one's feelings). Therefore, it appears that to have overwhelming sensations and not be able to identify them can increase confusion and anxiety.

Knowledge of the sensory issues that might be occurring in a client is critical for the success of any therapy, including CBT. The clinician needs to arrange the environment in such a way that it is tolerated by the client and promotes comfort. For example, the lighting may need to be dimmed or changed to nonfluorescent. Smells, such as perfumes or deodorants, may need to be minimized. If snacks are provided, texture and taste need to be considered. Therapists may need to ask their clients first, before engaging in any physical gestures, such patting them on the back for praise, handshakes, tapping their arms to gain attention, or hugs for comfort. Calming music or sounds can be played for clients who are very oversensitive to auditory stimulation. Other clients may be underresponsive to some sensations (e.g., pain), and the clinician may need to find ways to identify whether the client is indeed experiencing sensations that need to be addressed, and to help the client identify and express those experiences (e.g., help-seeking behaviors). The clinician may also need to help the client identify appropriate ways to satisfy sensory needs that are not disruptive or stigmatizing, yet may have a powerful effect in regulating their stress or anxiety. For example, the client may chew gum or manipulate a small object in his or her pocket to receive sensory input.

ADDITIONAL ASPECTS THAT MAY BE HELPFUL IN A CBT PROGRAM

A Workbook

CBT programs may benefit from a workbook in which participants record information and include any visual representations or supplemental information that may assist the client. By the same token, recording information in a workbook must be kept to a minimum due to the recognition that children and adolescents with ASD often have poor handwriting skills and prefer to listen, watch, and do rather than write. If there is a genuine aversion to writing, the clinician conducting the program can listen to the participant's spoken comments and answers, and write them in the workbook.

Between-Session Projects

Between each CBT session, a project can be completed that provides more information for the clinician and applies strategies in real-life situations. This information is usually discussed at the start of the subsequent session. Children with ASD often have an aversion to the concept of homework from negative school experiences (indeed, many neurotypical children also dislike homework), so the clinician conducting the CBT program needs to emphasize the importance of completing the project, and together with parents, clearly encourage children or adolescents to do so. There also needs to be good collaboration between home and school with regard to the CBT intervention goals (e.g., learning to identify and express emotions). It is important that teachers be aware of the program and the ways they can contribute to the child's knowledge base on achieving the target goals.

They can also help with the successful implementation and generalization of strategies.

Selection of Group Participants

If the program is using a group format, there may need to be careful selection of group participants. We recognize that children and adolescents with ASD are at risk of additional diagnoses or problematic behaviors, including externalizing behaviors such as impulsivity, hyperactivity, and oppositionality. Such challenging behaviors can impact the cohesion of the group. It is also important to consider the personality of each participant and his or her emotional and intellectual maturity, in order to maximize group cooperation, mutual support, and the possibility of the development of friendships within and after the group sessions. If a group format is used with children, the leaders should carefully consider the leader-to-participants ratio to allow effective monitoring and facilitation of group interactions and attention. The ratio can be adjusted, as needed, for children or adolescents who may be less hyperactive and more compliant in a small-group setting or those who may have more behavioral difficulties or be in a large-group setting.

The most recent prevalence study in the United States estimated that the ratio of boys to girls with an ASD is 5:1 (Centers for Disease Control, 2012). Should a girl with ASD be the only female in the group, she might feel uncomfortable and self-conscious. The strategies used in CBT are usually gender-neutral but there may be situations, such as being bullied by girls rather than boys, that require gender-specific strategies. Clinical experience has indicated that there can be advantages in having groups specifically for girls, if this is at all possible.

Time with Parents after Each Session

Researchers have noted the importance of including parents in CBT programs for children with ASD (see Reaven & Blakely-Smith, Chapter 5, this volume). It is helpful to set aside time at the end of each session to exchange information with the parents regarding their children's responses and abilities during the activities, to explain the project, and to seek information on particular issues that may be addressed in a subsequent session. Because criticism from family members may increase children's symptoms (Greenberg, Seltzer, Hong, & Orsmond, 2006), thus undermining success of the CBT program, it is also essential that family members be encouraged to respond positively and appropriately to the children's new abilities and understanding of emotion management, and to facilitate the successful application of strategies discovered during the program in real-life situations. Clinical experience has indicated that some family members of people with ASD may also have problems communicating emotion; thus, group discussion with parents may encourage solutions to problems experienced by other family members that have a positive influence on the emotional atmosphere at home and, consequently, the emotional equilibrium of the child or adolescent with ASD.

CONCLUDING COMMENTS

The modifications of CBT for children and adolescents with ASD are only minor adjustments and sometimes reflect good practice for any CBT program, regardless of the diagnosis of the client. However, clinical experience has indicated that the content and style of the therapy need to accommodate the unusual profile of abilities associated with ASD that is incorporated into the diagnostic criteria and recognized by clinicians who specialize in this area. It is also important to identify the personality of the person with ASD and how he or she has adapted to being different from peers. Some internalize their confusion and differences, tend to be socially withdrawn, and are too shy and reticent to interact with the clinician. In contrast, others may be intensely active and intrusive in social interactions, often unaware of social conventions and the potential to annoy others, including the clinician. However, the logical, practical, and structured approach of CBT suits the "mind-set" of those with higher-functioning ASD and may therefore be considered the therapy of first choice for clinicians working with clients with ASD who are not cognitively impaired and can benefit from addressing cognitive biases, deficits in affective knowledge, and social–behavioral competence.

REFERENCES

American Psychiatric Association. (2013). *Diagnostic and statistical manual of mental disorders* (5th ed.). Arlington, VA: Author.

Anderson, S., & Morris, J. (2006). Cognitive behavior therapy for people with Asperger syndrome. *Behavioural and Cognitive Psychotherapy, 34,* 293–303.

Attwood, T. (2007). *The complete guide to Asperger's syndrome.* London: Jessica Kingsley.

Attwood, T., Callesen, K., & Nielsen, A. (2008). *The CAT-kit Cognitive Affective Training.* Arlington, TX: Future Horizons.

Baron-Cohen, S. (1995). *Mind blindness: An essay on autism and theory of mind.* Cambridge, MA: MIT Press.

Baron-Cohen, S. (2000). Theory of mind and autism: A review. *International Review of Research in Mental Retardation, 23,* 170–184.

Beck, A. T., Rush, A. J., Shaw, B. F., & Emery, G. (1979). *Cognitive therapy of depression.* New York: Guilford Press.

Ben-Sasson, A., Cermak, S. A., Orsmond, G. I., Tager-Flusberg, H., Kadlec, M. B., & Carter, A. S. (2008). Sensory clusters of toddlers with autism spectrum disorders: Differences in affective symptoms. *Journal of Child Psychology and Psychiatry, 49,* 817–825.

Ben Shalom, D., Mostofsky, S. H., Hazlett, R. L., Goldberg, M. C., Landa, R. J., Faran, Y., et al. (2006). Normal physiological emotions but differences in expression of conscious feelings in children with high-functioning autism. *Journal of Autism and Developmental Disorders, 36,* 395–400.

Berthoz, S., & Hill, E. (2005). The validity of using self-reports to assess emotion regulation abilities in adults with autism spectrum disorder. *European Psychiatry 20,* 291–298.

Bishop, D. V. M. (1997). *Uncommon understanding: Development and disorders of language comprehension in children.* Hove, UK: Psychology Press.

Bishop, D. V. M., & Baird, G. (2001). Parent and teacher report of pragmatic aspects of communication: Use of the Children's Communication Checklist in a clinical setting. *Developmental Medicine and Child Neurology, 43,* 809–818.

Boucher, J., & Lewis, V. (1989). Memory impairments and communication in relatively able autistic children. *Journal of Child Psychology and Psychiatry, 33,* 99–122.

Carlson, C. L., & Tamm, L. (2000). Responsiveness of children with attention-deficit/hyperactivity disorder to reward and response cost: Differential impact on performance and motivation. *Journal of Consulting and Clinical Psychology, 68,* 73–83.

Centers for Disease Control and Prevention (CDC). (2012). Prevalence of autism spectrum disorders. *MMWR Surveillance Summary, 61*(SS03), 1–19.

Craske, M. G. (2010). *Cognitive-behavioral therapy.* Washington, DC: American Psychological Association.

Dalrymple, N. J. (1995). Environmental supports to develop flexibility and independence. In K. A. Quill (Ed.), *Teaching children with autism: Strategies to enhance communication and socialization* (pp. 243–264). New York: Delmar.

DuPaul, G. J., & Stoner, G. (2003). *ADHD in the schools* (2nd ed.). New York: Guilford Press.

Ellis, A. (1962). *Reason and emotion in psychotherapy.* Secaucus, NJ: Lyle Stuart.

Fein, D., Dixon, P., Paul, J., & Levin, H. (2005). Pervasive developmental disorder can evolve into ADHD: Case illustrations. *Journal of Autism and Developmental Disorders, 35,* 525–534.

Frith, U., & Happé, F. (1994). Autism: Beyond theory of mind. *Cognition, 50,* 115–132.

Frith, U., & Happé, F. (1999). Self-consciousness and autism: What is it like to be autistic? *Mind and Language, 14,* 1–22.

Golan, O., Ashwin, E., Granader, Y., McClintock, S., Day, K., Leggett, V., et al. (2010). Enhancing emotion recognition in children with autism spectrum conditions: An intervention using animated vehicles with real emotional faces. *Journal of Autism and Developmental Disorders, 40*(3), 269–279.

Goldstein, G., Johnson, C., & Minshew, N. (2001). Attentional processes in autism. *Journal of Autism and Developmental Disorders 31,* 433–440.

Grave, J., & Blissett, J. (2004). Is cognitive behavior therapy developmentally appropriate for young children?: A critical review of the evidence. *Clinical Psychology Review, 5*(3), 161–172.

Gray, C. A. (1995). Teaching children with autism to "read" social situations. In K. A. Quill (Ed.), *Teaching children with autism: Strategies to enhance communication and socialization* (pp. 219–242). New York: Delmar.

Greenberg, J. S., Seltzer, M. M., Hong, J., & Orsmond, G. I. (2006). Bidirectional effects of expressed emotion and behavior problems and symptoms in adolescents and adults with autism. *American Journal on Mental Retardation, 111,* 229–249.

Groden, J., & LeVasseur, P. (1995). Cognitive picture rehearsal: A system to teach self-control. In K. A. Quill (Ed.), *Teaching children with autism: Strategies to enhance communication and socialization* (pp. 287–303). New York: Delmar.

Harms, M. B., Martin, A., & Wallace, G. L. (2010). Facial emotion recognition in autism spectrum disorders: A review of behavioural and neuroimaging studies. *Neuropsychology Review, 20,* 290–322.

Hazell, P. (2006). Drug therapy for attention-deficit/hyperactivity disorder-like symptoms in autistic disorder. *Journal of Peadiatrics and Child Health, 43,* 19–24.

Hill, E. L. (2004). Executive dysfunction in autism. *Trends in Cognitive Sciences, 8,* 26–32.

Hill, E. L. (2008). Executive functioning in autism spectrum disorder: Where it fits in the causal model. In E. McGregor, M. Nunez, K. Cebula, & J. C. Gomez (Eds.), *Autism: An integrated view from neurocognitive, clinical, and intervention research* (pp. 145–166). Malden, MA: Blackwell.

Hobson, R. P. (2010). Explaining autism: Ten reasons to focus on the developing self. *Autism, 14,* 391–407.

Hopkins, I. (2011). Avatar assistant: Improving social skills in students with an ASD through a computer-based intervention. *Journal of Autism and Developmental Disorders, 41*(11), 1543–1555.

Kanner, L. (1943). Autistic disturbances of affective contact. *Nervous Child, 2,* 217–250.

Koegel, R. L., & Koegel, L. K. (2006). *Pivotal response treatments for autism.* Baltimore: Brookes.

LaCava, P. G., Golan, O., Baron-Cohen, S., & Smith Myles, B. (2007). Using assistive techonology to teach emotion recognition to students with Asperger syndrome. *Remedial and Special Education, 28,* 174–181.

Lang, R., Regester, A., Lauderdale, S., Ashbaugh, K., & Haring, A. (2010).

Treatment of anxiety in autism spectrum disorders using cognitive behavior therapy: A systematic review. *Developmental Neurorehabilitation, 13,* 53–63.

Liss, M., Mailloux, J., & Erchull, M. J. (2008). The relationships between sensory processing sensitivity, alexithymia, autism, depression, and anxiety. *Personality and Individual Differences, 45,* 255–259.

National Research Council. (2001). *Educating children with autism.* Washington, DC: National Academy Press.

Ollendick, T. H., Grills, A. E., & King, N. (2001). Applying developmental theory to the assessment and treatment of childhood disorders: Does it make a difference? *Clinical Psychology and Psychotherapy, 8,* 304–314.

Ozonoff, S., Cook, I., Coon, H., Dawson, G., Joseph, R. M., Klin, A., et al. (2004). Performance on Cambridge Neuropsychological Test Automated Battery subtests sensitive to frontal lobe function in people with autistic disorder: Evidence from the collaborative programs of excellence in autism network. *Journal of Autism and Developmental Disorders, 34,* 139–150.

Rotheram-Fuller, E., & MacMullen, L. (2011). Cognitive-behavioral therapy for children with autism spectrum disorders. *Psychology in the Schools, 48,* 263–271.

Silver, M., & Oakes, P. (2001). Evaluation of a new computer intervention to teach people with autism or Asperger syndrome to recognize and predict emotions in others. *Autism, 5,* 299–316.

Spencer, T. J., Biederman, J., & Wilens, T. (2000). Pharmacotherapy of attention deficit hyperactivity disorder. *Child and Adolescent Psychiatric Clinics of North America, 9,* 77–97.

Sturm, H., Fernell, E., & Gillberg, C. (2004). Autism spectrum disorders in children with normal intellectual levels: Associated impairments and subgroups. *Developmental Medicine and Child Neurology, 46,* 444–447.

Tanaka, J. T. (2010). Using computerized games to teach face recognition skills to children with autism spectrum disorder: The Let's Face It! program. *Journal of Child Psychology and Psychiatry, 51*(8), 944–952.

Tani, P., Joukamaa, M., Lindberg, N., Nieminen-von Wendt, T., Virkkala, J., Appelberg, B., et al. (2004). Asperger syndrome, alexithymia and sleep. *Neuropsychobiology, 49,* 64–70.

Twachtman-Cullen, D. (2000). More able children with autism spectrum disorders: Sociocommunicative challenges and guidelines for enhancing abilities. In A. M. Wetherby & B. M. Prizant (Eds.), *Autism spectrum disorders: A transactional developmental perspective* (pp. 225–249). Baltimore: Brookes.

Velting, O., Setzer, N., & Albano, A. (2004). Update on and advances in assessment and cognitive-behavioral treatment of anxiety disorders in children and adolescents. *Professional Psychology: Research and Practice, 35,* 42–54.

White, S. W., Kreiser, N. L., Pugliese, C. E., & Scarpa, A. (2012). Social anxiety mediates the effect of autism spectrum disorder characteristics on hostility in young adults. *Autism: The International Journal of Research and Practice, 16,* 453–464.

3

The Role of Assessment in Guiding Treatment Planning for Youth with ASD

Carla A. Mazefsky and Susan Williams White

Accurate assessment and diagnosis are critical to effective treatment planning. Assessment can inform several aspects of the treatment process, including identification of specific skills the child needs to learn or practice, measurement of treatment success, and identifying when treatment is not working and a new approach is needed (White, 2011). In addition, particularly for children with autism spectrum disorders (ASD), assessments are necessary to determine whether cognitive-behavioral therapy (CBT) is an appropriate form of treatment, and whether any modifications to the treatment delivery are necessary.

This chapter describes an approach to assessment in ASD that can be used to guide treatment planning. First, general considerations in assessment and how to choose and administer measures are discussed. Challenges with the use of self-report in high-functioning ASD (HFASD) are covered. The rest of the chapter includes a discussion of available measures, including their psychometric properties, utility in ASD, and any drawbacks. This begins with a discussion of diagnostic tools, including measures that diagnose ASD and can be used to assess psychiatric comorbidities in people with ASD. Measures that are useful in gauging response to intervention and those focusing on specific symptoms that are common treatment targets are then reviewed. The chapter concludes with a case example of how assessment can inform conceptualization and treatment planning for a child with ASD entering CBT.

CHOOSING AND ADMINISTERING MEASURES

Psychometric Properties

When choosing which assessment measure to use, it is important to consider the psychometric properties. Unfortunately, except for measures explicitly assessing symptoms of ASD, most standardization samples typically exclude children with ASD. Thus, some caution should always be taken when interpreting measures without information on psychometric properties for children with ASD, and preference should be given to those measures that have demonstrated reliability and validity in this sample. *Reliability* determines the consistency or stability of a specific measure, while *validity* determines the extent to which a test measures what it is intended to measure.

Use of Self-Report

The ideal approach to assessment is *multimethod*, utilizing a combination of continuous screening measures, structured and unstructured observation, and interviews, and multi-informant (e.g., parent-report, self-report, teacher-report, and clinician-rated measures). The assumption is that all sources provide unique and meaningful information to aid in the diagnostic process (Achenbach, McConaughy, & Howell, 1987; Jensen et al., 1999). For example, Jensen et al. (p. 1577) concluded that "for most conditions among 9- to 17-year-old children, both parent and child informants are necessary to obtain adequate diagnostic information, even though using only one informant may be appealing as more convenient or less costly."

Interpretation of multiple-informant assessments, however, can be difficult. Fairly low agreement among parent, teacher, and child ratings is common across clinical disorders and psychiatric symptoms (Achenbach et al., 1987; De Los Reyes & Kazdin, 2005; Reuterskiöld, Öst, & Ollendick, 2008). The discrepancy between parent- and child-report measures may be even more pronounced in children and adolescents with HFASD (Hurtig et al., 2009; Lopata et al., 2010; Mazefsky, Kao, Conner, & Oswald, 2011). The reasons for the low agreement are not well understood, but they may be associated with difficulty in providing accurate self-reports due to problems with verbal and nonverbal communication, inability to recognize thoughts and feelings, and poor emotional expression (Capps, Yirmiya, & Sigman, 1992; Leyfer et al., 2006).

Nonetheless, self-report should be obtained for verbal children with ASD whenever possible and may provide valuable information. A study focused on self-report psychiatric screening questionnaires found that the self-reports by adolescents with HFASD had as good as or even better internal reliability scores as the non-ASD standardization samples, suggesting that the adolescents understood what they were being asked and were able to answer the items in a consistent fashion (Mazefsky, Kao, et al., 2011). Furthermore, as expected, self-report scores in this study were higher for the comorbid than for the non-comorbid children with HFASD, albeit only by an average of half a standard deviation and despite lack of a significant difference. More research is needed to understand limitations in the validity of self-report by children with HFASD. For less verbal children, or children with reading difficulties, it may be helpful to read the items aloud or use visual graphics to accompany the rating scale.

ASSESSMENT PURPOSE

ASD Diagnosis

Although most often diagnosed by the age of 5 years (Centers for Disease Control and Prevention, 2009), identification and diagnosis of ASD can be delayed and may occur even in adulthood—a situation more common among very high-functioning people (White, Bray, & Ollendick, 2012). Earliest indicators of possible ASD include any behavioral regression or loss of language skills; lack of cooing, babbling, or other socially meaningful gestures by around 12 months of age; no single-word speech at 16 months; and a lack of two-word spontaneous phrase speech by 24 months of age (Johnson, Myers, & the American Academy of Pediatrics Council on Children with Disabilities, 2007). It is often these "red flag" indicators, as well as more subtle signs, such as a lack of social smiling or excessive interests in unusual objects or activities (National Institute of Mental Health, 2008), that prompt referral for diagnostic evaluation. However, for children with HFASD, it is often behavioral and emotional dysregulation that first prompts an evaluation (Mazefsky et al., 2012). Therefore, it is quite common for children with HFASD to receive mental health diagnoses first, before the ASD is recognized (e.g. Gilmour, Hill, Place, & Skuse, 2004). Thus, establishing whether an ASD is present may be the first step before initiating therapy, because it will probably affect the content, delivery, and course of the treatment.

Because children are often initially referred for evaluation for concerns that are not obviously indicative of an ASD (e.g., aggression, distractibility), broad-based rating scales that assesses for elevations across a range of problem domains may be quite helpful: The Behavior Assessment System for Children—Second Edition (BASC-2; Reynolds & Kamphaus, 2004) for ages 2–21 years is a well-validated, standardized scale used to assess a broad range of problem behaviors and adaptive skills. In its most recent revision, a Developmental Social Disorder (DSD) content scale was incorporated, which asks questions about behaviors indicative of ASD. Volker et al. (2010) found that the DSD scale had high sensitivity (98%) and specificity (95%), using a cutoff score of 60. The preschool version of the Child Behavior Checklist for ages 1½–5 years (CBCL; Achenbach & Rescorla, 2000) has a specific Pervasive Developmental Disorder (PDD) scale as well. Although the school-aged version of the CBCL (Achenbach & Rescorla, 2001) for ages 6–17 does not have a similar ASD scale, there is evidence that the school-age CBCL can be applied as a screening tool for ASD (Ooi, Rescorla, Ang, Woo, & Fung, 2011). Elevated scores on the Withdrawn, Social Problems, and Thought Problems scales of the CBCL best predict ASD diagnosis (Biederman et al., 2010; Mazefsky, Anderson, Conner, & Minshew, 2011). This also suggests that elevations on these and other scales on broad-based measures do not necessarily suggest that comorbidity is present. If a profile suggestive of possible ASD is obtained, follow-up with ASD-specific screening tools is recommended

Most of the psychometrically sound ASD screening measures described in Table 3.1 are paper-and-pencil questionnaires. Newer measures, however, are being developed in alternative formats to reduce problems inherent in questionnaires (e.g., response bias). For example, the Checklist for Autism Spectrum Disorder (CASD; Mayes, 2010) is a 15- to 20-minute parent interview followed by a clinician rating. The Autism Mental Status Examination (AMSE; Grodberg, Weinger, Kolevzon, Soorya, & Buxbaum, 2012) a brief observational tool comprised of just eight items rated by a clinician. Screening measures are typically completed by someone who knows the child well, usually a parent or teacher, in about 5–20 minutes. Results from screening measures should be carefully reviewed to determine whether further assessment is necessary. While most measures provide cutoff scores indicative of clinical degrees of concern, elevated scores that are below the cutoff should also be taken seriously, particularly in light of other observations or parent–teacher concerns.

Once the need for a more in-depth ASD evaluation has been determined, data should be obtained on multiple domains of behavior and functioning. Several practice parameters describing a staged approach to

TABLE 3.1. ASD Screening Measures

Name	Age range	Comments
Modified Checklist for Autism in Toddlers (M-CHAT; Robins, Fein, & Barton, 1999)	16–48 months	For early identification/designed to suggest the need for an evaluation; includes an overall score, as well as some items considered "critical" if failed; freely available.
Social Communication Questionnaire (SCQ; Rutter, Bailey, & Lord, 2003)	4–18 years	High degree of correspondence to the ADI-R; may miss some higher-functioning ASD; based on yes–no scores; child must have a mental age of at least 2 years.
Social Responsiveness Scale (SRS; Constantino & Gruber, 2005)	4–18 years[a]	Can detect HFASD and is used in studies of the broader autism phenotype as well; provides a continuous score, as well as ranges of severity.
Autism Screening Questionnaire (ASSQ; Ehlers, Gillberg, & Wing, 1999)	7–16 years	Designed for HFASD in particular; some items contain jargon and may be helpful to explain to the rater; freely available.
Checklist for Autism Spectrum Disorder (CASD; Mayes, 2010)	1–16 years	New measure with promising psychometric support; Intended to detect both lower- and higher-functioning ASD; different administration format.
Autism Quotient (AQ; Baron-Cohen, Wheelwright, Skinner, Martin, & Clubley, 2001)	Children through adults	Self-report screener for HFASD; overall score is psychometrically sound and good sensitivity; factor structure is less stable; clinically useful to discriminate social phobia and ASD in adults.

[a]Adult and preschool versions are now in prepublication.

screening, followed by more in-depth ASD assessment, have been developed (Filipek et al., 2000; Johnson et al., 2007). In addition to assessment of "core" ASD symptoms, any diagnostic evaluation for ASD should also include, at the least, full cognitive (IQ) testing and assessment of the person's adaptive behavior, as well as evaluation of receptive and expressive communication, given how common co-occurring intellectual disabilities and speech delays are in people with ASD. Initial diagnostic evaluation often involves a transdisciplinary team of professionals and may include assessment of neurological functioning, genetic testing, speech–hearing assessment, and assessment of the child's sensory profile (with an occupational therapist). Often, some of this information may be available from a child's individualized education plan (IEP).

No single tool or technique can be relied upon for diagnosis, but the two assessments most commonly used and considered the "gold standard" for diagnosis of ASD are the Autism Diagnostic Interview—Revised (ADI-R; Lord, Rutter, LeCouteur, 1994) and the Autism Diagnostic Observation Schedule (ADOS; Lord, Rutter, DiLavore, & Risi, 2002). The ADI-R is a lengthy (2+ hours) structured parental interview covering early development and both current and past behaviors. The ADOS, on the other hand, is a direct observational assessment designed to elicit behaviors that are characteristically absent (e.g., reciprocal communication) or present (e.g., restricted interests) in people with ASD. There are recently revised versions of both the ADI-R and ADOS for very young children (i.e., 12–30 months), and a new version of the ADOS (ADOS-2) is recently available. Both the ADOS and ADI-R require a significant amount of training to administer, and demonstration of reliability in administration and scoring procedures is required for use in research.

Although the ADOS and ADI-R are the most widely used and accepted ASD diagnostic tools, there are some alternative measures available. The Developmental, Dimensional, and Diagnostic Interview (3di; Skuse et al., 2004) is similar to the ADI-R but is computerized and provides, arguably, a more comprehensive psychiatric evaluation as well. The Childhood Autism Rating Scale (CARS; Schopler, Van Bourgondien, Wellman, & Love, 2010) is an alternative to the ADOS, since it provides a structured system for the clinician to rate the presence of ASD symptoms. The new second edition of the CARS also includes a specific high-functioning version in addition to the more standard version. However, it does not incorporate specific interaction probes as does the ADOS; rather it has a parent questionnaire to aid in gathering information to make the clinician rating.

Determining If CBT Is Appropriate

Information gathered as part of the ASD diagnostic process can be useful for decisions about whether CBT is an appropriate treatment. Both formal testing (e.g., IQ, adaptive) and observational data may guide the decision-making process. Unfortunately, there are no clear-cut guidelines, because CBT effectiveness has not been evaluated for those with comorbid intellectual disability. In general, one might assume that a minimal level of cognitive ability is required for the cognitive components of CBT (e.g., identifying erroneous thoughts), but processing difficulties (e.g., slow auditory processing) and executive function problems (e.g., rigid, rule-bound, and poor task flexibility), both of which are often seen in higher-functioning individuals with ASD, do not necessarily contraindicate CBT. They do, however, need to be considered in treatment delivery. Modifications may be necessary, such as allowing additional processing time, more repetitive and varied delivery of the same concepts, the addition of more visual cues, and extra practice. In addition, some adaptations of CBT are recommended for children with ASD regardless of functioning level, such as the use of a high-level structure, potential increases in the intervention dosage, peer involvement (particularly if targeting social skills), and careful matching of skills training to deficit areas (based on assessments) (see Attwood & Scarpa, Chapter 2, this volume; White, 2011).

Comorbid Psychiatric Diagnosis

Psychiatric comorbidity is a significant and critical problem of which all providers who work with individuals with ASD should be aware due to both its high rate of occurrence and its negative impact on functioning (e.g., Lefyer et al., 2006). However, the assessment of psychiatric comorbidity is quite complicated. When assessing an adolescent without ASD, it is often the best practice to begin assessment by talking with the the adolescent.With a young person with ASD, however, it may be preferable to interview the youth and parent jointly, or to interview the parent in lieu of interviewing the adolescent alone, especially if there are difficulties with self-reporting accurately, poor insight, or impaired verbal expression. In all cases, providers must use clinical judgment and try to gather information from multiple sources to arrive at final diagnoses.

There are few measures designed specifically to detect psychiatric comorbidity in ASD, and those that have been developed are in their infancy and therefore lack validation data. Interviews not specifically for individuals with ASD need to be reviewed carefully to make certain that symptoms that are part of ASD are not being misconceptualized as being due to a comorbid disorder (see Mazefsky & Handen, 2011). For example, it is important to consider whether symptoms suggestive of separation anxiety disorder stem from avoidance of unpleasant environmental factors (e.g., being teased, noisy environments, disruption in routine) that should be attributed to the ASD rather than interpreted as being related to interpersonal attachment to the caregiver. Or for social phobia, it is critical to determine whether the child's behaviors seem driven by fear of embarrassment and social humiliation or lack of social interest.

We summarize in Table 3.2 some of the available interviews for children that can be used as a guide in the detection of comorbid diagnoses or risk. With the exception of the Child and Adolescent Psychiatric Assessment (CAPA; Angold, Cox, Prendergast, Rutter, & Simonoff, 1995), which

TABLE 3.2. Psychiatric Interviews for Children Used in Assessing ASD

Name	Ages	Comments
Kiddie-Schedule for Affective Disorders & Schizophrenia (KSADS; Kaufman, Birmaher, Brent, Rao, & Ryan, 1996)	6–18 years	Semistructured interview with branching; present and lifetime versions; widely used in psychiatric research; must be administered by a clinically skilled interviewer; freely available at *www.wpic. pitt.edu/ksads*
Anxiety Disorders Interview Schedule–IV (ADIS-IV; Silverman & Albano, 1996)	7–17 years	Semistructured interview with branching; more in-depth assessment of anxiety disorders but briefer assessment of other concerns; must be administered by clinically skilled interviewer; purchased through Oxford University Press.
Child and Adolescent Psychiatric Assessment (CAPA; Angold et al., 1995)	8–18 years	Semistructured interview with branching; formal training through Duke University is required; involves obtaining information on behaviors in emotions in various settings that may be helpful for conceptualization and planning; free with approval at *http://devepi.duhs.duke.edu/ capa/html.*
Diagnostic Interview Schedule for Children (DISC; Shaffer, Fisher, Lucas, Dulcan, & Schwab-Stone, 2000)	9–17 years	Highly structured with branching; differentiates current (4 weeks), past year, and lifetime disorders; organized into six diagnostic sections (each section is "self-contained"); available in Spanish as well; can be administered by "lay" interviewers after a minimal training period.
Autism Comorbidity Interview (ACI; Lainhart et al., 2003)	Children and adults	Semistructured interview with branching; modification of the K-SADS for ASD with helpful differential diagnosis additions; fairly new instrument; provides subsyndromal and subthreshold diagnoses as well; must be administered by clinically skilled interviewer or clinician; presently available for research use with author permission.

only covers current (e.g., the past 3 months) symptoms, all of the other interviews assess for both current and past (lifetime) disorders. Definitions of *current* vary, though the past 3 months is most common. It is important to note that the Autism Comorbidity Interview (Lainhart, Leyfer, & Folstein, 2003) is the only interview included in Table 3.2 that was developed specifically for ASD/developmentally delayed populations.

Interviews are either highly structured (e.g., all specific probes must be used exactly) or semistructured (includes probes, but they do not need to be used verbatim). Semistructured interviews generally require more training and clinical skill to administer but are more flexible and may be a better match for ASD given that they allow the investigator to use language the child–parent will relate to and understand. Many diagnostic interviews involve a branching structure, with screening items administered first, and follow-up items administered only if the screening items indicate the possibility of a disorder being present. Thus, administration time can vary widely from child to child, but most psychiatric interviews are very time-intensive and take anywhere from 1 to 3 hours.

When making comorbid psychiatric diagnoses in children with ASD, clinicians should carefully consider underlying baseline functioning, how symptoms may overlap or stem from the ASD itself rather than a separate disorder, and potential differences in the presentation of psychiatric concerns in ASD when completing the differential diagnosis process (Mazefsky & Handen, 2011). One of the main challenges in diagnosing psychiatric disorders in individuals with ASD is the possibility of different presenting symptoms and difficulty in differentiating between impairment related to the underlying ASD and impairment due to a separate condition. While we do not want to miss true comorbid diagnoses, overdiagnosing comorbidity can be equally harmful, particularly due to the psychopharmacological treatment regimen indicated for certain diagnoses (e.g., bipolar disorder, attention-deficit/hyperactivity disorder [ADHD]). In later childhood and adolescence, it may be important to consider personality disorder and eating disorder diagnoses. Unfortunately, there are no specific screens for assessing these disorders in ASD, and more research in this area is needed. Developing a time line of symptom presentation is criticial in determining the most parsimonious explanation for behaviors and avoiding overdiagnosing symptoms that are a manifestation of ASD.

Nonepisodic disorders, such as ADHD, can be particularly difficult to tease apart from the underlying ASD. While there are no clear guidelines on best assessment approaches, a great deal has been written about the presentation of ADHD in ASD, as well as debates about how to best conceptualize these symptoms (Reiersen & Todd, 2008). Some important differential diagnostic considerations include inattention from lack of understanding, hearing impairment, transient behavioral reactions, or distractibility that is better thought of as part of ASD (e.g., due to sensory overstimulation or seeking, preoccupation with a special interest) (Mazefsky & Handen, 2011).

There are general rules of thumb in the differential diagnostic process specifically for episodic disorders such as depression and anxiety (Lainhart et al., 2003; Mazefsky & Handen, 2011):

- Symptoms should differ qualitatively or quantitatively (*an important and meaningful change*) from "baseline" functioning with the ASD.
  - In order to determine this, one must first establish how the individual is *at his or her best*, or in his *normal mood.*
  - With comorbidity, there may be new symptoms *or* a worsening of baseline behaviors–emotions.
  - There should be *additional* impairment related to the new or changed symptoms.
- It is important to make sure that the "additional" symptoms one is applying as evidence of a comorbid disorder make sense for the person with ASD (e.g., the symptom "purposefully annoys" others in oppositional defiant disorder assumes that one can detect when someone is annoyed, has the social cognition to determine what annoys the person, and intent to annoy).
- Symptoms counted as evidence of the existence of a comorbid disorder should co-occur temporally. It is rare to have simultaneous onset of two discrete disorders. Furthermore, often it becomes clear with probing that a pattern of inappropriate emotional responses might have been present throughout the child's life, rather than representing a new episode/disorder.

When there has been a significant change in behavior but a careful assessment rules out a comorbid disorder, a functional behavioral assessment (FBA) is often helpful to identify the underlying cause of the behavioral change and the appropriate treatment target. In brief, an FBA can include structured and unstructured observations with ratings of the target behavior, direct manipulation of an aspect of the environment to observe whether there is a change, or a variety of rating scales or interviews. The primary information that is ultimately gathered includes any triggers or antecedents to the event; a detailed and operationalized description of the behavior itself; any consequences that result from the behavior; and identifications of any situations, places, or times of day when the behavior is more likely to occur (for more information, see Alfieri, Burkley, & McGonigle, 2011; O'Neill, Horner, Albin, Sprague, Storey, & Newton, 1997).

Monitoring Diagnostic Changes

An obvious outcome measure for treatment is change in diagnostic status. This can be accomplished via readministration of the original diagnostic measures. In addition, global ratings of illness severity can be informative. A commonly used rating system, the Clinical Global Impression (CGI) scale, provides a 7-point metric for rating illness severity, global improvement or change, and therapeutic response. The Children's Global Assessment Scale (CGAS; Shaffer et al., 1983), a modification of the Global Assessment Scale, can be quite useful when administered by a skilled clinician who knows the child. It provides a single rating, from 1 *(most impaired)* to 100 *(healthiest)* to describe overall level of functioning and impairment. The fairly recent Developmental Disabilities Modification of the CGAS (DD-CGAS; Wagner et al., 2007) includes rating benchmarks designed specifically to gauge behaviors and domains of functioning that typically are problematic for children with ASD. Emerging evidence (Smith, Schry, & White, 2012) indicates that the DD-CGAS may be sensitive to change in adolescents with ASD.

Continuous Measures of Symptom Severity

It is often necessary to go beyond a categorical diagnosis to get a full picture of a child's functioning level and treatment needs. Even when an official comorbid diagnosis does not make sense, it still may be the case that treatment is necessary due to the interference of symptoms. Furthermore, continuous measures of various symptom domains can be helpful in determining outcome and tracking progress. It is recommended to use measures of adaptive behavior or overall functioning, as well as measures of the specific target symptoms.

Adaptive Behavior

In addition to the use of adaptive behavior information to determine a diagnosis of intellectual disability, adaptive behavior information may also be used to clarify an individual's level of impairment and the intensity of support that is required. Even among high-functioning children with ASD, it is common for overall adaptive behavior skills to be dramatically lower than one might expect based on intellectual ability (e.g., Mazefsky, Williams, & Minshew, 2008). Adaptive behavior assessment can assist in the development of goals and objectives for treatment by identifying areas of strength and weakness, and specific skills that require remediation. Finally, regular assessment of adaptive behavior can contribute to the monitoring of progress as an individual moves through treatment. This type of assessment must be done cautiously, however, given that most adaptive behavior indices span a fairly wide time frame—usually the past 6 months or so. Age-equivalent scores may be most useful in gauging treatment gains over the course of treatment (Williams et al., 2006). The most commonly used measures of adaptive behavior are summarized in Table 3.3.

TABLE 3.3. Adaptive Behavior Assessment Instruments

Name	Ages	Method of administration	Domains
Adaptive Behavior Assessment, Second Edition (Harrison & Oakland, 2003)	Birth to 89 years	Questionnaire	Communication, functional academics, self-direction, social skills, leisure skills, self-care, home or school living, community use, work, health/safety.
Scales of Independent Behavior—Revised (Bruininks, Woodcock, Weatherman, & Hill, 2010)	Infancy to 80+ years	Questionnaire or structured interview	Motor skills, social interaction and communication skills, personal living skills, community living skills, problem behaviors.
Vineland Adaptive Behavior Scales, Second Edition (Sparrow, Cicchetti, & Balla, 2005)	Birth to 90 years	Questionnaire or structured interview	Communication, daily living skills, socialization, motor skills, maladaptive behavior.

Social Skills and Social Cognition

It is both surprising and unfortunate that the field lacks a clear "gold standard" assessment tool for social disability as presented by people with ASD, given how central this deficit domain is to the diagnosis itself. Accurate assessment of the nature and severity of the social deficit is critical to treatment planning and to monitoring progress once treatment has begun (Gillis, Callahan, & Romanczyk, 2011). Perhaps the most frequently used parent-report quantitative measure of social skills is the Social Skills Rating System (SSRS; Gresham & Elliott, 1990) for ages 8–18 years. The SSRS was developed to help screen for social behavioral difficulties in typically developing children. Although not created for use with children with ASD, the SSRS has been used extensively in research to evaluate change in skills. Its ability to detect treatment progress in youth on the autism spectrum has not been firmly established, however (White, Koenig, & Scahill, 2007). The Social Responsiveness Scale (SRS; Constantino & Gruber, 2005), for ages 4–18, with preschool and adult versions that recently became available (SRS-2; Constantino, 2012), described earlier as an ASD diagnostic screening tool, provides a dimensional measure of severity of social deficits specifically designed for the ASD population. In addition to the Global Functioning Index, the SRS has five treatment subscales designed to evaluate change as a function of treatment. Several recent treatment outcome studies (Bass, Duchowny, & Llabre, 2009; Lopata et al., 2010; White, Albano, Johnson, Kasari, Ollendick, et al., 2010; White, Ollendick, et al., 2012) indicate that the SRS is sensitive to change with treatment in people with ASD. Wang, Sandall, Davis, and Thomas (2011) compared the SSRS and the Preschool and Kindergarten Behavior Scale (PKBS; Merrell, 1994) for ages 3–6 years and concluded that both are are psychometrically sound but neither measure appears sensitive to gauging treatment response in young children (36–76 months). A second ASD-specific measure, the Autism Social Skills Profile (ASSP; Bellini & Hopf, 2007) for ages 6–17 years, focuses exclusively on the child's present level of functioning (i.e., not other ASD core symptoms, such as repetitive behaviors). The ASSP may be useful in treatment planning and in providing information on deficits specific to ASD. It not yet commercially available, although the preliminary research on its use is promising (Bellini & Hopf, 2007). Two additional measures of social functioning include the self-reported Matson Evaluation of Social Skills with Youngsters (MESSY; Matson, Rotatori, & Helsel, 1983) for ages 4–18 years, and the fairly new Behavioral Assessment of Social Interactions in Young Children (BASYC; Callahan, Gillis, Romanczyzk, & Mattson, 2011) for ages 2–12 years. Finally, although options for observational/behavioral measures of social skills are presently limited, the Contextual Assessment of Social Skills (CASS; Ratto, Tumer-Brown, Rupp, Mesibov, & Penn, 2011) is a promising role-play measure of social functioning for adolescents and adults with HFASD.

It can also be helpful to assess specific aspects of social cognition, in addition to overall social skills. The construct of "theory of mind" has been well-studied in general, and people with ASD are often thought to have principal deficits in their ability to display a theory of mind. Baron-Cohen (1995) termed this deficit in theory of mind as "mindblindness," referring to deficient ability to mentalize about self and others as thinking beings with interpretable intentions, motives, and emotions. Theory of mind is a developmental phenomenon (Wellman, Cross, & Watson, 2001), and most typical children pass such false-belief tasks by age 3 to 4 years. People with ASD often, though inconsistently across sample and task, demonstrate impairments in such tasks (e.g., see Happé, 1995, for review). Success on theory of mind tasks, which is largely tied to verbal ability, in people with ASD is related to the sophistication of the task (Happé, 1995).

Among the many specific theory of mind tasks, the more common ones are variations of the Sally Ann task (e.g., Wimmer & Perner, 1983), in which the child is told a story of a girl (Sally Ann) who puts something in a certain place (e.g., a cupboard), another person moves it to a new location (e.g., a drawer) when she is away, then the child is asked where Sally Ann will look for the item. A child who responds that she will look for the item in the drawer has not mastered theory of mind on this false-belief task. There are other modalities, outside of false-belief tasks, for assessing theory of mind. One parent-report measure is the Theory of Mind Inventory (ToMI; Hutchins, Bonazinga, Prelock, & Taylor, 2008) for ages 2–17 years, developed specifically for parents of children with ASD. Lerner, Hutchins, and Prelock (2011) found that ToMI scores were positively correlated with parent-reported social skills and negatively correlated, as expected, with ASD symptoms in adolescents on the spectrum. A theory of mind test developed specifically for adults is The Awareness of Social Inference Test (TASIT; McDonald, Flanagan, Rollins, & Kinch, 2003) for ages 13–60 years, a three-part test that assesses social perception via videotaped social interaction vignettes. Although a bit lengthy (approximately 1 hour administration time), it has good psychometric data, including test–retest stability (McDonald et al., 2006), and has recently been used with adults with ASD (Ratto et al., 2011). An application of Happé's strange stories has been shown to be an effective measure of advanced theory of mind skills for younger (5- to 12-year-old) children with HFASD (O'Hare, Bremner, Nash, Happé, & Pettigrew, 2009).

Anxiety and Depression

As mentioned earlier, it is established that different raters (e.g., parent and child) often given highly discrepant symptom reports of psychiatric symptoms in children with ASD, and it is often the case that children and adolescents, even those who are cognitively higher functioning, underreport their symptoms (Mazefsky, Kao, et al., 2011; Russell & Sofronoff, 2005; White, Schry, & Maddox, 2012). Thus, it is particularly important not to stop assessing for the possibility of a psychiatric disorder when a self-report measure does not indicate risk, especially if other indicators, such as a decline in functioning, are present. A child's underreporting of symptoms may be useful information for treatment planning and suggest the need to focus on increasing self-awareness, including how to recognize and communicate about emotions. In order to monitor treatment progress, both parent- and self-report of psychiatric symptoms should be utilized when possible.

Overall, research at this point does not support recommending any particular self- or parent-report questionnaires for use in ASD populations as measures of anxiety and depression. Although there has been some pilot research on certain self-report measures in ASD samples (e.g., Mazefsky, Kao, et al., 2011; White, Schry, et al., 2012), the validity and reliability of most psychiatric screens have not been established for ASD samples. Some that have been used in research on anxiety in ASD include the Screen for Child Anxiety Related Emotional Disorders (SCARED; Birmaher et al., 1997) for ages 8–18, the Revised Child Manifest Anxiety Scale (RCMAS; Reynolds & Richmond, 1985) for ages 6–19 years, the Multidimensional Anxiety Scale for Children (MASC; March, 1998) for ages 8–19 years, and the Pediatric Anxiety Rating Scale (PARS; Research Units of Pediatric Psychopharmacology [RUPP] Anxiety Study Group, 2002) for ages 6–17, which all have both parent- and self-report versions. The Child Depression Inventory (CDI; Kovacs, 1992) for ages 7–17 is an option for depression, as is the Mood and Feelings Questionnaire (MFQ; Costello & Angold, 1988) for ages 8–18, though the MFQ is more widely used in research than in clinical settings and does not provide cutoff scores. Both the SCARED and MFQ are freely available.

General Behavior Problems

Presenting concerns frequently involve behavioral problems such as aggression and perseverative behaviors, and so forth. While some children with ASD meet criteria for oppositional defiant disorder, this diagnosis should be conservatively applied, because it may lead to a misconceptualization of behaviors. Often, externalizing behaviors among children with ASD stem from a combination of emotional distress and skills deficits (e.g., frustration stemming from communication difficulties, misinterpreting a social situation and lashing out). Given the overlap of symptoms, the measures most commonly used to measure behavioral problems also include scales related to the "core" ASD symptoms. For example, one of the most widely used measures, the Aberrant Behavior Checklist (ABC; Aman & Singh 1986), provides scores for irritability, agitation, crying, lethargy, social withdrawal, stereotypical behavior, noncompliance, and inappropriate speech. It has separate norms for Community and Residential versions and can be used for individuals ages 5–51 years. Another commonly used option is the Pervasive Developmental Disorder Behavior Inventory (PDDBI; Cohen & Sudhalter, 2005) for children ages 1 year, 6 months to 12 years, 5 months, which asseses ASD symptoms, as well as arousal regulation, fear, and aggression.

CASE EXAMPLE: ASSESSMENT AND CONCEPTUALIZATION FOR CBT

The following abbreviated assessment and case conceptualization are derived from real data with identifying information removed or changed to protect confidentiality.

Brief Intake

Grace, a 13-year-old Asian American female, was referred for psychiatric evaluation and treatment. Presenting concerns, per her own report and that of her adoptive parents, included difficulty making new friends and getting along with people at school, lacking confidence, and getting picked on. Grace reported that she wanted to "fit in," but her mother said she misunderstood others. She had a previous diagnosis of Asperger syndrome based on DSM-IV-TR criteria from a community clinician.

A physically healthy youngster, Grace had no notable problems developmentally, physically, or otherwise. All developmental milestones were met on time. She was taking her first steps and using single words by about 12 months of age. She was in the eighth grade at the time of this intake, with a formal service plan (i.e., a 504 Plan) at her school. She received extra time on in-class tests. Grace excelled academically, maintaining a 3.9 grade point average (GPA). She experienced considerable anxiety about academics, however, which interfered with her home and family life. She refused to miss school, even when ill, and her studies impeded her participation in family activities.

Grace was not taking any medications but previously had been prescribed Celexa for depression and anxiety (discontinued the previous year). Her mother reported that it was not helpful, and they discontinued it because of the negative side effects. There was no reported history of abuse or legal problems, and no evidence of thought disorder or suicidal ideation. Grace stated that her primary goal with therapy was to learn how to initiate conversations, develop four to 10 good friends, and reduce her anxiety. Her mother's treatment goal was for Grace to have at least one friend with whom she could talk, and to reduce her anxiety about schoolwork.

Assessments

Anxiety Disorders Interview Schedule—Parent/Child (ADIS-C/P)
Autism Diagnostic Interview—Revised (ADI-R)
Autism Diagnostic Observation Schedule—Module 3 (ADOS: 3)

Multidimensional Anxiety Scale for Children (MASC)
Social Responsiveness Scale (SRS)
Vineland Adaptive Behavior Scales—Second Edition
Wechsler Abbreviated Scale of Intelligence (WASI)

Results

The ADI-R was completed with Grace's mother. Based on her responses, Grace obtained scores above the diagnostic threshold in the domains of Qualitative Abnormalities in Reciprocal Social Interaction; Qualitative Abnormalities in Communication; and Restricted, Repetitive, and Stereotyped Patterns of Behavior. Some of the specific behaviors noted in the interview included a lack of interest in peers (when she was younger), no same-age friends, a lack of shared enjoyment and spontaneous seeking to direct others' attention or interest, and inappropriate facial expressions and social responses. Grace also, per her mother's report, has difficulty with nonverbal communication (e.g., pointing, nodding), has never been able to engage easily in reciprocal give-and-take conversations, and often uses unusual phrasing or words. There was not, however, evidence of abnormality or concern with Grace's development prior to 36 months of age. On the ADOS, Grace obtained a Communication + Social Interaction total score of 8, which is above the cutoff score of 7, indicative of likely ASD. During the ADOS, Grace used language appropriately and did not display any echolalia or idiosyncratic speech. She did, however, speak in a flat tone of voice throughout the assessment. She rarely offered information about herself or her interests and never asked the examiner personally appropriate questions. She was inconsistent in her eye contact and demonstrated a limited range of facial expressions; but she did seem to enjoy the interaction with the examiner. Grace's SRS Total T-score of 63 falls in the mild to moderate range, suggesting clinically significant difficulty with reciprocal social behavior. Scores in this range are characteristic of high-functioning children with ASD.

On the ADIS-C/P, Grace's highest obtained Clinician Severity Ratings (CSRs) were on Social Phobia (6), Generalized Anxiety Disorder (6), Separation Anxiety Disorder (4), and Obsessive–Compulsive Disorder (3). On the MASC, Grace obtained elevated scores on the Social Anxiety scale (T-score = 70) and the Separation Anxiety scale (T-score = 74). Her Physical Symptoms and Harm Avoidance scale scores were not elevated, at 54 and 44, respectively. Grace's total score on the MASC was 64, which is above average, though her Social Anxiety and Separation Anxiety scale scores were very much above average. The worries and fears Grace reported in these domains seemed to have a fairly recent onset, supporting the conceptualization of these issues as comorbid problems rather than as symptoms or manifestations of the ASD itself.

Her estimated Verbal IQ on the WASI was 123, in the high average range. Her adaptive behavior scores on the Vineland, were variable, falling from moderately low to moderately high ranges: In the Communication domain, she obtained a standard score of 116; in Daily Living Skills, her score was 83; and in Socialization, her total score was 82. Grace's overall Adaptive Behavior Composite score of 92 was considerably below her assessed cognitive ability. Grace's cognitive ability and adaptive behavior, though variable, did not contraindicate use of CBT as a treatment.

Diagnostic Impressions

Grace met diagnostic criteria for Asperger syndrome, social anxiety disorder, and generalized anxiety disorder (GAD) using DSM-IV-TR (American Psychiatric Association, 2000) criteria. Although she achieved a clinically elevated score on the ADIS-C/P for separation anxiety disorder, this was not diagnosed, because symptoms appeared to occur exclusively when separated from her parents in social situations (e.g., not when they were leaving the home), and were therefore thought to be better captured under the social phobia diagnosis. Her subthreshold CSR for OCD did not appear to warrant diagnosis, because the behavioral symptoms were better subsumed under social phobia and GAD.

Treatment Plan

Primary concerns related to worrying about what peers thought of her and being fearful that she was too quiet (specifically, that others would think she was odd or weird because she was quiet) indicated that social anxiety was a primary target for treatment. Grace was hypersensitive to peers' judgments of her and intensely fearful of anything indicating failure (e.g., an A– or social ridicule) in her mind. Although she desperately wanted friends in school and struggled to interact with her peers, Grace generally avoided doing so, which prevented her from making friends despite her highly likable personal qualities. Based on the results of this assessment, it was recommended that Grace receive a course of individual CBT, in the hope that this approach would strengthen the cohesion of the family and her parents could be taught to "coach" her to refrain from behaviors maintaining the anxious avoidance, while also helping her build age-appropriate coping and self-help skills. Psychoeducation on ASD and anxiety disorders, instruction on how to identify and challenge some automatic negative thinking that likely exacerbated her anxiety, methods for practicing appropriate social skills, and strategies for reducing her anxious feelings were recommended topics to be addressed in therapy. Some of the specific interpersonal approaches to be taught and practiced included how to initiate conversation with peers using appropriate conversational skills (e.g., elaborating on what the other person says), and facing fears without distraction (i.e., exposure). It was hypothesized that Grace entertained many unhelpful (e.g., "distorted") thoughts and assumptions that served to strengthen her anxiety and subsequent avoidance, including a tendency to jump to conclusions (e.g., assuming the worst will happen) and filtering (e.g., noticing and attending to only evidence for "bad" or threatening situations, while overlooking evidence of positive situations/events). These distortions were not formally assessed, but the evaluator shared them as "hypotheses to be explored further," and both Grace and her parents concurred that they seemed accurate.

SUMMARY

Assessment provides a crucial foundation for conceptualization, treatment planning, and monitoring of treatment progress. When working with potential clients with ASD, the first step is often to establish the ASD diagnosis and characterize the level of impairment, as well as strengths and weaknesses across core diagnostic symptoms, cognition, and adaptive behavior. The field has made great progress in this area, and many measures now aid in ASD diagnosis, though often a fair amount of ASD-specific expertise is still required. Other types of assessment in ASD, particularly related to comorbidity and continuous measures of social dysfunction and psychiatric symptoms, remain in their infancy. Differential diagnosis of comorbid disorders in ASD is quite complex, and because the majority of measures are not ASD-specific, they do not directly point to some of the key considerations. There remains no "gold standard" for quantitative measures of social disability, anxiety, and depression in ASD. In part because of this state of the field, and in partly because of complexities related to self-report, assessment in ASD should be as multimethod and multi-informant as possible, with the ultimate conceptualization stemming from a synthesis of all available information and clinical judgment.

ACKNOWLEDGMENTS

This chapter was supported by grants from the National Institute of Child Health and Human Development (No. 1K23 HD060601; Carla A. Mazefsky, Principal Investigator) and the National Institute of Mental Health (No. 1K01MH079945-01;

Susan Williams White, Principal Investigator). We would like to thank and acknowledge Taylor Day, Shivani Patel, and Dana Schreiber at the University of Pittsburgh for their contributions to this chapter.

REFERENCES

Achenbach, T. M., McConaughy, S. H., & Howell, C. T. (1987). Child/adolescent behavioral and emotional problems: Implications of cross-informant correlations for situational specificity. *Psychological Bulletin, 101*(2), 213–232.

Achenbach, T. M., & Rescorla, L. A. (2000). *Manual for the ASEBA preschool forms and profiles*. Burlington: University of Vermont, Research Center for Children, Youth, and Families.

Achenbach, T. M., & Rescorla, L. A. (2001). *Manual for the ASEBA school-age forms and profiles*. Burlington: University of Vermont, Research Center for Children, Youth, and Families.

Alfieri, J. B., Burkley, R., & McGonigle, J. J. (2011). Functional behavior assessment (FBA). In M. J. Lubetsky, B. L. Handen, & J. J. McGonigle (Eds.), *Autism spectrum disorder* (pp. 115–122). New York: Oxford University Press.

Aman, M., & Singh, N. (1986). *Aberrant Behavior Checklist: Manual*. East Aurora, NY: Slosson Educational Publications.

Angold, A., Cox, A., Prendergast, M., Rutter, M., & Simonoff, E. (1995). The Child and Adolescent Psychiatric Assessment (CAPA). *Psychological Medicine, 25*, 739–753.

Baron-Cohen, S. (1995). *Mindblindness: An essay on autism and theory of mind*. Cambridge, MA: MIT Press.

Baron-Cohen, S., Wheelwright, S., Skinner, R., Martin, J., & Clubley, E. (2001). The Autism-Spectrum Quotient (AQ): Evidence from Asperger syndrome/high-functioning autism, males and females, scientists and mathematics. *Journal of Autism and Developmental Disorders, 31*, 5–17.

Bass, M. M., Duchowny, C. A., & Llabre, M. M. (2009). The effect of therapeutic horseback riding on social functioning in children with autism. *Journal of Autism and Developmental Disorders, 39*(9), 1261–1267.

Bellini, S., & Hopf, A. (2007). The development of the autism social skills profile: A preliminary analysis of psychometric properties. *Focus on Autism and Other Developmental Disabilities, 22*(2), 80–87.

Biederman, J., Petty, C. R., Fried, R., Wozniak, J., Micco, J. A., Henin, A., et al. (2010). Child Behavior Checklist clinical scales discriminate referred youth with autism spectrum disorder: A preliminary study. *Journal of Developmental and Behavioral Pediatrics, 31*(6), 485–490.

Birmaher, B., Khetarpal, S., Brent, D., Cully, M., Balach, L., Kaufman, J., et al. (1997). The Screen for Child Anxiety Related Emotional Disorders (SCARED): Scale construction and psychometric characteristics. *Journal of the American Academy of Child and Adolescent Psychiatry, 36*, 545–553.

Bruininks, R. H., Woodcock, R. W., Weatherman, R. F., & Hill, B. K. (2010). *Scales of Independent Behavior—Revised*. San Antonio, TX: Harcourt Assessment.

Callahan, E. H., Gillis, J. M., Romanczyk, R. G., & Mattson, R. E. (2011). The behavioral assessment of social interactions in young children: An examination of convergent and incremental validity. *Research in Autism Spectrum Disorders, 5,* 768–774.

Capps, L., Yirmiya, N., & Sigman, M. (1992). Understanding of simple and complex emotions in non-retarded children with autism. *Journal of Child Psychology and Psychiatry, 33*(7), 1169–1182.

Centers for Disease Control and Prevention. (2009). *Autism spectrum disorders: Data and statistics* [Data file]. Retrieved from *www.cdc.gov/ncbddd/autism/data.html.*

Cohen, I. L., & Sudhalter, V. (2005). *The PPD Behavior Inventory.* Lutz, FL: Psychological Assessment Resources.

Constantino, J. N. (2012). The Social Responsiveness Scale—second edition. Los Angeles: Western Psychological Services.

Constantino, J. N., & Gruber, C. P. (2005). *The Social Responsiveness Scale manual.* Los Angeles: Western Psychological Services.

Costello, E. J., & Angold, A. (1988). Scales to assess child and adolescent depression: Checklists, screens, and nets. *Journal of the American Academy of Child and Adolescent Psychiatry, 27,* 726–737.

De Los Reyes, A., & Kazdin, A. E. (2005). Informant discrepancies in the assessment of childhood psychopathology: A critical review, theoretical framework, and recommendations for further study. *Psychological Bulletin, 131*(4), 483–509.

Ehlers, S., Gillberg, C., & Wing, L. (1999). A screening questionnaire for Asperger syndrome and other high-functioning autism spectrum disorders in school age children. *Journal of Autism and Developmental Disorders, 29,* 129–141.

Filipek, P. A., Accardo, P. J., Ashwal, S., Baranek, G. T., Cook, E. H., Jr., Dawson, G., et al. (2000). Practice parameter: Screening and diagnosis of autism—Report of the quality standards subcommittee of the American Academy of Neurology and Child Neurology Society. *Neurology, 55,* 468–479.

Gillis, J. M., Callahan, E. H., & Romancyzk, R. G. (2011). Assessment of social behavior in children with autism: The development of the Behavioral Assessment of Social Interactions in Young Children. *Research in Autism Spectrum Disorders, 5*(1), 351–360

Gilmour, J., Hill, B., Place, M., & Skuse, D. (2004). Social communication deficits in conduct disorders: A clinical and community survey. *Journal of Child Psychology and Psychiatry, 45,* 967–978.

Gresham, F. M., & Elliott, S. N. (1990). *Social Skills Rating System: Manual.* Circle Pines, MN: American Guidance Service.

Grodberg, D., Weinger, P. M., Kolevzon, A., Soorya, L., & Buxham, J. D. (2012). Brief report: The Autism Mental Status Examination: Development of a brief autism-focused exam. *Journal of Autism and Developmental Disorders, 42*(3), 455–459.

Happé, F. G. E. (1995). The role of age and verbal ability in the theory of mind task performance of subjects with autism. *Child Development, 66*(3), 843–855.

Harrison, P., & Oakland, T. (2003). *Adaptive Behavior Assessment System—Second Edition.* San Antonio, TX: Harcourt Assessment.

Hurtig, T., Kuusikko, S., Mattila, M.-L., Haapsamo, H., Elbeling, H., Iussila, K., et al. (2009). Multi-informant reports of psychiatric symptoms among high-functioning adolescents with Asperger syndrome or autism. *Autism, 13*(6), 583–598.

Hutchins, T., Bonazinga, L., Prelock, P. A., & Taylor, R. S. (2008). Beyond false beliefs: The development and psychometric evaluation of the Perceptions of Children's Theory of Mind Measure—Experimental Version (PCToMM-E). *Journal of Autism and Developmental Disorders, 38*(1), 143–155.

Jensen, P. S., Rubio-Stepic, M. A., Canino, G., Bird, H. R., Dulcan, M. K., Schwab-Stone, M. E., et al. (1999). Parent and child contributions to diagnosis of mental disorders: Are both informants always necessary? *Journal of the American Academy of Child and Adolescent Psychiatry, 38,* 1569–1579.

Johnson, C. P., Myers, S. M., & the American Academy of Pediatrics Council on Children with Disabilities. (2007). Identification and evaluation of children with autism spectrum disorders. *Pediatrics, 120*(5), 1183–1215.

Kaufman, J., Birmaher, B., Brent, D., Rao, U., & Ryan, N. (1996). *The Schedule for Affective Disorders and Schizophrenia for School-Age Children.* Pittsburgh: University of Pittsburgh Medical Center.

Kovacs, M. (1992). *The Children's Depression Inventory (CDI) technical manual update.* Toronto: Multi-Health Systems.

Lahey, B. B. (1999). Parent and child contributions to diagnosis of mental disorders: Are both informants always necessary? *Journal of the American Academy of Child and Adolescent Psychiatry, 38,* 1569–1579.

Lainhart, J. E., Leyfer, O. T., & Folstein, S. E. (2003). *Autism Comorbidity Interview—Present and Lifetime version (ACI-PL).* Salt Lake City: University of Utah.

Lerner, M. D., Hutchins, T. L., & Prelock, P. A. (2011). Brief report: Preliminary Evaluation of the Theory of Mind Inventory and its relationship to measures of social skills. *Journal of Autism and Developmental Disorders, 41*(4), 512–517.

Leyfer, O. T., Folstein, S. E., Bacalman, S., Davis, N. O., Dinh, E., Morgan, J., et al. (2006). Comorbid psychiatric disorders in children with autism: Interview development and rates of disorders. *Journal for Autism and Developmental Disorders, 36,* 849–861.

Lopata, C., Thomeer, M. L., Volker, M. A., Toomey, J. A., Nida, R. E., Lee, G. K., et al. (2010). RCT of a manualized social treatment for high-functioning autism spectrum disorders. *Journal of Autism and Developmental Disorders, 40,* 1297–1310.

Lord, C., Rutter, M., DiLavore, P. C., & Risi, S. (2002). *Autism Diagnostic Observation Schedule.* Los Angeles: Western Psychological Services.

Lord, C., Rutter, M., & Le Couteur, A. (1994). Autism Diagnostic Interview—Revised: A revised version of a diagnostic interview for caregivers of individuals with possible pervasive developmental disorders. *Journal of Autism and Developmental Disorders, 24,* 659–685.

Matson, J. L., Rotatori, A. F., & Helsel, W. J. (1983). Development of a rating scale to measure social skills in children: The Matson Evaluation of Social

Skills with Youngsters (MESSY). *Behaviour Research and Therapy, 21*(4), 335–340.

March, J. S. (1998). *Multidimensional Anxiety Scale for Children manual.* North Tonawanda, NY: Multi-Health Systems.

Mayes, S. D. (2010). *Checklist for Autism Spectrum Disorder (CASD).* Wood Dale, IL: Stoelting.

Mazefsky, C. A., Anderson, R., Conner, C. M., & Minshew, N. J. (2011). *Child Behavior Checklist* scores for school-aged children with autism: Preliminary evidence of patterns suggesting the need for referral. *Journal of Psychopathology and Behavioral Assessment, 33,* 31–37.

Mazefsky, C. A., & Handen, B. L. (2011). Addressing behavioral and emotional challenges in school-aged children with ASD. In M. J. Lubetsky, B. L. Handen, & J. J. McGonigle (Eds.), *Autism spectrum disorder* (pp. 253–270). New York: Oxford University Press.

Mazefsky, C. A., Kao, J., Conner, C., & Oswald, D. P. (2011). Preliminary caution regarding the use of psychiatric self-report measures with adolescents with high-functioning autism spectrum disorders. *Research in Autism Spectrum Disorders, 5,* 164–174.

Mazefsky, C. A., Oswald, D. P., Day, T., Eack, S., Minshew, N. J., & Lainhart, J. E. (2012). ASD, a comorbid psychiatric disorder, or both?: Psychiatric diagnoses in high-functioning adolescents with ASD. *Journal of Clinical Child and Adolescent Psychology, 41*(4), 516–523.

Mazefsky, C. A., Williams, D. L., & Minshew, N. J. (2008). Variability in adaptive behavior in autism: Evidence for the importance of family history. *Journal of Abnormal Child Psychology, 36,* 591–599.

McDonald, S., Bornhoften, C., Shum, D., Long, E., Saunders, C., & Neulinger, K. (2006). Reliability and validity of "The Awareness of Social Inference Test" (TASIT): A clinical test of social perception. *Disability and Rehabilitation, 28*(4), 1529–1542.

McDonald, S., Flanagan, S., Rollins, J., & Kinch, J. (2003). TASIT: A new clinical tool for assessing social perception after traumatic brain injury. *Journal of Head Trauma Rehabilitation, 18,* 219–238.

Merrell, K. W. (1994). *The preschool and kindergarten behavior scales.* Austin, TX: PRO-ED.

National Institute of Mental Health. (2008). *Autism spectrum disorders: Pervasive developmental disorders.* Retrieved from *www.nimh.nih.gov/health/publications/autism/index.shtml.*

O'Hare, A. E., Bremner, E. L., Nash, M., Happé, F., & Pettigrew, L. M. (2009). A clinical assessment tool for advanced theory of mind performance in 5 to 12 year olds. *Journal of Autism and Developmental Disorders, 39,* 916–928.

O'Neill, R., Horner, R., Albin, R., Sprague, J., Storey, K., & Newton, J. (1997). *Functional assessment and programme development for problem behaviour: A practical handbook.* Pacific Grove, CA: Brooks/Cole.

Ooi, Y. P., Rescorla, L., Ang, R. P., Woo, B., & Fung, D. S. S. (2011). Identification of autism spectrum disorders using the Child Behavior Checklist in Singapore. *Journal of Autism and Developmental Disorders, 41,* 1147–1156.

Ratto, A. B., Tumer-Brown, L., Rupp, B. M., Mesibov, G. B., & Penn, D. L. (2011). Development of the Contextual Assessment of Social Skills (CASS): A role play measure of social skill for individuals with high-functioning autism. *Journal of Autism and Developmental Disorders. 41*, 1277–1286.

Reiersen, A., & Todd, R., (2008). Co-occurence of ADHD and autism spectrum disorders: Phenomenology and treatment. *Expert Review of Neurotherapeutics, 8*(4), 657–669.

Reynolds, C. R., & Kamphaus, R. W. (2004). *Behavior Assessment System for Children—Second Edition.* Circle Pines, MN: American Guidance Service.

Reynolds, C. R., & Richmond, B. O. (1985). *Revised Children's Manifest Anxiety Scale manual.* Los Angeles: Western Psychological Services.

Research Units of Pediatric Psychopharmacology (RUPP) Anxiety Study Group. (2002). The Pediatric Anxiety Rating Scale (PARS): Development and psychometric properties. *Journal of the American Academy of Child and Adolescent Psychiatry, 41*(9), 1061–1069.

Reuterskiöld, L., Öst, L., & Ollendick, T. (2008). Exploring child and parent factors in the diagnostic agreement on the Anxiety Disorders Interview Schedule. *Journal of Psychopathology and Behavioral Assessment, 30*(4), 279–290.

Robins, D., Fein, D., & Barton, M. (1999). *The Modified Checklist for Autism in Toddlers (M-CHAT).* Storrs: University of Connecticut.

Russell, E., & Sofronoff, K. (2005). Anxiety and social worries in children with Asperger syndrome. *Australian and New Zealand Journal of Psychiatry, 39*(7), 633–638.

Rutter, M., Bailey, A., & Lord, C. (2003). *Social Communication Questionnaire.* Los Angeles, CA: Western Psychological Services.

Schopler, E., Van Bourgondien, M. E., Wellman, G. J., & Love, S. R. (2010). *Childhood Autism Rating Scale* (2nd ed.). Los Angeles: Western Psychological Services.

Shaffer, D., Fisher, P., Lucas, C. P., Dulcan, M. K., & Schwab-Stone, M. E. (2000). NIMH Diagnostic Interview Schedule for Children Version IV (NIMH DISC-IV): Description, differences from previous versions, and reliability of some common diagnoses. *Journal of the American Academy of Child and Adolescent Psychiatry, 39*(1), 28–38.

Shaffer, D., Gould, M. S., Brasic, J., Ambrosini, P., Fisher, P., Bird, H., et al. (1983). A Children's Global Assessment Scale (CGAS). *Archives of General Psychology, 40*(11), 1228–1231.

Silverman, W. K., & Albano, A. M. (1996). *Anxiety Disorders Interview Schedule (ADIS-IV) Child and Parent Interview Schedules.* New York: Graywind.

Smith, L. A., Schry, A. R., & White, S. W. (2012, May). *The DD-CGAS as a tool for the assessment of global functioning in treatment outcome research in ASD.* Poster presented at the international meeting for Autism Research, Toronto, ON.

Sparrow, S. S., Cicchetti, C. V., & Balla, D. A. (2005). *Vineland Adaptive Behavior Scales* (2nd ed.) (Vineland-II). San Antonio, TX: Psychological Corporation.

Skuse, D., Warrington, R., Bishop, D., Chowdhury, U., Lau, J., Mandy, W., et al. (2004). The Developmental, Dimensional and Diagnostic Interview (3di): A novel computerized assessment for autism spectrum disorders. *Journal of the American Academy of Child and Adolescent Psychiatry, 43*(5), 548–558.

Volker, M. A., Lopata, C., Smerbeck, A. M., Knoll, V. A., Thomeer, M. L., Toomey, J. A., et al. (2010). BASC-2 PRS profiles for students with high-functioning autism spectrum disorders. *Journal of Autism and Developmental Disorders, 40*, 188–189.

Wagner, A., Lecavalier, L., Arnold, L. E., Aman, M. G., Scahill, L., Stigler, K. A., et al. (2007). Developmental Disabilities Modification of Children's Global Assessment Scale (DD-CGAS). *Biological Psychiatry, 61*(4), 504–511.

Wang, H. T., Sandall, S. R., Davis, C. A., & Thomas, C. J. (2011). Social skills assessment in young children with autism: A comparison evaluation of the SRSS and PKBS. *Journal of Autism and Developmental Disorders, 41*(11), 1487–1495.

Wellman, H. M., Cross, D., & Watson, J. (2001). Meta-analysis of theory-of-mind development: The truth about false belief. *Child Development, 72*(3), 665–684.

White, S. W. (2011). *Social skills training for children with Asperger syndrome and high-functioning autism.* New York: Guilford Press.

White, S. W., Albano, A., Johnson, C., Kasari, C., Ollendick, T., Klin, A., et al. (2010). Development of a cognitive-behavioral intervention program to treat anxiety and social deficits in teens with high-functioning autism. *Clinical Child and Family Psychology Review, 13*, 77–90.

White, S. W., Bray, C. B., & Ollendick, T. H. (2012). Examining shared and unique aspects of social anxiety disorders and autism spectrum disorder using factor analysis. *Journal of Autism and Developmental Disorders, 42*(5), 874–884.

White, S. W., Koenig, K., & Scahill, L. (2007). Social skills development intervention in children with autism spectrum disorders: A review of the intervention research. *Journal of Autism and Developmental Disorders, 37*, 1858–1868.

White, S. W., Ollendick, T., Albano, A., Oswald, D., Johnson, C., Southam-Gerow, M., et al. (2012). Randomized controlled trial: Multimodal anxiety and social skill intervention for adolescents with autism spectrum disorder. *Journal of Autism and Developmental Disorders, 43*(2), 382–394.

White, S. W., Schry, A. R., & Maddox, B. B. (2012). Brief report: The assessment of anxiety in high-functioning adolescents with autism spectrum disorder. *Journal of Autism and Developmental Disorders, 42*(6), 1138–1145.

Williams, S. K., Scahill, L., Vitiello, B., Aman, M. G., Eugene, L. E., McDougle, C. J., et al. (2006). Risperidone and adaptive behavior in children with autism. *Journal of the American Academy of Child and Adolescent Psychiatry, 45*, 431–439.

Wimmer, H., & Perner, J. (1983). Beliefs about beliefs: Representation and constraining function of wrong beliefs in young children's understanding of deception. *Cognition, 13*(1), 103–128.

PART II

ANXIETY AND BEHAVIOR PROBLEMS

4

Cognitive–Behavioral Therapy for Anxiety Disorders in Youth with ASD

Emotional, Adaptive, and Social Outcomes

SHULAMITE A. GREEN AND JEFFREY J. WOOD

HISTORICAL BACKGROUND
AND SIGNIFICANCE OF THE TREATMENT

Youth with autism spectrum disorders (ASD) are substantially more likely to have anxiety disorders than typically developing (TD) youth (e.g., Bellini, 2004; Guttmann-Steinmetz, Gadow, DeVincent, & Crowell, 2010; Russell & Sofronoff, 2005), youth with externalizing disorders, such as conduct disorder (Green, Gilchrist, Burton, & Cox, 2000) or attention-deficit/hyperactivity disorder (ADHD; Gadow, DeVincent, Pomeroy, & Azizian, 2005), and youth with intellectual disability (Brereton, Tonge, & Einfeld, 2006). Rates of anxiety disorders in ASD have been reported as 30% or higher (e.g., de Bruin, Ferdinand, Meesters, de Nijs, & Verheij, 2007; Leyfer et al., 2006) with some studies reporting rates as high as 87% (Muris, Steerneman, Merckelbach, Holdrinet, & Meesters, 1998). Anxiety is particularly common in youth with high-functioning ASD (HFASD), which is ASD without co-occurring intellectual disability (e.g., Sukhodolsky et al., 2008).

Cognitive-behavioral therapy (CBT) is an evidence-based treatment for TD youth with anxiety disorders, and there is emerging evidence that, with adaptations, it can be effective for youth with ASD as well. This chapter briefly reviews the background of presentation of anxiety in youth with ASD, the basic components of ASD, and current evidence for the use of CBT with this population, then examines in depth how CBT is adapted for youth with ASD. Finally, an in-depth description of an individual CBT program with potential efficacy for youth with ASD, Behavioral Interventions for Anxiety in Children with Autism (BIACA), is presented.

Anxiety in ASD

The reason for such high rates of anxiety in individuals with ASD is not fully understood. The validity of an anxiety diagnosis as a comorbid disorder in individuals with ASD is still in question, and it is possible that the high rates are due to inaccurate differential diagnosis or phenotypic overlap rather than true comorbidity (e.g., Wood & Gadow, 2010). For example, social avoidance may be due to lack of social interest (a symptom of ASD) or anxiety in social situations (a symptom of social phobia). Similarly, the restricted and repetitive interests common to ASD may overlap with symptoms of obsessive–compulsive disorder (OCD).

Some recent evidence supports anxiety as a distinct syndrome that varies in individuals with ASD. For example, parent and teacher ratings of DSM-IV-TR symptoms have been shown to cluster into similar generalized anxiety disorder (GAD) factors for children with and without ASD (Lecavalier, Gadow, DeVincent, Houts, & Edwards, 2009). Furthermore, several of the same gene polymorphisms have been found to be associated with anxiety in both TD individuals and individuals with ASD (e.g., Gadow, DeVincent, & Schneider, 2009; Gadow, Roohi, DeVincent, Kirsch, & Hatchwell, 2009). Finally, youth with ASD and anxiety disorders respond well to cognitive-behavioral interventions similar to the evidence-based treatments for TD youth with anxiety disorders (e.g., Wood, Drahota, Sze, & Har, 2009). These interventions are reviewed in detail in this chapter.

Assuming that the high rates of anxiety in individuals with ASD are not solely due to poor differential diagnosis, ASD may put an individual at particular risk for anxiety because of the substantial life stress created by having this disorder (Wood & Gadow, 2010). Life for an individual with ASD can be unpredictable, stressful, and overwhelming due to the constant pressure to conform in daily activities such as school and social interactions, difficulty in understanding others' mental states, and sensitivity to environmental sensory stimuli (Ben-Sasson et al., 2008; Gillott & Standen, 2007). Additionally, individuals with ASD show cortisol patterns similar to those seen in individuals with chronic stress (Corbett, Mendoza, Wegelin,

Carmean, & Levine, 2008). Anxiety might also be a mediator of the relationship between ASD and symptom severity; for example, ASD might put some people at risk for social anxiety, which leads them to avoid social situations and exacerbates their social skills deficits (cf. Bellini, 2004, 2006; Chang, Quan, & Wood, in press; Pfeiffer, Kinnealey, Reed, & Herzberg, 2005; Sukholdolsky et al., 2008). Potentially, anxiety may also function as a moderator such that individuals with ASD and anxiety have worse functional outcomes than those with ASD but without anxiety (Wood & Gadow, 2010).

Additionally, individuals with ASD may have neurobiological risk for an overactive fear response. There is some evidence that youth with ASD have larger amygdalar volumes than TD children and that amygdalar volume is positively related to severity of anxiety and social–communication symptoms (Amaral, Schumann, & Nordahl, 2008; Juranek et al., 2006).

Research indicates that anxiety is associated with additional functional impairment for youth with ASD and co-occurring high anxiety, including greater deficits in social competence (Bellini, 2004, 2006; Pfeiffer et al., 2005; Sukholdolsky et al., 2008), functional academics (Pfeiffer et al., 2005), externalizing behaviors (Kim, Szatmari, Bryson, Streiner, & Wilson, 2000), sensory sensitivity (Ben-Sasson et al., 2008), and repetitive behaviors and autism symptoms (Sukhodolsky et al., 2008). Thus, an effective treatment for anxiety in youth with ASD has wide implications for the overall functioning of this population. Indeed, there is some evidence that CBT for anxiety in ASD can simultaneously decrease other impairments, such as core autism symptoms and daily living skills deficits (Drahota, Wood, Sze, & Van Dyke, 2011; Wood, Drahota, Sze, Van Dyke, et al., 2009).

CBT for Anxiety

The effectiveness of CBT for anxiety disorders in TD children and adolescents has been demonstrated consistently across a number of studies and age groups (e.g., Albano & Kendall, 2002; Compton et al., 2004). CBT for anxiety is based on the premise that anxiety can be an appropriate, protective response to real danger but that individuals with anxiety disorders have an excessive, maladaptive response to situations that are not truly dangerous to them (Kendall, 1993). This maladaptive response is a combination of anxious behaviors, feelings, and thoughts. For example, children who feel anxious about an upcoming class presentation might be motivated to prepare more, whereas children with an anxiety disorder might feel so excessively fearful that they refuse to do the presentation. The anxiety response is accompanied by physiological, autonomic arousal that prepares the individual for a "fight-or-flight" response, and by a distorted cognitive appraisal of the situation, such as "Everyone in class is laughing at me and thinking I'm dumb." Avoidance of the feared situation causes the feelings of anxiety to decrease in the short term, which then reinforces the individual to continue avoiding. However, avoidance maintains the anxiety, because only experiencing the feared situation and learning that the feared consequence does not occur, or if it does occur, that it is not catastrophic, can teach the individual that it truly is not dangerous. CBT for youth with anxiety disorders targets these maladaptive thoughts, feelings, and behaviors by providing children with the coping strategies needed to change their distorted appraisals and reduce their physiological arousal to a level at which they are gradually able to face the feared stimuli.

Kendall and colleagues developed the first manualized CBT treatment for youth with major anxiety disorders, called the *Coping Cat program* (Kendall, Kane, Howard, & Siqueland, 1990). This intervention comprises psychoeducation, relaxation training, cognitive restructuring, hierarchical exposure, and contingent reinforcement across 16 weekly sessions. In this program, therapists work with children to recognize their anxious feelings, physiological reactions, and maladaptive thoughts in anxiety-provoking situations. Children are taught coping skills such as positive self-talk and relaxation exercises. Therapists create a hierarchy of feared situations and gradually expose the children to increasingly anxiety-provoking situations, while facilitating use of the coping skills to ensure that children's anxiety responses decrease at each level of the hierarchy before they move to the next level. This basic treatment model has been replicated and demonstrated to be effective across different sites, ages, and treatment modalities (i.e., group and individual treatment; Compton et al., 2004).

PRACTICAL CONSIDERATIONS IN IMPLEMENTING CBT WITH CHILDREN WITH ASD

It is necessary to adapt CBT to accommodate the special needs of youth with ASD (e.g., more concrete and visual thought processes, lower attention span). Some of the more common adaptations are described here:

Increasing Affective Education

Youth with ASD often have great difficulty recognizing and interpreting their own emotions, which makes it hard for them to know when they are anxious. Because recognizing anxiety is an important component of

CBT that allows children to use the coping strategies they learned to regulate their anxiety, it has been recommended that CBT for youth with ASD include a greater focus on affective education (e.g., Attwood, 2003; Anderson & Morris, 2006). Thus, CBT protocols directed at children with ASD often simplify and reinforce the connection among physiological feelings, anxious thoughts, and anxiety-related behaviors, and add additional practice in recognizing facial expressions related to anxiety.

While most CBT programs for children include some affect recognition procedures, these components must be adapted for youth with ASD by providing very basic education about what emotions are, why they are important, and how to recognize an emotion (e.g., Attwood, 2003; White et al., 2010). Youth with ASD require greater practice at recognizing emotions, and Attwood (2003) recommends techniques to make emotions more concrete, such as drawing individual emotions and creating a scrapbook for the emotion, with pictures that elicit the emotion for the client. Sofronoff, Attwood, and Hinton (2005) use a metaphor of the child as a scientist or astronaut exploring a new planet and collecting cues about what emotions the people there might be feeling.

Increasing Use of Visual Approaches

CBT protocols for youth with ASD also emphasize use of visual aids to accommodate the often more visual and concrete learning styles of children with ASD. These approaches may include drawing exercises, cartoons, or videos (e.g., Lang, Regester, Lauderdale, Ashbaugh, & Haring, 2010; Reaven et al., 2008; White et al., 2010). For example, Reaven et al. (2008) used worksheets and multiple-choice lists to teach basic CBT concepts. Later in this intervention, children created their own movies in which they face their anxiety and cope in different contexts. White et al. (2010) also used worksheets with visual structure to help with the learning process, for example, outlines of bodies, so that children can indicate where in their bodies they feel the anxious sensation, and thought bubbles in which children write in anxious thoughts they are having. Wood, Drahota, Sze, Har, et al. (2009) used a series of cartoons to help youth recognize physiological symptoms of anxiety and anxious thoughts, and generate coping thoughts. The youth in this intervention were then encouraged to draw their own cartoons, based on their own experiences of anxiety.

Emphasizing Behavioral Aspects

Despite modifications to make the cognitive aspects of CBT more concrete, many children with ASD still have trouble fully understanding their own thoughts and feelings (e.g., Lang et al., 2010). Therefore, adaptations of CBT involve emphasizing the behavioral aspects of anxiety, with the recognition that even if youth do not fully acknowledge or understand their own anxiety, they can still benefit from the reduction in anxious avoidance enabled through exposure to feared but benign stimuli. As an example, compared to the approximately eight sessions (out of 16) of exposure therapy in the Coping Cat program for typical children, the Wood, Drahota, Sze, Har, et al. (2009) intervention for ASD has a modular therapy approach that often entails 12 sessions (out of 16) of exposure therapy. In this intervention, children gain most of their practice in using coping skills (e.g., positive self-statements and relaxation) during the process of *in vivo* exposure. Additionally, parents are trained in recognizing the antecedents of their children's anxiety-related behaviors and how to change the consequences to reduce avoidance and promote positive coping (e.g., through the use of positive reinforcement).

Incorporating Special Interests

Youth with ASD often have difficulties with social engagement, attention, and motivation. Incorporating their special interests into activities can significantly increase their social interest and participation (e.g., Baker, Koegel, & Koegel, 1998). Many CBT adaptations incorporate the special or repetitive interests common to individuals with ASD into CBT activities and reinforcement systems to establish rapport and increase participation and motivation. Wood, Drahota, Sze, Har, et al. (2009) integrate special interests into the cartoon drawings and example scenarios used to teach CBT concepts. A child who has a preoccupation with pirates, for example, might draw a pirate who is anxious because he is about to sail in rough seas, and discuss his anxious and coping thoughts around this fear. Additionally, children are sometimes encouraged to think about or do something related to their special interest as a coping strategy or to self-reinforce (e.g., Attwood, 2003).

Increasing Parent Involvement

Modifications to CBT usually include substantial parent involvement (e.g., Lang et al., 2010; Reaven, 2011; White et al., 2010). Parent psychoeducation often includes information about ASD, such as the particular risk for anxiety in this population and the connection between independence in self-help skills and decreased anxiety. Parents are taught to be coaches or co-therapists, and participate in the intervention by encouraging exposures, coping strategies, and self-help skills, and by providing reinforcement. Some programs also include parent training to target parents' responses to children's difficult behaviors, encourage use of reinforcers and positive interactions, and address family stress. Parents of children with ASD may be especially likely to be overprotective of their children, so therapists may work with parents to increase gradually their children's independence and adaptive skills (e.g., Reaven, 2011; Wood, Drahota, Sze, Har, et al., 2009).

Targeting Co-Occurring Difficulties in ASD

ASD-related deficits in social skills, communication, and adaptive behavior can exacerbate anxiety. For example, youth who lack appropriate social behaviors may be teased, and begin to avoid social situations, which further exacerbates their social discomfort. Likewise, communication difficulties and lack of emotion understanding can cause difficulty in reading social cues and make social situations unpredictable. Some adaptations of CBT for anxiety in ASD include additional modules to target these co-occurring symptoms, and there is emerging evidence of the effectiveness of CBT for anxiety in improving these symptoms (e.g., Wood, Drahota, Sze, Van Dyke, et al., 2009). In these modifications, children with ASD are prepared for social exposures with social skills training, such as learning when to make eye contact, how to use the appropriate tone of voice and social greetings, and how to maintain a conversation (Lang et al., 2010). Some adaptations also include group components focused on practicing social skills (White, Ollendick, Scahill, Oswald, & Albano, 2009) or fear hierarchies that include steps toward making friends (Wood, Drahota, Sze, Har, et al., 2009). Other aids for ASD-related deficits, such as self-help skills, can also be added to hierarchies (e.g., Drahota et al., 2011).

BIACA: OVERVIEW OF SESSIONS

The BIACA intervention, adapted from the *Building Confidence* CBT program (Wood & McLeod, 2008) for children ages 7–14 with ASD, includes not only anxiety-focused cognitive restructuring and behavior exposure components, but also modules to target social skills, adaptive skills, and stereotyped interests. These modules were added because, as noted earlier, anxiety in youth with ASD is linked to increased functional impairment, particularly deficits in adaptive functioning and social skills. There is likely a transactional nature to this relationship: Deficits in self-help skills contribute to a feeling of lack of self-efficacy and independence, which exacerbates anxiety, and anxiety makes youth more likely to avoid socializing and completing self-help tasks. For example, a child with separation anxiety avoids taking out the trash because he is anxious when he leaves the house without his parent, and his inability to accomplish this task leads to feelings of inadequacy and helplessness that further exacerbate his anxiety. Likewise, social skills deficits can make social situations difficult and unrewarding, which leads to avoidance and increased social anxiety. Given the transactional nature of these problems, treating them simultaneously is likely to be lead to better overall outcomes for youth with ASD than addressing them separately. The intervention comprises 16 weekly, 90-minute sessions; approximately 30 minutes of this time is spent with the child and 60 minutes, with the parent or family.

Case Study

Examples from the following case study illustrate implementation of the most commonly used modules. A. K. (name changed to protect identity) was an 8-year-old boy diagnosed with high-functioning autism who met criteria for separation anxiety disorder (SAD) and social phobia (SP). A. K. followed his mother around the house and was fearful of being in rooms of the house by himself, particularly his bedroom and a back bedroom upstairs, claiming there was a "ghost" there. A. K. went to sleep in his mother's bed or on the couch in the living room every night and wet the bed almost every night. A. K.'s mother rarely left him with a friend or relative, because he would become extremely anxious and worry that something bad would happen to him or to his mother while they were apart (e.g., getting kidnapped). In addition to these symptoms of anxiety, A. K. had major deficits in adaptive skills: He did not bathe on his own, dress himself, use the toilet on his own, order his own food in a restaurant, or do any chores around the house.

Cognitive Modules

PSYCHOEDUCATION

Treatment begins with psychoeducation about anxiety and its relationship with ASD. Both parents and children are provided information about what causes and maintains anxiety, and how it is linked to ASD. Children are engaged through discussions and games based on their interests. Parents engage in a more detailed discussion with therapists about the antecedents and consequences of their children's anxiety.

REWARD SYSTEM

Therapists emphasize to parents the importance of reinforcements for their children, and they work with children and parents to establish a reward system. The reward system varies based on the child's developmental level and interests but often takes the form of a token economy, in which children can earn stickers or points for homework and for exposures both in session and at home. A certain number of these can be traded in for both a larger reward that is decided on in advance and daily, home-based privileges such as access to television.

Referring to our case example, A. K.'s reinforcement plan included earning electronics time at the end of the day for each sticker earned that day, and extra electronics time on the weekend if he completed a certain number of exposures during the week. The therapist provided A. K. with "Transformers" stickers for completing activities or exposures in therapy, based on his special interest in this topic.

KICK PLAN

Children are introduced to cognitive restructuring and the rationale for *in vivo* exposure through the KICK plan, an acronym that helps them remember steps they can take to reduce their anxiety. The *K* stands for "Knowing I'm nervous." In this step, children are taught to identify emotions using pictures, cartoons, and role play with their therapist. The physiological symptoms of anxiety are discussed, and the therapist uses cartoon and drawing activities to help children practice recognizing these symptoms.

In the second step of the KICK plan, is *I* for "Icky thoughts" or "Irritating thoughts" (depending on children's developmental level). In this step, children are encouraged to identify anxious thoughts of children experiencing anxiety in cartoons, then their own anxious situations. For example, for a child who is afraid of the dark, the therapist can use a cartoon of a child looking frightened in bed a night. The therapist helps the child generate possible anxious thoughts, such as "There is a monster under my bed," or "A burglar might come in the window." For most children, the Socratic method is used (e.g., the therapist might ask, "What kinds of scary things might this boy worry are under his bed? and "What else might he be afraid of when he's alone in the dark?" These kinds of questions give hints and structure for a general class of answers, while encouraging the children to reflect and process the topic at a semantically based, meaning-laden level of thought.

In the C step, for "Calm thoughts," children are encouraged to challenge the "icky thoughts" by asking (1) how likely they are to happen and/ or (2) how bad would it really be if they did happen? For the earlier example of the child scared of the dark, the therapist would teach the children the skill, through the Socratic method, of asking themselves questions, such as "How likely is it that there are monsters under the bed? Have I ever seen a monster under the bed? Have I ever seen a monster at all?" Humor is also used (e.g., "Even if monsters did exist, why would they want to live under a bed with all the dust down there?"). These questions can help the children create coping statements for themselves, such as "Monsters aren't real; scientists have proven that, so there's nothing to fear under my bed." Similarly, a child who is afraid of reading in front of the class might have the anxious thought, "The other kids will laugh at me." The child would then learn to challenge that type of thinking by both assessing issues of probability and posing the general question "How bad would it be?" and questions such as, "How long would they laugh at me?"; "Will they remember my reading forever?"; "Would the laughter make me sick?" Related coping thoughts that the therapist would help the child generate with Socratic questioning might include "They might laugh for a few minutes, but then they will forget about it" or "Their laughter can't really hurt me."

The final K stands for "Keep practicing." In this step, children are taught the importance of gradually exposing themselves to their fears, a concept that helps to prepare them for the exposures in the next stage of treatment. For example, they discuss the method most children use to learn a complex and potentially dangerous activity such as swimming (i.e., taking small steps, mastering each new level with confidence before moving on to more difficult steps). Furthermore, therapists aid children in explaining each stage of the KICK plan to their parents, to help them consolidate their knowledge and to keep parents apprised of what their children are learning.

In our case example, A. K. had an interest in fishing, so the therapist presented a cartoon of a fisherman who fell overboard and aided A. K. in thinking through "Knowing I'm nervous" (e.g., a fearful facial expression), what "Icky thoughts" he may be having (e.g., "I will drown"), and what "Calm thoughts" he could use to make himself feel better (e.g., "I know how to swim," "My crew will pull me aboard soon"). After he explained the KICK plan to his mother, she encouraged A. K. to use the KICK plan at home by putting the acronym up on his bedroom wall and reminded him to think of calm thoughts when he became anxious.

Behavioral/Exposure Modules

DEVELOPING A HIERARCHY

Therapists work with parents and children together to come up with a list of feared situations and a fear rating for each. The therapist creates a hierarchy for each target anxiety behavior in the order of the anxiety level each situation causes. For example, a child who has a fear of speaking in front of a group might first practice reading a sentence to the therapist, then gradually work up to a full text, with the therapist asking questions about it. The child would then gradually work toward reading the text to a parent, a group of family members, a stranger, and then a group of strangers. Finally, the child might read the text, making mistakes deliberately to decrease the fear of making mistakes in front of others. Other common exposures for social phobia include saying hello to salespeople or peers, ordering food at a restaurant, or calling a peer on the phone. Exposures for separation anxiety may consist of staying in bed alone for increasing amounts of time or going into a room in the house without a parent. Exposures for generalized anxiety sometimes involve exposure to the target of the worry, such as thinking about, talking about, or drawing the worry (a natural disaster, failing a test, etc.) to promote habituation and a sense of control.

EXPOSURES

Exposures are assigned for homework and also *in vivo,* in session. Before each exposure, the therapist and child create a KICK plan and a reward plan for the situation to ensure they will have the appropriate coping skills and motivation to succeed. Before and after each step of the exposure, the child is asked to rate his or her anxiety, and exposures continue until the child's anxiety has decreased significantly. Parents are often asked to observe some of the *in vivo* exposures in session, so the therapist can model for the parent how to motivate the child to perform and structure the exposure to allow the child to be successful.

Regarding our case example, in-session exposures with A. K. focused on increasingly challenging scenarios that involved speaking to strangers. The therapist first practiced appropriate nonverbal and conversational skills (e.g., eye contact, smiling, creating a script of what to say) with A. K., then aided A. K. in practicing these skills with his mother, a familiar research assistant, and an unfamiliar research assistant. The therapist took A. K. around the university campus and encouraged him to speak to students about a topic of interest (e.g., asking them whether they had seen the *Transformers* movie and how much they had liked it). A. K. was initially

extremely anxious and avoidant of this task, but as he spoke to more students his anxiety decreased, he had shorter intervals between approaching
students, and he expressed enjoyment (e.g., "I think he liked me!").

A. K. was assigned home-based exposures to increase the time he spent
in his own room and bed. His mother provided reinforcements to him first
for increasing time spent in his room alone during the day; then at night,
first with the door open and his mother outside, then with the door closed,
with his mother down the hall, and finally with her downstairs. His mother
then began encouraging him to spend increasing amounts of time in his
own bed at night. After A. K. reached about 15 minutes of time in his
own bed, he began to fall asleep on his own. He was given extra reinforcers any mornings he woke up in his own bed and praised for being "a big
kid." A. K. was encouraged to use coping skills during these exposures, for
example, generating calm thoughts to respond to his anxiety about ghosts.
By the end of treatment, A. K. went upstairs to his room on his own every
night to put on his pajamas and woke up in his own bed three or four nights
a week. Ending treatment at this level of progress—partial remission of a
symptom—can happen with some anxiety symptoms because of the slow
pace of systematic desensitization some children need to be comfortable;
however, often even partial remission represents clinical improvement that
can continue in a steady, linear fashion after treatment is finished.

PARENT TRAINING

In addition to modeling exposures, therapists also provide skills to parents to help their children be successful in home- and community-based
exposures. These include planned ignoring (e.g., ignoring their children's
anxious behaviors), reinforcement, and problem-solving skills. Parents are
taught to use the CALM system when they are frustrated with their children: Catch your breath, Accept your child's negative feelings, Label your
child's emotions, Model coping skills. The CALM technique has been used
in both neurotypical and ASD-specific versions of the BIACA program
(Wood & McLeod, 2008; Wood, Drahota, Sze, Har, et al., 2009).

PLAYDATES

Therapists discuss the importance of playdates with parents and children.
Children are taught how to be a good host in a very concrete, step-by-step
manner. Skills include asking the guest to choose what to play, staying
with the guest at all times, complimenting the guest, and smiling during
activities with the guest. Therapists also teach children how to invite a

guest over; how to make a phone call, what to say on the phone, and how to respond if the friend says no. For children who feel anxiety about any of these steps, therapists use the KICK plan and a gradual hierarchy to help reduce the anxiety.

Therapists help parents brainstorm a list of friends who are appropriate for their child and might be interested in being friends. Depending on the child's abilities, this might include other children at school, children in extracurricular activities, younger children, or other children with disabilities. Parents are encouraged to schedule regular playdates and to coach their child to be a good host during the playdate.

SOCIAL COACHING

Therapists travel to the school or into the community to conduct *in vivo* social coaching with children. Therapists help children to develop a goal for the social interaction immediately beforehand (e.g., saying hello to someone, eating lunch with someone, or joining in on a game). Therapists identify discussion topics and important nonverbal behaviors, and role-play the interaction with the child directly before entering the social situation. Therapists also teach parents to act as social coaches for their children.

MENTORING

Therapists work with parents to identify a younger "buddy" for the child to mentor. The purpose of the mentoring relationship is to build the child's self-confidence, possibly leading to a friendship with a younger child in a way that does not lower the child's self-esteem. The therapist teaches the child how to interact with the mentee in an appropriate way and establish a reinforcement system, if necessary.

SCHOOL INVOLVEMENT

When possible, the therapist meets with the child's teacher to establish a behavioral reward program at school, to review the child's social coaching plan and model social coaching for the teacher, and to explore mentoring opportunities at the school.

Adaptive Skills Module

Therapists provide parents with psychoeducation about the relationship between anxiety and self-help skills, and the necessity of allowing children independence to increase their self esteem and self efficacy. Parents are encouraged to give their children increasing independence in self-help tasks, with a gradual hierarchy and reinforcement system, similar to the homework anxiety exposures. Parents choose at least three age-appropriate skills to work on throughout the course of the intervention (dressing, bathing, preparing breakfast, etc.).

Referring back to our case example, because of A. K.'s deficits in self-help skills, a portion of multiple parent sessions focused on improving these skills. The therapist provided for A. K.'s mother a sticker chart to use each week, with three self-help skills that gradually increased in difficulty (e.g., first just running his own bath, building up to finally taking a bath on his own, with his mother checking on him no more than once).

Stereotyped Interests Module

This module is used with children whose stereotyped interests cause functional impairments, such as interference with making friends. Therapists provide parents with psychoeducation about interests and activities that are developmentally appropriate for the child's age, and brainstorm with parents the steps to reduce manifestations of nonappropriate interests (e.g., fire hydrants; traffic lights) in public places, replacing them with more developmentally appropriate topics or interests. Children are not encouraged to give up special interests but to moderate their focus on them around other children in order to facilitate social interactions.

Termination

At the 16th session, children's progress is celebrated with a "party" involving snacks, a certificate, and a small gift. Therapists review progress with children and parents, focusing on their positive accomplishments. Therapists review with parents the parenting skills they have learned and urge them to continue using these skills to conduct exposures and encourage their children's coping skills in the future.

RESEARCH TO DATE ON THE TREATMENT

Wood, Drahota, Sze, Har, et al. (2009), which examined the efficacy of BIACA, is to date the only published randomized controlled trial of an individual CBT treatment for anxiety in ASD. In this study, 40 children ages 7–11 years with ASD and a comorbid anxiety disorder were randomized to an individual treatment condition or a wait-list control condition. Children were diagnosed with SAD, SP, or OCD using the Anxiety Disorders Interview Schedule—Child and Parent versions (ADIS-C/P; Silverman & Albano, 1996).

In addition to the ADIS-C/P, outcomes were also measured using the Multidimensional Anxiety Scale for Children (MASC; March, Parker, Sullivan, Stallings, & Conners, 1997) and the Clinical Global Impression—Improvement scale. At posttreatment, compared to children in the wait-list condition, children in the immediate treatment condition had greater decreases in ADIS-C/P Clinical Severity Rating scores, and 64.3% of treatment completers did not meet criteria for any anxiety disorder compared to 9.1% of wait-list completers. Additionally, 92.9% of children in the immediate treatment condition met CGI criteria for positive treatment response (i.e., were rated as *very much improved* or *very improved*), compared to 9.1% of children in the wait-list condition. Child-reported MASC scores decreased similarly in both groups, but parent-reported MASC scores decreased significantly more in the immediate treatment group.

Ten participants randomized to CBT (of 17 who initially started treatment) returned for a 3-month follow-up. Of these, 80% did not meet criteria for any anxiety disorder, and 90% maintained their positive treatment response scores on the CGI-I. There were no significant differences in parent- or child-reported MASC scores between posttreatment and follow-up, indicating that, on this measure as well, children maintained gains over the 3-month follow-up period. Furthermore, subsequent studies showed that children in the immediate treatment condition had fewer autism symptoms (Wood, Drahota, Sze, Van Dyke, et al., 2009) and better daily living skills (Drahota et al., 2011) than children in the wait-list group, and that these improvements correlated with improvements in anxiety.

Additional Evidence for CBT Targeting Youth with ASD and Anxiety

In addition to the published BIACA studies, there have been four additional, published group studies of CBT for youth with ASD and co-occurring anxiety disorders (Chalfant, Rapee, & Carroll, 2007; Reaven et al., 2008; Scarpa & Reyes, 2011; Sofronoff et al., 2005). These studies are reviewed in the following section, and additional details are presented in Table 4.1.

Sofronoff et al. (2005) compared child-only and child + parent CBT

TABLE 4.1. Clinical Trials of Treatments for Anxiety in Youth with ASD

Authors (year)	n	Age (years)	Diagnosis	Control	Sessions	Adaptations	Outcomes
Chalfant et al. (2007)	47	8–13	ASD	Randomized wait-list	Nine 2-hour weekly group sessions, three 2-hour monthly booster sessions—child and parent groups	Program extended, more visual aids and worksheets, more relaxation and exposure, exposures as homework, simplified cognitive activities	71.4% no longer met criteria for anxiety disorder, 0% in wait-list group, greater reduction in self-reported internalizing thoughts, self-reported anxiety, RCMAS scores, SCAS; no change in externalizing symptoms.
Reaven et al. (2008)	33	8–10 and 11–14	ASD	3-month wait-list	Twelve 90-minute weekly groups	Token reinforcement, visual structure and routine, worksheets, made own movie, video modeling, parent participation	Significant decrease in parent- but not child-rated SCARED.
Scarpa & Reyes (2011)	11	5–7	ASD	Wait-list	Nine 60-minute weekly groups	Shorter sessions, songs, stories, and activities, parent training, parent psychoeducation group, use of "toolbox" metaphor for coping strategies	Decrease in "outbursts," Increase in child-reported emotion regulation strategies, increase in parent confidence, reduction in negative/lability scores.
Sofronoff et al. (2005)	71	10–12	Asperger syndrome	Child only, child and parent, wait-list	Six 2-hour weekly sessions	Child as scientist/explorer, use of "toolbox" metaphor for coping strategies	Child and parent showed greatest decreases on SCAS-P, SAD, social worries, greater feeling of parent competency.
Wood, Drahota, Sze, Har, et al. (2009)	40	7–11	ASD	Randomized wait-list	Sixteen 90-minute individual split between child, parent, family	Parent training, improving daily living skills, addressing social skills, at home, school, in public, peer buddy and mentoring	Thirteen of 14 met CGI criteria for positive treatment response as opposed to two of 22 in wait-list condition; significant decrease in CSR scores and parent- but not child-reported MASC.

groups to a wait-list control. Weekly sessions focused mainly on teaching and practicing cognitive coping strategies. The beginning of treatment focused on emotion recognition and exploration. Subsequent sessions used the premise of a "toolbox" to provide children with different coping strategies to deal with difficult emotions. Coping strategies included physical activity, relaxation, social interaction, participation in or thought about enjoyed activities, and use of coping thoughts. Parents of children in the child + parent condition attended parent groups, where they were trained to encourage their children to use the coping skills learned in group and to complete home-based activities.

Anxiety symptoms were measured with the Spence Child Anxiety Scale—Parent version (SCAS-P; Nauta et al., 2004), the Social Worries Questionnaire—Parent (SWQ-P; Spence, 1995), and an anxiety scenario for which the children had to generate coping strategies. Overall, children in both treatment groups had a greater improvement in anxiety symptoms than children in the wait-list group, and children in the child + parent group showed even greater improvement than children in the child-only group. Most of the improvement was evident only at 6-week follow-up rather than posttreatment. The child + parent group may have shown the greatest improvement at follow-up, because the parents were encouraging new skills and experiences during this time. It should be noted that while direct exposure was not part of the intervention, because parents in the child + parent condition were encouraged to coach their children through anxiety-provoking situations, they may have been more likely than parents of children in the child-only condition to expose their children to these types of situations.

Scarpa and Reyes (2011) further adapted the intervention used in Sofronoff et al. (2005) as a preventative intervention for children ages 5–7 years with ASD. Anxiety was not an inclusion criteria for this study. As in the intervention by Sofronoff et al., the first two sessions focused on emotion understanding and recognition, and subsequent sessions used the "toolbox" metaphor to teach different types of coping strategies to deal with anxiety. To accommodate the needs of younger children, sessions were shortened and the overall treatment was lengthened, to nine 1-hour sessions. Therapists used a very structured session routine, as well as songs, stories, and visually based activities to engage the younger children. Additionally, the intervention included a simultaneous parent group that focused on psychoeducation, and parents were able to watch the child sessions. Posttreatment, compared to a wait-list group, children in the immediate treatment group reported a greater number of emotion regulation strategies in response to stories about anxiety-provoking situations.

Parents reported higher levels of confidence in their own and their children's ability to manage their anxiety, and greater decreases in their children's Negativity/Lability scores on an emotion regulation checklist. While results showed that children had gained skills to cope with anxiety, as of yet there is no long-term follow-up to determine the efficacy of this intervention for preventing anxiety.

Chalfant et al. (2007) randomly assigned children with HFASD to a group CBT condition or a wait-list condition. The CBT protocol was based on the "Cool Kids" (Lyneham, Abbott, Wignall, & Rapee, 2003) intervention but adapted for children with ASD, using visual materials, structured worksheets, an extended program, and more emphasis on the concrete components of CBT such as relaxation and exposure. However, exposure sessions focused on planning exposure exercises as homework rather than in session. Parents attend a concurrent group that included psychoeducation, anxiety coping exercises, exposure planning, parent management training, and relapse prevention.

Posttreatment, 71.4% of the CBT group, compared to 0% of the wait-list group, no longer met criteria for a primary anxiety disorder. The posttreatment diagnostic interview was administered by the study therapists, introducing some ambiguity into these results. Children in the CBT condition had greater reductions in self-reported anxiety on the SCAS and the Revised Children's Manifest Anxiety Scale (RCMAS, Reynolds & Richmond, 1978), Internalizing Thoughts on the RCMAS and the Children's Automatic Thoughts Scale (CATS; Schniering & Rapee, 2002), and parent- and teacher-reported Externalizing Difficulties on the Strengths and Difficulties Questionnaire (SDQ; Goodman, 1997).

Reaven et al. (2008) also compared a group CBT treatment to a wait-list control, although the groups were not randomly assigned. The intervention focused on anxiety recognition, cognitive restructuring, coping strategies, and graded exposure. It was adapted for children with ASD through additional structure and visual approaches such as worksheets, a token reinforcement program, and parent participation. Video was also incorporated into the program; therapists used videos to model coping in anxiety-provoking situations and also helped children create their own videos about "facing your fears." The parent component included psychoeducation, discussion of parenting styles and overprotection, and identification of target behaviors for the graded exposures.

Children in the treatment group had significantly greater decreases in parent-rated anxiety symptoms on the SCARED than children in the wait-list group. There were no group differences in child-reported SCARED scores at posttreatment.

FUTURE DIRECTIONS

CBT appears to be a promising treatment for anxiety in youth with ASD, which has important implications for developmental outcomes in this population given the high prevalence of anxiety and the functional impairment associated with it. Youth with ASD are able to participate in CBT, although certain adaptations such as increasing visual aids and structure, as well as simplifying the cognitive aspects, can help engage them in topics that are normally difficult for them, such as emotion recognition. However, while adaptations allow children to participate in the cognitive aspects of the program, the exposures are the most important components of treatment, as demonstrated by Kendall et al. (1997). Kendall and colleagues tested the efficacy of the initial eight cognitively focused sessions of Coping Cat and found them to be ineffective without the subsequent sessions of exposure. Thus, CBT, when adapted for the special needs of youth with ASD, is potentially effective at decreasing anxiety in this population, but more replication is necessary to establish the efficacy of these programs.

The current research highlights the multisymptom presentation of youth with ASD and anxiety, in terms of both multiple anxiety disorders and other comorbid disorders and impairments. Significant parent involvement is necessary in treatment, in part to teach parents skills for enhancing their child's treatment response. As shown by Sofronoff et al. (2005), children whose parents are involved in the CBT intervention improve more than those without the parent component. Most of the improvement in Sofronoff et al. occurred between posttreatment and follow-up, suggesting that parents' ongoing encouragement of their children's coping strategies contributed to their reduction in anxiety as much as (if not more so) than the child-focused treatment per se.

Furthermore, the complexity of presentation of youth with ASD and anxiety is consistent with a multitarget approach to therapy. Anxiety, ASD symptoms, and deficits in adaptive and social skills may have a transactional relationship, in that each problem maintains and exacerbates the others. As reviewed earlier, the BIACA program, developed by Wood, Drahota, Sze, Van Dyke, and colleagues (2009; Drahota et al., 2011), includes modules to improve adaptive and social skills in an anxiety-focused treatment, and the initial clinical trial was suggestive of improvements in both of these areas, as well as anxiety.

Limitations and Future Directions

To date, there are few randomized controlled trials of CBT for youth with ASD and anxiety, and no trials using an active treatment comparison.

Finding an appropriate active treatment comparison is difficult, because there are few alternatives to treating anxiety in youth with ASD, but a comparison of CBT to medication would be useful. Additionally, given the ASD-symptom-related outcomes of CBT, comparisons of CBT to other, non-anxiety-related treatments for ASD, such as social skills groups, are needed.

The CBT trials are also limited in their measurement of anxiety; as yet no studies have examined objective or physiological measures of anxiety, such as behavior avoidance tasks, eye tracking, or psychophysiological (e.g., skin conductance, heart rate) measures. Rather, studies tend to rely on parent or child report of anxiety, which may be biased toward reporting improvement after weeks of therapy. Furthermore, given the difficulty children with ASD have with introspection and emotion recognition, and the difficulty parents may have separating anxiety symptoms from other ASD-related symptoms, additional measures are needed. Coping strategy generation tests, such as the scenario "James and the Math Test" used by Sofronoff et al. (2005), are more objective assessments of outcome but measure coping strategies learned rather than anxiety symptoms. Future studies should include such objective measures of anxiety, as have studies of CBT with TD children (e.g., Kendall, 1994) to further establish the efficacy of CBT for anxiety in ASD.

Finally, additional evidence is needed for the long-term effectiveness of CBT for anxiety in youth with ASD. While long-term positive outcomes have been demonstrated up to 6 years posttreatment for TD youth (Compton et al., 2004), the longest follow-up time for CBT in youth with ASD is 6 months (Reaven, 2011; White et al., 2009). CBT, usually a relatively brief treatment, operates under the model of teaching children and their parents skills to prevent and cope with anxiety in the future rather than "curing" them of anxiety. Especially given the complexity and severity of presentation of youth with ASD and anxiety, a longer follow-up to determine how children and parents continue to use these skills would be helpful.

REFERENCES

Albano, A. M., & Kendall, P. C. (2002). Cognitive behavioural therapy for children and adolescents with anxiety disorders: Clinical research advances. *International Review of Psychiatry, 14,* 129–134.

Amaral, D. G., Schumann, C. M., & Nordahl, C. W. (2008). Neuroanatomy of autism. *Trends in Neuroscience, 31*(3), 137–145.

Anderson, S., & Morris, J. (2006). Cognitive behaviour therapy for people with Asperger syndrome. *Behavioural and Cognitive Psychotherapy, 34,* 293–303.

Attwood, T. (2003). Framework for behavioral interventions. *Child and Adolescent Psychiatric Clinics of North America, 12*, 65–86.

Baher, M. J., Koegel, R. L., & Koegel, L. K. (1998). Increasing the social behavior of young children with autism using their obsessive behaviors. *Research and Practice for Persons with Severe Disabilities, 23*(4), 300–308.

Bellini, S. (2004). Social skill deficits and anxiety in high-functioning adolescents with autism spectrum disorders. *Focus on Autism and Other Developmental Disabilities, 19*, 78–86.

Bellini, S. (2006). The development of social anxiety in adolescents with autism spectrum disorders. *Focus on Autism and Other Developmental Disabilities, 21*, 138–145.

Ben-Sasson, A., Cermak, S. A., Orsmond, G. I., Tager-Flusberg, H., Kadlec, M. B., & Carter, A. S. (2008). Sensory clusters of toddlers with autism spectrum disorders: Differences in affective symptoms. *Journal of Child Psychology and Psychiatry, 49*(8), 817–825.

Birmaher, B., Khetarpal, S., Brent, D., Cully, M., Balach, L., Kaufman, J., et al. (1997). The Screen for Child Anxiety Related Emotional Disorders (SCARED): Scale construction and psychometric characteristics. *Journal of the American Academy of Child and Adolescent Psychiatry, 36*(4), 545–553.

Brereton, A. V., Tonge, B. J., & Einfeld, S. L. (2006). Psychopathology in children and adolescents with autism compared to young people with intellectual disability. *Journal of Autism and Developmental Disorders, 36*, 863–870.

Chalfant, A. M., Rapee, R., & Carroll, L. (2007). Treating anxiety disorders in children with high functioning autism spectrum disorders: A controlled trial. *Journal of Autism and Developmental Disorders, 37*, 1842–1857.

Chang, Y., Quan, J., & Wood, J. J. (2012). Effects of anxiety disorder severity on social functioning in children with autism spectrum disorders. *Journal of Developmental and Physical Disabilities, 24*, 235–245.

Compton, S. N., March, J. S., Brent, D., Albano, A. M., Weersing, V. R., & Curry, J. (2004). Cognitive-behavioral psychotherapy for anxiety and depressive disorders in children and adolescents: An evidence-based medicine review. *Journal of the American Academy of Child and Adolescent Psychiatry, 43*(8), 930–959.

Corbett, B. A., Mendoza, S., Wegelin, J. A., Carmean, V., & Levine, S. (2008). Variable cortisol circadian rhythms in children with autism and anticipatory stress. *Journal of Psychiatry and Neuroscience, 33*(3), 227–234.

de Bruin, E. I., Ferdinand, R. F., Meester, S., de Nijs, P. F. A., & Verheij, F. (2007). High rates of psychiatric co-morbidity in PDD-NOS. *Journal of Autism and Developmental Disorders, 37*, 877–886.

Drahota, A., Wood, J. J., Sze, K., & Van Dyke, M. (2011). Effects of cognitive behavioral therapy on daily living skills in children with high-functioning autism and concurrent anxiety disorders. *Journal of Autism and Developmental Disorders, 41*, 257–265.

Gadow, K. D., DeVincent, C. J., Pomeroy, J., & Azizian, A. (2005). Comparison of DSM-IV symptoms in elementary school-aged children with PFF versus clinic and community samples. *Autism, 9*, 392–415.

Gadow, K. D., DeVincent, C. J., & Schneider, J. (2009). Comparative study of children with ADHD only, autism spectrum disorder + ADHD, and chronic multiple tic disorder + ADHD. *Journal of Attention Disorders, 12,* 474–485.

Gadow, K. D., Roohi, J., DeVincent, C. J., Kirsch, S., & Hatchwell, E. (2009). Association of COMT (Val158Met) and BDNF (Val66Met) gene polymorphisms with anxiety, ADHD and tics in children with autism spectrum disorder. *Journal of Autism and Developmental Disorders, 39,* 1542–1551.

Gillott, A., & Standen, P. J. (2007). Levels of anxiety and sources of stress in adults with autism. *Journal of Intellectual Disabilities, 11*(4), 359–370.

Goodman, R. (1997). The Strengths and Difficulties Questionnaire: A research note. *Journal of Child Psychology and Psychiatry, 38*(5), 581–586.

Green, J., Gilchrist, A., Burton, D., & Cox, A. (2000). Social and psychiatric functioning in adolescents with Asperger syndrome compared with conduct disorder. *Journal of Autism and Developmental Disorders, 30,* 279–293.

Guttman-Steinmetz, S., Gadow, K. D., DeVincent, C. J., & Crowell, J. (2010). Anxiety symptoms in boys with autism spectrum disorder, attention-deficit-hyperactivity disorder, or chronic multiple tic disorder and community controls. *Journal of Autism and Developmental Disorders, 40*(8), 1006–1016.

Juranek, J., Filipek, P. A., Berenji, G. R., Modahl, C., Osann, K., & Spence, M. A. (2006). Association between amygdala volume and anxiety level: Magnetic resonance imaging (MRI) study in autistic children. *Journal of Child Neurology, 21,* 1051–1058.

Kendall, P. C. (1993). Cognitive-behavioral therapies with youth: Guiding theory, current status, and emerging developments. *Journal of Consulting and Clinical Psychology, 61*(2), 235–247.

Kendall, P. C. (1994). Treating anxiety disorders in children: Results of a randomized clinical trial. *Journal of Consulting and Clinical Psychology, 62,* 200–210.

Kendall, P. C., Flannery-Schroeder, E., Panichelli-Mindel, S. M., Southam-Gerow, M., Henin, A., & Warman, M. (1997). Therapy for youths with anxiety disorders: A second randomized clinical trial. *Journal of Consulting and Clinical Psychology, 65,* 366–380.

Kendall, P. C., Kane, M., Howard, B., & Siqueland, L. (1990). *Cognitive-behavioral treatment of anxious children: Treatment manual.* (Available from Philip C. Kendall, Department of Psychology, Temple University, Philadelphia, PA)

Kim, J. A., Szatmari, P., Bryson, S. E., Streiner, D. L., & Wilson, F. J. (2000). The prevalence of anxiety and mood problems among children with autism and Asperger syndrome. *Autism, 4*(2), 117–132.

Lang, R., Regester, A., Lauderdale, S., Ashbaugh, K., & Haring, A. (2010). Treatment of anxiety in autism spectrum disorders using cognitive behaviour therapy: A systematic review. *Developmental Neurorehabilitation, 13*(1), 53–63.

Lecavalier, L., Gadow, K. D., DeVincent, C. J., Houts, C., & Edwards, M. C. (2009). Deconstructing the PDD clinical phenotype: Internal validity of the DSM-IV. *Journal of Child Psychology and Psychiatry, 50,* 1246–1254.

Leyfer, O. T., Folstein, S. E., Bacalman, S., Davis, N. O., Dinh, E., Morgan, J., et al. (2006). Comorbid psychiatric disorders in children with autism: interview development and rates of disorders. *Journal of Autism and Developmental Disorders, 36,* 849–861.

Lyneham, H. J., Abbott, M. J., Wignall, A., & Rapee, R. M. (2003). *The Cool Kids family program—Therapist manual.* Sydney: Macquarie University.

March, J. S., Parker, J. D. A., Sullivan, K., Stallings, P., & Conners, K. (1997). The Multidimensional Anxiety Scale for Children (MASC): Factor structure, reliability, and validity. *Journal of the American Academy of Child and Adolescent Psychiatry, 36,* 554–565.

Muris, P., Steerneman, P., Merckelbach, H., Holdrinet, I., & Meesters, C. (1998). Comorbid anxiety symptoms in children with pervasive developmental disorders. *Journal of Anxiety Disorders, 12*(4), 387–393.

Nauta, M. H., Scholing, A., Rapee, R., Abbott, M., Spence, S., & Waters, A. (2004). A parent report measure of children's anxiety: Psychometric properties and comparison with child-report in a clinic and normal sample. *Behaviour Research and Therapy, 42,* 813–839.

Pfeiffer, B., Kinnealey, M., Reed, C., & Herzberg, G. (2005). Sensory modulation and affective disorders in children and adolescents with Asperger's disorder. *American Journal of Occupational Therapy, 59,* 335–345.

Reaven, J. (2011). The treatment of anxiety symptoms in youth with high-functioning autism spectrum disorders: Developmental considerations for parents. *Brain Research, 1380,* 255–263.

Reaven, J. A., Blakeley-Smith, A., Nichols, S., Dasari, M., Flanigan, E., & Hepburn, S. (2008). Cognitive-behavioral group treatment for anxiety symptoms in children with high-functioning autism spectrum disorders: A pilot study. *Focus on Autism and Other Developmental Disabilities, 24*(27). 27–37.

Reynolds, C. R., & Richmond, B. O. (1978). What I think and feel: A revised measure of children's manifest anxiety. *Journal of Abnormal Child Psychology, 6,* 271–280.

Russell, E., & Sofronoff, K. (2005). Anxiety and social worries in children with Asperger syndrome. *Australian and New Zealand Journal of Psychiatry, 39*(7), 633–638.

Scarpa, A., & Reyes, N. M. (2011). Improving emotion regulation with CBT in young children with high functioning autism spectrum disorders: A pilot study. *Behavioural and Cognitive Psychotherapy, 39*(4), 495–500.

Schniering, C. A., & Rapee, R. M. (2002). Development and validation of a measure of children's automatic thoughts: The Children's Automatic Thoughts Scale. *Behaviour Research and Therapy, 40,* 1091–1109.

Silverman, W. K., & Albano, A. M. (1996). *The Anxiety Disorders Interview Schedule for DSM-IV—Child and Parent versions.* San Antonio, TX: Graywind.

Sofronoff, K., Attwood, T., & Hinton, S. (2005). A randomized controlled trial of a CBT intervention for anxiety in children with Asperger syndrome. *Journal of Child Psychology and Psychiatry, 46*(11), 1152–1160.

Spence, S. H. (1995). *Social skills training: Enhancing social competence with children and adolescents.* Windsor, Berkshire, UK: NFER-Nelson.

Sukhodolsky, D. G., Scahill, L., Gadow, K. D., Arnold, L. E., Aman, M. G., McDougle, C. J., et al. (2008). Parent-rated anxiety symptoms in children with pervasive developmental disorders. Frequency and association with core autism symptoms and cognitive functioning. *Journal of Abnormal Child Psychology, 36,* 117–128.

White, S. W., Albano, A. M., Johnson, C. R., Kasari, C., Ollendick, T., Klin, A., et al. (2010). Development of a cognitive-behavioral intervention program to treat anxiety and social deficits in teens with high-functioning autism. *Clinical Child and Family Psychological Review, 13,* 77–90.

White, S. W., Ollendick, T., Scahill, L., Oswald, D., & Albano, A. M. (2009). Preliminary efficacy of a cognitive-behavioral treatment program for anxious youth with autism spectrum disorders. *Journal of Autism and Developmental Disorders, 39,* 1652–1662.

Wood, J. J., Drahota, A., Sze, K., Har, K., Chiu, A., & Langer, D. A. (2009). Cognitive behavioral therapy for anxiety in children with autism spectrum disorders: A randomized, controlled trial. *Journal of Child Psychology and Psychiatry, 50*(3), 224–234.

Wood, J. J., Drahota, A., Sze, K. M., Van Dyke, M., Decker, K., Fujii, C., et al. (2009). Brief report: Effects of cognitive behavioral therapy on parent-reported autism symptoms in school-age children with high-functioning autism. *Journal of Autism and Developmental Disabilties, 39,* 1608–1612.

Wood, J. J., & Gadow, K. D. (2010). Exploring the nature and function of anxiety in youth with autism spectrum disorders. *Clinical Psychology Science and Practice, 17*(4), 281–292.

Wood, J. J., & McLeod, B. D. (2008). *Child anxiety disorders: A family-based treatment manual for practitioners.* New York: Norton.

5

Parental Involvement in Treating Anxiety in Youth with High-Functioning ASD

JUDY REAVEN AND AUDREY BLAKELEY-SMITH

HISTORICAL BACKGROUND AND SIGNIFICANCE OF THE TREATMENT

Children with autism spectrum disorders (ASD) are at high risk for developing co-occurring psychiatric conditions, and anxiety symptoms are among the most common mental health symptoms these youth experience (de Bruin, Ferdinand, Meester, de Nijs, & Verheij, 2007; Leyfer et al., 2006; Simonoff et al., 2008; Skokauskas & Gallagher, 2012). While anxiety disorders are estimated to occur in 2.2–27% of the general pediatric population, rates of occurrence in youth with ASD are reported to be as much as two times higher (Costello, Egger, & Angold, 2005). In fact, in a recent meta-analysis reviewing psychiatric comorbidity in young people (under age 18) with ASD, over 39% of youth across studies met criteria for at least one DSM-IV-TR anxiety diagnosis (van Steensel, Bogels, & Perrin, 2011). While information regarding the occurrence of specific anxiety disorders in the ASD population has been somewhat variable, the most frequently identified anxiety disorder was specific phobia (29.8%), followed by obsessive–compulsive disorder (17.4%) and social anxiety disorder (16.6%) (van Steensel et al., 2011).

Anxiety disorders appear to be at least as impactful and interfering in day-to-day functioning as other psychiatric disorders, markedly affecting family processes, peer relationships, and academic function, including school attendance (Rapee, Schniering, & Hudson, 2009). The presence of anxiety symptoms has also been shown to be negatively associated with social competence and popularity, and positively associated with victimization (Giora, Gega, Landau, & Marks, 2005). In addition, without intervention, anxiety symptoms in typically developing children may persist into adulthood (Hudson, Krain & Kendall, 2001), contributing to the development of additional psychiatric conditions, such as depression or other mood disorders (Rapee et al., 2009). Given the vulnerability of children with ASD, anxiety symptoms may have a similar long-term impact, further signaling the critical importance of treating anxiety symptoms in children with ASD.

Developmental Considerations

Research on the nature and course of anxiety in typically developing children has indicated that anxiety in early childhood frequently involves separation from attachment figures, the dark, and personal safety, with anxiety surrounding social issues emerging in early to midadolescence, and obsessive–compulsive disorder emerging in mid- to late adolescence (Alfano, Beidel, & Turner, 2006; Barrett, 2000; Kessler, Chiu, Demler, Merikangas, & Walters, 2005). For individuals with ASD, the course of anxiety across development is still unclear; however, the overall developmental trajectory of anxiety symptoms is characterized by increases in symptoms from toddlerhood to childhood, decreases in symptoms from childhood to young adulthood, then increases again from young to older adulthood (Davis et al., 2011). Younger children with ASD and those with less developed cognitive abilities may experience milder anxiety, while adolescents may experience more social anxiety (Farrugia & Hudson, 2006; White, Oswald, Ollendick, & Scahill, 2009). The changing course and nature of anxiety across childhood may be impacted by the development of *metacognition* (i.e., thinking about thinking), as well as by a family's cultural context and background (Barrett, 2000).

Identifying the presence of anxiety in children with ASD is complicated by the challenge of determining which symptoms are unique to ASD and which may be associated with a co-occurring anxiety disorder (White et al., 2009). *Diagnostic overshadowing* (i.e., attributing symptoms to the developmental disability rather than to a co-occurring psychiatric condition; Reiss, Levitan & Szyszko, 1982) and *psychosocial masking* (i.e., the difficulty individuals with developmental disabilities have in reporting their psychiatric symptoms; Fuller & Sabatino, 1998) may further complicate the diagnostic process. Finally, challenges in child self-report of anxiety symptoms have been reported, with children with ASD endorsing fewer symptoms of anxiety than their parents endorse (Blakeley-Smith, Reaven, Ridge, & Hepburn, 2012; Mazefsky, Kao, & Oswald, 2011; White, Schry, & Maddox, 2012); this finding is in direct contrast to what is typically observed in general pediatric populations. Despite this under-reporting of symptoms, there is some evidence to suggest that in clinical populations of children with HFASD and anxiety, children's reports of anxiety symptoms are still significantly elevated and parent–child agreement is no worse than that observed in the general pediatric population (Blakeley-Smith et al., 2012). The continued use of multi-informant report is thus recommended, with child self-report considered complementary to parent-report.

Parents of children with ASD are therefore in the challenging position of reporting more symptoms of anxiety than their children identify and assuming responsibility for encouraging participation in treatment that their children do not consider necessary. For parents of adolescents with ASD, this journey may be made more difficult by adolescents' natural desire to assert independence, while simultaneously managing their own worries regarding the transition to adulthood. In addition, a parent's journey with his or her child can be a time-intensive struggle to secure community supports for the child through adulthood. For adolescents with ASD and anxiety, frustration often mounts as their symptoms of social anxiety emerge and their social skills lag behind their social ambitions. Their parents may further compound the problem by recommending that their teen participate in yet another treatment (Marcus, Kunce, & Schopler, 1999; White et al., 2010). Thus, the complex and evolving dynamic between youth with ASD and their parents becomes critical to understand.

Factors Contributing to the Development of Anxiety in Youth with ASD: A Road Map for Treatment Direction

Many factors have been implicated in the development of anxiety symptoms for youth in the general population, and there is no reason to believe that the development of anxiety in children with ASD is any less complex. Although a comprehensive review of the etiological factors that contribute to the development of anxiety is beyond the scope of this chapter, it is worth highlighting the combination of genetic influences, temperament, cognitive biases, parenting style and parental anxiety, social learning paradigms, and the presence of negative or traumatic life events that are potentially influential in symptom development. For example, a withdrawn and behaviorally inhibited temperamental style has been considered to be a risk factor for the development of anxiety symptoms later in life, perhaps because of the connection between behavioral inhibition and avoidant coping (Rapee et al., 2009). Research exploring the impact of cognitive biases suggests that anxious children, relative to nonanxious peers, tend to interpret ambiguous or mildly aversive situations as more negative and dangerous because they overestimate danger and underestimate their ability to cope (Creswell, Schniering, & Rapee, 2005). However, it is unclear whether these cognitive biases precede the development of anxiety symptoms in children or are a result of anxious behavior. Vicarious learning may also contribute to anxious behavior in that a parent, sibling, or peer acting in a fearful manner toward specific objects may influence others to develop similar fear reactions (Rapee et al., 2009). Finally, the presence of acute life stressors, as well as chronic adversities, can lead to the onset of anxious symptoms for some children (Allen, Rapee, & Sandberg, 2008).

Several researchers have begun to explore the nature and development of anxiety in children with ASD, focusing on factors thought to contribute to anxiety in typical populations such as those previously described, as well as factors that may be unique to youth with ASD (e.g., the interplay between anxiety and core deficits of ASD). In a study examining cognitive factors in adolescents with ASD and anxiety, Farrugia and Hudson (2006) reported correlations among anxiety symptoms, negative automatic thoughts, and behavioral problems in teens with ASD, as well as increased negative automatic thoughts, relative to participants in the comparison groups (nonclinical adolescents and adolescents with anxiety disorders). Bellini (2006) and Wood and Gadow (2010) have explored models of anxiety development, considering the role of core deficits. Bellini (2006) explored the relationship between physiological arousal and social deficits in teens with ASD and concluded that physiological arousal combined with social deficits likely contribute to the self-reported symptoms of social anxiety in the teens. Wood and Gadow (2010) postulated that anxiety in children with ASD may occur when stressors such as peer rejection, victimization, and social confusion occur as a result of the core deficits of ASD, which may in turn contribute to general negative affect, including anxiety. Symptoms of anxiety may lead to increases in behavioral problems, personal distress, and increased avoidance of social situations. Wood and Gadow (2010) further state that the presence of anxiety symptoms may exacerbate the severity of core ASD deficits, implying a reciprocal relationship between these conditions.

Parent Mental Health

Parental anxiety and parenting style are often referenced in the general literature as additional factors that contribute to the development of anxiety in children. Anxious parents are more likely to have anxious children, although the exact mechanism of transmission of symptoms from one generation to the other is unclear and complicated by shared genetic influence (Rapee et al., 2009). Thus, in addition to potential genetic transmission, parental anxiety may actively influence the learning experiences the parent provides to a child (Field, Cartwright-Hatton, Reynolds, & Creswell, 2008). For example, *interpretation bias* (e.g., the tendency to interpret ambiguous situations as threatening and dangerous) between parents and children is significantly and positively correlated (Creswell et al., 2005). In addition, parental modeling of fearful and/or avoidant responses to specific stimuli may also lead to anxiety reactions in their offspring (Creswell, Willetts, Murray, Singhal, & Cooper, 2008). Furthermore, the presence of maternal anxiety may contribute to maternal overreporting of anxious symptoms in their offspring, although anxious symptoms in children cannot be completely explained by reporter bias (Frick, Silverthorn, & Evans, 1994). Finally, many anxiety treatment programs require parents to help their children to engage in exposure activities (e.g., directly facing feared stimuli). Encouraging children to face fears may be difficult for anxious parents, who themselves may find the activities hard to execute (Creswell & Cartwright-Hatton, 2007).

In the emerging body of literature exploring the nature of anxiety in children with ASD, the role of parental anxiety and/or parenting behaviors in the development of anxious symptoms is conspicuously absent. The primary focus on the biological basis of ASD and child-driven effects may in part be an artifact of early research, in which parents, particularly mothers of children with ASD, were depicted as contributing to symptom development (Baker, Smith, Greenberg, Seltzer, & Taylor, 2011; Bettelheim, 1967). Though Bettelheim's work has long since been discredited, the damage that resulted from his early work may have led researchers away from exploring how the family environment may influence the developmental course for children with ASD (Baker et al., 2011; Greenberg, Seltzer, Hong, & Orsmond, 2006). However, emerging evidence suggests that parental behavior may in fact influence the autism phenotype throughout development and deserves more attention than it has been afforded in the past (Baker et al., 2011). It is important to emphasize that thoughtful discussion about parenting factors that may be associated with anxious symptoms in youth with ASD is not the same as assigning blame. Rather, parents may be the untapped yet crucial agents of change their children need when they support skills development, foster generalization of new skills, and even help to prevent the onset of anxiety symptoms. Thus, delineation of the parent's role in the treatment of anxiety would be an important contribution to the growing body of literature on intervention programs for youth with ASD.

The presence of psychiatric symptoms in parents of youth with ASD is one area of research that has received attention. For example, it is known that parents of children with ASD generally present with more psychiatric symptoms than parents of typically developing children or children with other developmental disabilities (Murphy et al., 2000; Rao & Beidel, 2009). Furthermore, research on the broader autism phenotype has indicated that parents and other family members may experience increases in traits such as anxiety, impulsivity, irritability, shyness, aloofness, and eccentric behaviors (Murphy et al., 2000). Interestingly, some traits in parents (e.g., deficits in social functioning) have been found to precede the child's diagnosis of ASD, while other traits appear to occur subsequent to the birth of a child with ASD (e.g., anxiety symptoms), suggesting that the presence of a child with ASD may trigger or exacerbate social difficulties, anxiety, and similar traits in parents (Murphy et al., 2000).

In addition to their increased rates of psychiatric symptoms, it is also well known that parents of children with ASD experience high rates of stress and caregiver strain (Orsmond, Seltzer, Greenberg, & Krauss, 2006). Although there may be many reasons for high caregiver stress, a number of studies have implicated the presence of child maladaptive behaviors, particularly when compared with other child factors such as ASD severity or deficits in adaptive behavior (Baker, Blacher, Crnic, & Edelbrock, 2002; Estes et al., 2008; Lecavalier, Leone, & Wiltz, 2006). Interestingly, child cognitive ability does not appear to contribute to parental stress as much as child problem behavior. In a study that specifically explored stress in families of children with high-functioning ASD, high levels of parenting stress were directly related to child factors such as hyperactivity, highly demanding behaviors, and disturbed mood. Thus, strong intellectual ability in this group of youth did not appear to mitigate the stress involved in raising a child with ASD (Rao & Beidel, 2009).

Although the etiology of maladaptive behaviors in children with ASD is unclear, challenging behaviors likely develop as a result of multiple variables, such as genetic influence and other biologically based factors; learning history; environmental variables; and the presence of core deficits in areas of social, communication, and play behaviors. Although the exact nature of the relationship between problem behaviors and mental health symptoms in children with ASD is unknown, it is likely that symptoms of anxiety and depression may in part underlie observed behavioral outbursts in children with ASD (Reaven, 2011; Myles & Southwick, 2005). It is also very common for children with ASD to have multiple psychiatric diagnoses (Reaven, Blakeley-Smith, Culhane-Shelburne, & Hepburn, 2012), further contributing to their complex behavioral presentation. Therefore, this psychiatric complexity and ensuing maladaptive behaviors may in large part contribute to increases in parenting stress. In fact, Hastings (2003) argues that challenging behaviors in children with ASD may lead to increases in parenting stress because of a disruption in parenting behaviors, which may inevitably lead to ongoing difficulties with managing the child's challenging behaviors over time. Furthermore, parenting self-efficacy has been demonstrated to mediate the relationship between parental anxiety–depression and child behavior problems (Rezendes & Scarpa, 2011). In other words, parental stress related to the behavioral challenges of a child with ASD may negatively affect parents' confidence in their ability to manage these problem behaviors, and exacerbate their own mood–anxiety symptoms.

Parental Expressed Emotion and Problem Behaviors

Further impacting the parent–child relationship for families of children with ASD may be high levels of expressed emotion (EE), defined as "high levels of criticism and/or marked emotional overinvolvement by one family member towards another with an illness or disability" (Greenberg et al., p. 230). Research has indicated that high EE levels occur in between 25% and 33% of mothers of children with developmental disabilities, rates that are lower than for mothers of children with psychiatric disorders, but higher than for mothers of typically developing children (Orsmond et al., 2006). Some have speculated that high levels of EE may be the product of extended periods of caregiving and/or may occur in the presence of difficult problem behaviors (Dossetor, Nicol, Stretch, & Rajkhowa, 1994; Orsmond et al., 2006). In a study examining the relationship between mothers and adolescents and young adults with ASD, Orsmond and colleagues (2006) found that specific characteristics of the individual with ASD, in combination with maternal characteristics, were predictive of a more positive parent–child relationship. For example, children with ASD who had few maladaptive behaviors and also had mothers with an optimistic outlook were more likely to have a warm and positive relationship with each other than were children and mothers with more negative characteristics. Other research has demonstrated that maternal warmth, praise, and relationship quality were related to reductions in behavior problems (both internalizing and externalizing behaviors) and reductions in core ASD symptoms (e.g., repetitive behaviors; Smith, Greenberg, Seltzer, & Hong, 2008). Conversely, high levels of EE in mothers of individuals with ASD were associated with increasing levels of maladaptive behaviors and/or more severe autism symptoms over time (Greenberg et al., 2006). Increased severity of internalizing, externalizing, and asocial problem behaviors were related to high levels of overall maternal EE in the sample of mothers and adolescent–adult children with ASD. More than half of the participants in this study (57%) were given a diagnosis of intellectual disability. Thus, the extent to which these associations might be true for a sample of participants with average or better intellectual ability is unknown.

Treatment research targeting EE is limited, although some studies have demonstrated that EE can be modified via psychoeducational group interventions, at least for families of individuals with schizophrenia (Tarrier et al., 1988). Family-based interventions for individuals with ASD that specifically target EE and parental criticism may be essential, because the ongoing effects of parental EE into adulthood may be detrimental (Greenberg et al., 2006). In fact, research has shown that there may be a strong positive association between high levels of parental criticism and problem behaviors in adult children with ASD, and that the trajectories of each of the factors are positively linked over time (Baker et al., 2011). Treatment implications based on this finding may be that intervention targeting *either* parental criticism *or* maladaptive behaviors could result in positive changes in family functioning.

Finally, it is important to note that although families of children with ASD are significantly stressed, not all families display high levels of EE; in fact, results from Greenberg et al. (2006) suggest that the number of families of children with ASD exhibiting high EE levels is lower than what would be expected for families of children with equally serious illnesses or disabilities. The relatively small number of families in some studies may reflect family strengths and/or effective coping techniques. The relatively low levels of parental criticism in these samples, coupled with studies highlighting the positive ways that mothers can influence their children's development (e.g., via maternal warmth and praise), may also serve to dispel the antiquated negative characterizations of mothers of children with autism (Greenberg et al., 2006; Smith et al., 2008). Thus, it is essential that future treatment programs harness family strengths and positive perceptions within ongoing treatment for families of children with ASD.

Parental Involvement in the Treatment
of Childhood Anxiety

The general pediatric literature has examined how parents may be incorporated into treatment programs, what their involvement entails, and whether their involvement leads to better child outcomes than primarily child-focused programs. For example, the earliest cognitive-behavioral therapy (CBT) programs for the treatment of childhood anxiety focused on an individual child, with parent involvement occurring primarily in the form of several adjunct parent meetings over the course of the 16 weekly therapy sessions (Kendall, 1994). Later CBT programs for childhood anxiety began to include a family component as part of the intervention package (Barrett, Dadds, & Rapee, 1996; Cobham, Dadds, & Spence, 1998). Family-based interventions developed in part because the results of early efficacy trials indicated that individual, child-focused interventions led to significant reductions in anxiety for approximately 50–80% of children, with 20–50% of child participants remaining symptomatic (Ginsburg & Schlossberg, 2002). Thus, the inclusion of parents aimed to further improve children's response to existing CBT interventions.

Much variability exists among family-based intervention programs for youth anxiety, making it difficult to compare results (Rapee et al., 2009). However, in general, the content has typically included a combination of the following key elements or treatment goals: (1) psychoeducation and presentation of a CBT model of anxiety and treatment; (2) contingency management (i.e., rewarding courageous behaviors and extinguishing excessive anxiety); (3) increasing parents' awareness of their own anxiety symptoms and the extent to which they may inadvertently contribute to the development and maintenance of child anxiety symptoms; (4) directly treating parental anxiety (e.g., parent anxiety management [PAM; Cobham et al., 1998]); (5) teaching parents to model effective problem solving and proactive responses in reaction to their own anxiety; (6) modifying parents' dysfunctional cognitions; (7) improving the parent–child relationship; and (8) teaching both parents (when possible) to work together as a co-parenting team (Ginsburg & Schlossberg, 2002; Reaven & Hepburn, 2006).

The results of studies comparing child-focused individual CBT to various forms of family-based CBT have yielded mixed results. One study reported more statistically significant reductions in anxiety symptoms after participation in family-based treatment programs than after individual child CBT (Barrett et al., 1996), whereas another found no added benefit of more intensive parent participation but reported value in conceptualizing parents as collaborators rather than co-clients (Kendall, Hudson,

Gosch, Flannery-Schroeder, & Suveg, 2008). It appears, however, that the value of more intensive parent participation is observed when certain child-specific factors are at play. For example, Barrett and colleagues (1996) found that females and younger children (ages 7–10) responded better to family-based CBT than to individual CBT, but there was no significant difference between conditions for older children (ages 11–14). Furthermore, when "autistic features" were assessed in typically developing child participants with clinical anxiety symptoms,[1] results indicated that children with "moderate" autistic features on the SRS-P were significantly more likely to improve from participation in family CBT than individual CBT (Puleo & Kendall, 2011). The authors noted that the differences in treatment outcome may be related to more at-home exposure practice. Thus, without family support, the cognitive inflexibility of children with autism-related symptoms may make it difficult to fully access standard individual CBT interventions.

Research has also examined the impact of parent-specific factors such as parent anxiety on child treatment outcome. A large body of research demonstrates that parental anxiety negatively impacts outcome (Creswell & Cartwright-Hatton, 2007; Creswell et al., 2008). In an early study, Cobham and colleagues (1998) compared the impact of individual CBT plus PAM and CBT alone. The efficacy of CBT was greatly reduced when child participants had an anxious parent. Furthermore, adding the PAM component increased efficacy of individual CBT for children with one or more anxious parents, but not for children whose parents were not anxious. Subsequent studies have questioned whether it is in fact parental anxiety that should be the target of family-based interventions for childhood anxiety, or whether interventions should target specific parenting behaviors (e.g., maternal overinvolvement; maternal expression of fear) associated with parental anxiety (Creswell et al., 2008). Further work on treatments that target these specific mechanisms would be useful.

Finally, some of the most recent research on the efficacy of CBT for childhood anxiety has shifted from focusing on youth treatment outcome to exploring the bidirectional and reciprocal influence of the parent–child relationship (Silverman, Kurtines, Jaccard, & Pina, 2009). Rather than examining the improvements in youth outcome as a result of interventions targeting parental anxiety or behavior, Silverman and colleagues (2009) tested the alternative supposition that reductions in youth anxiety would positively impact parent variables. In their efficacy trial, participants (ages

---

[1] "Autistic features" were assessed using the Social Responsiveness Scale—Parent version (SRS-P; Constantino & Gruber, 2005).

7–16) who received CBT with minimal parent involvement and those who received CBT with active parent involvement evidenced significant improvements in anxiety. However, there were no significant differences in youth anxiety when parenting variables alone were directly targeted. Furthermore, when youth anxiety was targeted and symptom improvement resulted, all measured parent variables showed statistically significant improvements. Taken together, these results provide initial support for a bidirectional consideration of parent-to-youth and youth-to-parent influence. Similar studies have not been conducted with families of children with ASD, although the extent to which improved outcomes for youth with ASD influence parent variables may reflect an important area of investigation. Clearly, further research is needed to explore the dynamic relationship between parenting factors and child behaviors.

To summarize, research examining parental involvement in the treatment of childhood anxiety in the typically developing population generally suggests that family-based interventions may reduce anxiety symptoms at least as well as child-focused CBT programs. We would also expect parental involvement to be most important for younger children and for parents who acknowledge their own anxious symptoms (Creswell & Cartwright-Hatton, 2007; Rapee et al., 2009). The degree to which parental anxiety rather than parenting behaviors and/or features of the parent–child relationship is specifically targeted is unclear, because these variables have yet to be systematically studied. Finally, studying the bidirectional nature of the parent–child relationship in the development and maintenance of anxiety symptoms may further inform directions for youth anxiety treatment programs.

PRACTICAL CONSIDERATIONS

The Parents' Role in the Treatment of Children with High-Functioning ASD

Whereas the preceding section focused exclusively on work with typically developing youth who present with anxiety, this section reviews interventions for children with ASD. Although a similar body of research does not yet exist for children with HFASD, the critical importance of including parents of children with ASD in their treatment has been emphasized (Moree & Davis, 2010; Reaven, 2011). In fact, parents may play a larger and more constant role than they ordinarily play for typically developing offspring given the severity and chronicity of the core deficits and other social, developmental, or behavioral challenges of children with ASD (Reaven, 2011).

Assuming the roles of advocate, teacher, cheerleader, and friend, in addition to parent, may be part and parcel of parenting a child with ASD. Helping their children and adolescents navigate school, manage friendships, obtain vocational experiences, live independently, and establish self-advocacy skills represents only a portion of the burden and responsibility that parents may experience as their children with ASD move into adolescence and young adulthood. Moreover, the ongoing nature of the parenting role for families of children with ASD does not allow a lessening of parental responsibilities. The presence of psychiatric symptoms likely exacerbates an already complex picture, thus making these common developmental tasks even more difficult to achieve (Reaven, 2011).

Four randomized controlled trials using modified CBT for the treatment of anxiety symptoms in youth with ASD have been conducted, in addition to our own work (see below). Three of the studies incorporated parents into their intervention programs (Chalfant, Rapee, & Carroll, 2007; Sofronoff, Attwood, & Hinton, 2005; Wood et al., 2009), while one program did not include parents in the treatment, citing this as a limitation (Sung et al., 2011). Descriptions of parent involvement in these studies are relatively brief, making it difficult to assess the core features of the parent curriculum, as well as the amount of parent involvement required. Sofronoff et al. (2005) suggest that it is important to work with parents as "co-therapists." In their study of children between ages 10 and 12 with HFASD and anxiety, therapists worked with parents in all aspects of the treatment, specifically, teaching parents to encourage their children to use coping strategies in different anxiety-provoking situations and to complete home based projects. Results indicated that when children were randomized to one of three conditions (wait-list control, intervention for child only, intervention for child and parent), parent-reported anxiety symptoms in child participants significantly decreased for both intervention groups, along with significant increases in child-generated positive coping strategies when presented with anxiety-provoking situations. Even greater decreases in parent-reported anxiety symptoms were apparent in the intervention condition that included parent involvement, suggesting that active parent involvement appeared to enhance the usefulness of the treatment program.

Chalfant et al. (2007) also included parents in their adaptation of the Cool Kids program (Lyneham, Abbott, Waignall, & Rapee, 2003). Although originally developed for typically developing children with anxiety, Cool Kids was modified for the learning styles of children with HFASD. The parent component of the intervention focused on anxiety education that involved teaching relaxation strategies, cognitive restructuring exercises, graded exposure, parent management training, and relapse prevention. Parent sessions were conducted concurrently with the child program. Children (ages 8–13) were randomly assigned to either the CBT intervention or to a wait-list control group. Results indicated that children and their parents who participated in the CBT program demonstrated significant reductions in anxiety symptoms relative to children in the wait-list condition.

In the randomized trial by Wood et al. (2009), children with ASD and co-occurring anxiety were enrolled in a 16-week individual treatment program. Each session lasted 90 minutes (30 minutes with the child; 60 minutes with the parents/family). The authors modified the Building Confidence CBT program (Wood & McLeod, 2009) for children with ASD. Parents were taught to support *in vivo* exposures, as well as to use positive reinforcement and communication skills to encourage independence and autonomy in their children. Parents also acted as coaches around the development of friendship skills and adaptive behavior. Results indicated that even in the presence of high levels of psychiatric comorbidity, children who were randomized to the active CBT condition displayed significant positive treatment outcomes.

In a paper detailing their treatment program for adolescents with HFASD, the Multimodal Anxiety and Social Skills Intervention (MASSI), White et al. (2010) emphasize the importance of parent and family involvement. In the treatment program, parents act as "coaches" for exposure activities, thereby promoting skills generalization. Parents participate in the last 15–20 minutes of each session and receive regular communication from the therapist, who describes target skills and provides suggestions for enhancing skills development at home. In addition, ongoing feedback and input are obtained from parents regarding treatment progress. This empirical work, as well as descriptions of developing interventions for youth with ASD, document the importance of including parents in treatment programs.

Facing Your Fears: Group Therapy for Managing Anxiety in Children with High-Functioning ASD

Facing Your Fears (FYF; Reaven, Blakeley-Smith, Nichols, & Hepburn, 2011) is a 14-week, group CBT program targeting anxiety symptoms in children ages 7–14 with HFASD.[2] Clinical and research experience has

---

[2] *HFASD* in this study refers to children who are verbally fluent (Verbal IQ > 80) and meet criteria for an ASD.

indicated that youth with ASD typically present with anxiety in combination with a number of other psychiatric symptoms and conditions. FYF is designed for youth with ASD and multiple psychiatric comorbid conditions, but for whom anxiety symptoms are most prominent. Children are considered eligible if their anxiety symptoms are consistent with a diagnosis of either generalized anxiety disorder, social anxiety disorder, separation anxiety, or specific phobia. Our research program used the Anxiety Disorders Interview Schedule—Parent version (ADIS-P; Silverman & Albano, 1996), a semistructured psychiatric interview administered to parents to obtain information regarding clinical symptoms. Once child participants meet criteria for a specific anxiety disorder, clinician severity ratings are assigned to each diagnosis. Primary diagnoses are determined by selecting the diagnosis with the highest severity rating. Children with specific phobias are eligible provided they meet diagnostic criteria for an additional anxiety diagnosis. Sessions typically comprise four to five multifamily groups, each lasting approximately 1½ hours. Each session occurs within one of three main modalities: large-group activities (parents and children together); parent–child dyadic work; and small-group activities (children and parents meet in separate concurrent groups). FYF was originally designed to be delivered using a group modality; however, it is a program that can easily be modified for individual delivery. Given that research in the general pediatric population indicates comparable outcomes for children with anxiety who participate in individual CBT and those who participate in group CBT (Rapee, Wignall, Hudson, & Schniering, 2000), it is possible that a similar outcome pattern could be observed in the ASD population.

FYF was written and developed specifically for children with ASD. However, FYF incorporates important components of existing empirically supported programs for typically developing children (e.g., Coping Cat; Kendall & Hedtke, 2006), while making appropriate adaptations for youth with HFASD. Standard CBT components such as graded exposure, somatic management, cognitive self-control, and a focus on improving emotion regulation were included in the FYF intervention (Kendall, 1994; Silverman, Pina, & Viswesvaran, 2008). Modifications of traditional CBT activities were made to meet the cognitive, linguistic, and social needs of children with ASD, in line with previous recommendations (Moree & Davis, 2010; Reaven et al., 2009). A token reinforcement program, providing visual structure and support, and establishing a predictable routine for each session were included in the program to enhance the accessibility of the content for youth with ASD. Multiple-choice lists, written examples of core concepts, hands-on activities, an emphasis on creative outlets for expression, a focus on strengths and special interests, multiple opportunities for repetition and practice, and video self-modeling were used throughout the FYF program (Reaven et al., 2011).

FYF was originally created for implementation by mental health professionals with diverse training backgrounds, including clinicians with experience in working with youth with ASD but less familiarity with CBT for anxiety, as well as clinicians familiar with CBT but less experienced with the ASD population. To meet the needs of the anticipated heterogeneity of the professionals using this program, FYF was written in a detailed, step-by-step manner, complete with "helpful hints" sections intended to guide clinicians through common problems and to provide suggestions for working with youth with ASD and anxiety. As with other manualized programs, clinicians are encouraged to deliver content as written, but in a flexible manner (Kendall & Beidas, 2007).

In the FYF intervention, parents attend every session for the duration of the intervention (14 weeks), and for the full 90 minutes, because they are viewed as critical to children's success in treatment. They are also encouraged to use each other as sources of support, encouragement, and information. The parent component of FYF includes (1) psychoeducation of anxiety disorders and introduction to the basic principles of CBT; (2) identification of the child's specific anxiety symptoms; (3) management strategies for handling emotion dysregulation; (4) identification of target behaviors in preparation for graded exposure assignments; (5) discussion of parental anxiety and parenting style, and how these factors affect parenting a child with anxiety; and (6) discussion of the social and communicative challenges inherent in ASD, and how these challenges may lead to a protective parenting style (Reaven et al., 2011). The concepts of adaptive protection and excessive protection are introduced to parents as a way to characterize common parental responses to children's anxious behavior. That is, *adaptive protection* occurs when a child presents with marked areas of developmental, physical, or emotional challenge (e.g., ASD) and a caregiver consciously titrates the child's exposure to challenging environmental events in order to create success experiences for the child. Parents who engage in adaptive protection encourage brave behavior but provide appropriate parental protection as needed, particularly in light of a child's cognitive or social challenges. *Excessive protection*, on the other hand, is a parental response that may limit a child's exposure to anxiety-provoking situations through avoidant behavior, *even* when the child possesses the necessary skills for success. Allowing children to avoid anxious situations consistently can limit the opportunities to generate and practice effective coping strategies for handling anxiety-provoking situations in the future.

At the heart of successful reduction of anxiety symptoms, especially for children with special needs, may be parents' ability to help their children face fears, through the creative implementation of children's exposure hierarchies. Together, parents, children, and therapists rank-order anxiety-provoking stimuli from *mild levels of anxiety* to *high levels of anxiety*, and encourage children to face their fears a little at a time, beginning with a low level of fear. Much of the parent group sessions focus on ensuring parental understanding and implementation of these core concepts (Reaven et al., 2011). Beginning with therapist modeling of conducting exposure hierarchies, a "transfer of control" from the therapist to the parent occurs over time (Silverman et al., 1999) as parents are encouraged to conduct exposure hierarchies in session, then at home.

FYF: SESSION BY SESSION

Group sessions for the children are carefully paced, interactive, and activity-based. As with other CBT programs (Kendall & Hedtke, 2006; March & Mulle, 1998), the FYF intervention can be divided into two 7-week blocks. The first half of treatment involves introduction to anxiety symptoms, with an emphasis on the individual expression in each participant, as well as an overview of common CBT principles and strategies. The second half of treatment includes a focus on the implementation and generalization of specific tools and strategies to treat anxious symptoms (e.g., graded exposure).

In Sessions 1 and 2, children and parents become comfortable with the group format and participate in a series of activities designed to expand children's emotion vocabulary (Attwood, 2004) and to identify children's worries and anxiety-induced physiological symptoms. In Session 3, children and parents are encouraged to externalize or objectify anxious symptoms through the creation of "worry bugs" and "helper bugs" that represent worry and challenging worry, respectively. In this way, child and parents learn to separate the anxious symptoms from the child, so that they may align together to form a "team" to manage anxiety (March & Mulle, 1998; White & Epston, 1990). In Sessions 4 and 5, tools such as deep breathing, expansion of daily calming activities, recognition of automatic negative thoughts ("active minds"; Garland & Clark, 1995), and development of positive coping statements ("helpful thoughts") are introduced and taught to families, so that they can manage and even resist anxious symptoms. Families are taught that anxiety or worry comes and goes, and that they can have some control over reducing symptoms. The children and their parents use a *stress-o-meter* to measure anxiety and heighten awareness of calm and relaxed states versus periods of high stress or anxiety. The stress-o-meter incorporates color zones (e.g., red, yellow, and green), with an 8-point scale to connote the degree of an individual's subjective experience of anxiety. The stress-o-meter is also used as a tool to facilitate emotion regulation; together with their parents, children develop a plan for "getting to green," or moving from the red zone *(high levels of anxiety)* to the yellow *(medium levels of anxiety),* and eventually to the green zone *(completely calm).* "Show and tell" is incorporated at the end of every group, beginning in Session 4, to allow participants to "show off" special interests and strengths and to expand the focus beyond anxiety related symptoms or activities.

In Sessions 6 and 7, graded exposure is introduced to the families via videotaped examples of children "facing their fears" in a variety of situations (e.g., facing fears of dogs, fears of talking on the telephone). Following the video viewing, parent–child pairs create a hierarchy of anxiety-provoking situations, targeting specific fears or worries (at home and/or school or group) that interfere with day-to-day functioning. Children are rewarded for engaging in *graded-exposure tasks* (i.e., facing fears a little at a time) conducted both in session and in other settings (e.g., home, school).

Because social impairments likely underlie some of the specific anxiety symptoms, FYF embeds social skills development within the context of each group treatment session. For example, child participants regularly practice greeting peers and adults; speaking in front of a group; conversational skills, including commenting and asking questions; sharing personal information, including emotional expression with the group; and working cooperatively with other group members to complete a group project. Additionally, specific social skills are taught in conjunction with exposure practice, where applicable. For example, if a child has a fear of talking to people, then the intervention would likely include not only exposure steps of increasing difficulty (greeting a familiar peer, greeting a teacher, having a conversation with a peer, talking to a stranger, etc.) but also coaching on *how* to greet others, suggestions for improving conversational skills, and so forth.

Sessions 8–13 are essentially identical in content, as children and parents participate in graded exposure practice in each of these sessions, providing stress-o-meter ratings prior to, during, and after each exposure task. After the exposure practice is completed, children rate how well the exposure went and note what they might do differently next time. Children and parents then meet separately; parents spend time with the facilitators troubleshooting exposure hierarchies and other relevant challenges, while the children write, direct, and star in a series of short *Facing Your Fears* videos depicting children facing their fears in a variety of contexts. The primary purpose of the video activity is to enhance generalization of skills across settings through the repetition of key concepts (Kendall & Hedtke, 2006). In Session 14, a "graduation" session, families are encouraged to bring other family members to celebrate the end of group. *Facing Your Fears* videos are viewed and distributed (where appropriate), and both children and parents review core components of FYF. Awards and graduation certificates are given to all youth participants. Finally, a booster session is offered 4–6 weeks after the final session. In the booster session, updates regarding the children's progress are obtained, along with a final review of core treatment components.

FYF—Adolescent Version

An adolescent version of FYF (FYF-A) was subsequently developed to meet the unique developmental needs of teens with ASD and their families. Similar to the original FYF program, the 14 multifamily group sessions include an introduction to anxiety symptoms and common CBT strategies for treatment of anxiety, as well as in-session opportunities to practice implementation of the strategies (e.g., graded exposure). Modifications unique to the adolescent version of FYF, including: (1) a specific social skills module; (2) parent–teen dyadic work to identify primary anxiety diagnoses and related goals; (3) technology incorporated in the form of a personalized digital assistant (e.g., iPod Touch); (4) a greater number of in-session exposure practices; and (5) a parent curriculum, focused on the unique developmental challenges of adolescence. The group format of FYF-A allows for much parent-to-parent input and discussion.

Clinical observations during the pilot program of FYF-A revealed that some of the parent–teen dyads were characterized by high levels of parental EE; that is, frequent parental criticism that may be related to long-standing adolescent behavioral challenges (Greenberg, et al., 2006). Anecdotally, this high level of parental EE appeared to occur more frequently in the older adolescent dyadic pairings, and was less noticeable in younger cohorts (i.e., ages 8–13). In an attempt to ameliorate these negative interactions, opportunities for positive interaction between parents and teens were encouraged and created by emphasizing teen strengths and increasing the understanding that frequent displays of teen resistance could be related to long histories of social rejection rather than lack of motivation or interest (Reaven, 2011; Reaven et al., 2012; White et al., 2010). Research is needed to determine whether EE mediates treatment outcome for adolescents with ASD and anxiety, as well as which specific treatment components can improve parent–teen relations and complement the active ingredients of CBT.

RESEARCH TO DATE ON THE TREATMENT

In the following section, results from three treatment trials exploring the initial efficacy of FYF/FYF-A in treating anxiety symptoms in children with high functioning ASD are presented: (1) a pilot study that compared parent and child participation in a 12-week version of FYF for children with ASD to a wait-list group (Reaven et al., 2009); (2) a randomized clinical trial that compared treatment as usual (TAU) with parent and child participation in FYF (Reaven et al., 2012); and (3) a pilot study examining FYF-A for adolescents with ASD (Reaven et. al., 2012). Impact of the treatment package was assessed in all three studies by examining the reduction in parent-reported anxiety symptoms in youth.

In the initial pilot study, 33 children with HFASD and their parents participated in the 12-week FYF program. Parent–child pairs were assigned either to FYF or to the wait-list control condition on a first come, first serve basis. Results indicated significantly greater reductions in parent-reported anxiety symptoms on the Screen for Child Anxiety Related Emotional Disorders (SCARED; Birmaher et al., 1999) for children who participated in the FYF program than for children in the wait-list control condition, with a large effect size (Cohen's $d = 1.03$). This initial pilot study had several limitations, including lack of random assignment, lack of a control condition for the intervention, and poor parent completion of outcome measures (Reaven et al. 2009). These limitations were addressed in the second, more rigorous trial described below.

The second study, a randomized clinical trial, was conducted to further examine the efficacy of FYF (Reaven et al., 2012). The intent-to-treat (ITT) sample included 50 children ages 8–14 (and their parents) with HFASD and clinically significant symptoms of anxiety. Participants were randomly assigned to either FYF or TAU. Parents completed a "gold standard" anxiety assessment interview (Anxiety Disorders Inventory Schedule for Children—Parent version; ADIS-P; Silverman & Albano, 1996) pre- and posttreatment, with an independent clinical evaluator (ICE) who was blind to the participant's treatment condition. Three outcome variables were analyzed for the ITT sample, including clinician severity ratings, diagnostic status of the anxiety diagnoses, and the Clinical Global Impressions—Improvement scale (CGI-I; National Institute of Mental Health, 1970), a 1- to 7-point rating scale assigned by the ICE regarding the overall impression of improvement (i.e., 1 indicated *very much improved*; 4 indicated *no change;* and 7 indicated *very much worse*). Results indicated significant reductions in anxiety and interference for participants in the FYF condition and fewer anxiety diagnoses compared to participants in TAU.

Furthermore, 50% of participants in the FYF condition demonstrated clinically meaningful improvement in anxiety symptoms, as indicated by CGI-I ratings of 1 or 2, compared with only 8.7% of children in the TAU group (Cohen's d = 1.03). Six-month follow-up data indicated that postintervention reductions were maintained over time. Limitations included relatively small sample size and the lack of an attention control group.

In the third study we extended the FYF intervention to a high-functioning adolescent sample. Twenty-four adolescents ages 13–18 (and their parents) participated in the pilot study (Reaven et al., 2012). Parents completed the ADIS-P (Silverman & Albano, 1996) pre- and posttreatment. Adolescents and their parents participated in the 14-week FYF-A program. Results indicated significant reductions in anxiety severity and interference posttreatment, with low rates of anxiety maintained at 3-month follow-up. The results also indicated that nearly 46% of teens had a clinically meaningful improvement in anxiety symptoms based on the CGI-I for the primary diagnosis, while 33% of teens were *somewhat improved,* and for 21% of teens the symptoms status remained the same (Cohen's d = 0.9). No teen participants' symptoms worsened after treatment. Although initial findings from this pilot study suggest that FYF-A may be effective in reducing anxiety symptoms, the findings are very preliminary. More research is needed and should include a more rigorous treatment design (i.e., random assignment, control group) before more definitive conclusions can be offered.

CONCLUSIONS AND FUTURE DIRECTIONS

The results of the three treatment trials conducted to date using FYF/FYF-A suggest that a group CBT program developed specifically for youth with ASD may be effective in managing anxiety symptoms. Significant reductions in anxiety followed participation in the FYF treatment program across all three studies. In addition, large effect sizes were observed across the three FYF studies described. Although limitations remain, these findings are promising and generally in line with results from other treatment programs (Chalfant et al., 2007; Wood et al., 2009).

We believe parent involvement to be integral to the FYF/FYF-A programs. The parent curriculum for the FYF programs was derived from previous research on family-based programs in the typically developing population. However, the content and "dosage" for parent participation in treatment programs for youth with ASD and co-occurring anxiety have yet to be examined empirically. Head-to-head comparisons of individually oriented CBT (minimal parent involvement) and family-based CBT approaches for youth with ASD would provide important information regarding the content of treatment programs and the nature of parent participation. Varying the key content of the parent curriculum would also prove helpful in further understanding *what* should be targeted when parents are involved in treatment. Furthermore, the extent to which parent mental health status (i.e., parental anxiety) impacts youth outcome for individuals with ASD has also been empirically investigated, but represents an important next step. The bidirectional influence that others have discussed (Silverman et al., 2009) would be key to explore for youth with ASD and their families, because the results from such studies could significantly influence treatment outcome and the direction of future research.

REFERENCES

Alfano, C. A., Beidel, D. C., & Turner, S. M. (2006). Cognitive correlates of social phobia among children and adolescents. *Journal of Abnormal Child Psychology, 34*, 189–201.

Allen, J. L., Rapee, R. M., & Sandberg, S. (2008). Severe life events and chronic adversities as antecedents to anxiety in children: A matched control study. *Journal of Abnormal Child Psychology, 36*, 1047–1056.

Attwood, T. (2004). *Exploring feelings: Cognitive behavior therapy to manage anxiety.* Arlington, TX: Future Horizons.

Baker, B. L., Blacher, J., Crnic, K. A., & Edelbrock, C. (2002). Behavior problems and parenting stress in families of three-year-old children with and without developmental delays. *American Journal on Mental Retardation, 107*, 433–444.

Baker, J. K., Smith, L. E., Greenberg, J. S., Seltzer, M. M., & Taylor, J. L. (2011). Change in maternal criticism and behavior problems in adolescents and adults with autism across a seven-year period. *Journal of Abnormal Psychology, 120*, 465–475.

Barrett, P. M. (2000). Treatment of childhood anxiety: Developmental aspects. *Clinical Psychology Review, 20*, 479–494.

Barrett, P. M., Dadds, M. R., & Rapee, R. M. (1996). Family treatment of childhood anxiety: A controlled trial. *Journal of Consulting and Clinical Psychology, 64*, 333–342.

Bellini, S. (2006). The development of social anxiety in adolescents with autism spectrum disorders. *Focus on Autism and Other Developmental Disabilities, 21*, 138–145.

Bettelheim, B. (1967). *The empty fortress: Infantile autism and the birth of the self.* New York: Free Press.

Birmaher, B., Brent, D., Chiapetta, L., Bridge, J., Monga, S., & Baugher, M.

(1999). Psychometric properties of the Screen for Child Anxiety Related Emotional Disorders (SCARED). *Journal of the American Academy of Child and Adolescent Psychiatry, 38,* 1230–1236.

Blakeley-Smith, A., Reaven, J., Ridge, K., & Hepburn, S. (2012). Parent–child agreement of anxiety symptoms in youth with autism spectrum disorders. *Research in Autism Spectrum Disorders, 6,* 707–716.

Chalfant, A. M., Rapee, R., & Carroll, L. (2007). Treating anxiety disorders in children with high functioning autism spectrum disorders: A controlled trial. *Journal of Autism and Developmental Disorders, 37,* 1842–1857.

Cobham, V. E., Dadds, M. R., & Spence, S. H. (1998). The role of parental anxiety in the treatment of childhood anxiety. *Journal of Consulting and Clinical Psychology, 66,* 893–905.

Constantino, J., & Gruber, C. (2005). *Social Responsiveness Scale (SRS) manual.* Los Angeles, CA: Westerns Psychological Services.

Costello, E., Egger, H., & Angold, A. (2005). 10-year research update review: The epidemiology of child and adolescent psychiatric disorders: I. Methods and public health burden. *Journal of the American Academy of Child and Adolescent Psychiatry, 44,* 972–986.

Creswell, C., & Cartwright-Hatton, S. (2007). Family treatment of child anxiety: Outcomes, limitations and future directions. *Clinical Child and Family Psychology Review, 10,* 232–252.

Creswell, C., Schniering, C. A., & Rapee, R. M. (2005). Threat interpretation in anxious children and their mothers: Comparison with nonclinical children and the effects of treatment. *Behaviour Research and Therapy, 43,* 1375–1381.

Creswell, C., Willetts, L., Murray, L., Singhal, M., & Cooper, P. (2008). Treatment of child anxiety: An exploratory study of the role of maternal anxiety and behaviours in treatment outcome. *Clinical Psychology and Psychotherapy, 15,* 38–44.

Davis, T. E., III, Hess, J. A., Moree, B. N., Fodstad, J. C., Dempsey, T., Jenkins, W. S., et al. (2011). Anxiety symptoms across the lifespan in people diagnosed with autistic disorder. *Research in Autism Spectrum Disorders, 5,* 112–118.

de Bruin, E. I., Ferdinand, R. F., Meester, S., de Nijs, P. F., & Verheij, F. (2007). High rates of psychiatric co-morbidity in PDD-NOS. *Journal of Autism and Developmental Disorders, 37,* 877–886.

Dossetor, D. R., Nicol, A. R., Stretch, D. D., & Rajkhowa, S. J. (1994). A study of expressed emotion in the parental primary carers of adolescents with intellectual impairment. *Journal of Intellectual Disability Research, 38,* 487–499.

Estes, A., Munson, J., Dawson, G., Koehlere, E., Zhou, X.-H., & Abbott, R. (2009). Parenting stress and psychological functioning among mothers of preschool children with autism and developmental delay. *Autism, 13,* 375–387.

Farrugia, S., & Hudson, J. (2006). Anxiety in adolescents with asperger syndrome: Negative thoughts, behavioral problems, and life interference. *Focus on Autism and Other Developmental Disabilities, 21,* 25–35.

Field, A. P., Cartwright-Hatton, S., Reynolds, S., & Creswell, C. (2008). Future directions for child anxiety theory and treatment. *Cognition and Emotion, 22,* 385–394.

Frick, P., Silverthorn, P., & Evans, C. (1994). Assessment of childhood anxiety using structured interviews: Patterns of agreement among informants and association with maternal anxiety, *Psychological Assessment, 6,* 372–379.

Fuller, C. G., & Sabatino, D. A. (1998). Diagnosis and treatment considerations with comorbid developmentally disabled populations. *Journal of Clinical Psychology, 54,* 1–10.

Garland, E., & Clark, S. (1995). *Taming worry dragons: A manual for children, parents and other coaches.* Vancouver: British Columbia's Children's Hospital.

Ginsburg, G. S., & Schlossberg, M. C. (2002). Family-based treatment of childhood anxiety disorders. *International Review of Psychiatry, 14,* 143–154.

Giora, A., Gega, L., Landau, S., & Marks, I. (2005). Adult recall of having been bullied in attenders of an anxiety disorder unit and attenders of a dental clinic: A pilot controlled study. *Behaviour Change, 22,* 44–49.

Greenberg, J. S., Seltzer, M. M., Hong, J., & Orsmond, G. I. (2006). Bidirectional effects of expressed emotion and behavior problems and symptoms in adolescents and adults with autism. *American Journal on Mental Retardation, 111,* 229–249.

Hastings, R. P. (2003). Child behaviour problems and partner mental health as correlates of stress in mothers and fathers of children with autism. *Journal of Intellectual Disability Research, 47,* 231–237.

Hudson, J. L., Krain, A. L., & Kendall, P. C. (2001). Expanding horizons: Adapting manual-based treatments for anxious children with comorbid diagnoses. *Cognitive and Behavioral Practice, 8,* 338–346.

Kendall, P. C. (1994). Treating anxiety disorders in children: Results of randomized clinical trial. *Journal of Counseling and Clinical Psychology, 62,* 100–110.

Kendall, P. C., & Beidas, R. S. (2007). Smoothing the trail for dissemination of evidence-based practices for youth: Flexibility within fidelity. *Professional Psychology: Research and Practice, 38,* 13–20.

Kendall, P. C., & Hedtke, K. (2006). *Coping Cat workbook* (2nd ed.). Ardmore, PA: Workbook.

Kendall, P. C., Hudson, J. L., Gosch, E., Flannery-Schroeder, E., & Suveg, C. (2008). Cognitive-behavioral therapy for anxiety disordered youth: A randomized clinical trial evaluating child and family modalities. *Journal of Consulting and Clinical Psychology, 76,* 282–297.

Kessler, R. C., Chiu, W. T., Demler, O., Merikangas, K. R., & Walters, E. E. (2005). Prevalence, severity, and comorbidity of 12-month DSM-IV disorders in the National Comorbidity Survey Replication. *Archives of General Psychiatry, 62,* 617–627.

Lecavalier, L., Leone, S., & Wiltz, J. (2006). The impact of behaviour problems on caregiver stress in young people with autism spectrum disorders. *Journal of Intellectual Disability Research, 50,* 172–183.

Leyfer, O. T., Folstein, S. E., Bacalman, S., Davis, N. O., Dinh, E., Morgan, J., et al. (2006). Comorbid psychiatric disorders in children with autism: Interview development and rates of disorders. *Journal of Autism and Developmental Disorders, 36,* 849–861.

Lyneham, H., Abbott, M., Wignall, A., & Rapee, R. (2003). *The Cool Kids family program—therapist manual.* Sydney, Australia: Macquarie University.

March, J. S., & Mulle, K. (1998). *OCD in children and adolescents: A cognitive-behavioral treatment manual.* New York: Guilford Press.

Marcus, L., Kunce, L., & Schopler, E. (1999). Working with families. In D. Cohen & F. Volkmar (Eds.), *Handbook of autism and pervasive developmental disorders* (pp. 631–649). New York: Wiley.

Mazefsky, C. A., Kao, J., & Oswald, D. P. (2011). Preliminary evidence suggesting caution in the use of psychiatric self-report measures with adolescents with high-functioning autism spectrum disorders. *Research in Autism Spectrum Disorders, 5,* 164–174.

Moree, B. N., & Davis, T. E., III. (2010). Cognitive-behavioral therapy for anxiety in children diagnosed with autism spectrum disorders: Modification trends. *Research in Autism Spectrum Disorders, 4,* 346–354.

Murphy, M., Bolton, P. F., Pickles, A., Fombonne, E., Piven, J., & Rutter, M. (2000). Personality traits of the relatives of autistic probands. *Psychological Medicine, 30,* 1411–1424.

Myles, B. S., & Southwick, J. (2005). *Asperger syndrome and difficult moments: Practical solutions for tantrums, rage, and meltdowns* (2nd ed.). Shawnee Mission, KS: Autism Asperger.

National Institute of Mental Health. (1970). *CGI: Clinical Global Impressions.* In W. Guy & R. R. Bonato (Eds.), *Manual for the ECDEU Assessment Battery 2* (rev. ed., pp. 1–6). Chevy Chase, MD: National Institute of Mental Health.

Orsmond, G. I., Seltzer, M. M., Greenberg, J. S., & Krauss, M. W. (2006). Mother–child relationship quality among adolescents and adults with autism. *American Journal on Mental Retardation, 111,* 121–137.

Puleo, C., M., & Kendall, P. C. (2010). Anxiety disorders in typically developing youth: Autism spectrum symptoms as a predictor of cognitive-behavioral treatment. *Journal of Autism and Developmental Disorders, 41,* 275–286.

Rao, P. A., & Beidel, D. C. (2009). The impact of children with high-functioning autism on parental stress, sibling adjustment, and family functioning. *Behavior Modification, 33,* 437–451.

Rapee, R., Wignall, A., Hudson, J., & Schniering, C. (2000). *Treating anxious children and adolescents: An evidence-based approach.* Oakland, CA: New Harbinger.

Rapee, R. M., Schniering, C. A., & Hudson, J. L. (2009). Anxiety disorders during childhood and adolescence: Origins and treatment. *Annual Review of Clinical Psychology, 5,* 311–341.

Reaven, J. (2011). The treatment of anxiety symptoms in youth with high-functioning autism spectrum disorders: Developmental considerations for parents. *Brain Research, 1380,* 255–263.

Reaven, J., Blakeley-Smith, A., Culhane-Shelburne, K., & Hepburn, S. (2012). Group cognitive behavior therapy for children with high-functioning autism spectrum disorders ad anxiety: A randomized trial. *Journal of Child Psychology and Psychiatry, 53,* 410–419.

Reaven, J., Blakeley-Smith, A., Leuthe, E., Moody, E., & Hepburn, S. (2012). Facing your fears in adolescence: Cognitive-behavior therapy for high-functioning autism spectrum disorders and anxiety. *Autism Research and Treatment, 42,* 2013–2020.

Reaven, J., Blakeley-Smith, A., Nichols, S., Dasari, M., Flanigan, E., & Hepburn, S. (2009). Cognitive behavioral group treatment for anxiety symptoms in children with high-functioning autism spectrum disorders: A pilot study. *Focus on Autism and Other Developmental Disabilities, 24,* 27–37.

Reaven, J., Blakeley-Smith, A., Nichols, S., & Hepburn, S. (2011). *Facing your fears: Group therapy for managing anxiety in children with high-functioning autism spectrum disorders.* Baltimore: Brookes.

Reaven, J., & Hepburn, S. (2006). The parent's role in the treatment of anxiety symptoms in children with high-functioning autism spectrum disorders. *Mental Health Aspects of Developmental Disabilities, 9,* 73–80.

Reiss, S., Levitan, G. W., & Szyszko, J. (1982). Emotional disturbance and mental retardation: Diagnostic overshadowing. *American Journal of Mental Deficiency, 86,* 567–574.

Rezendes, D. L., & Scarpa, A. (2011). Associations between parental anxiety/depression and child behavior problems related to autism spectrum disorders: The roles of parenting stress and parenting self-efficacy. *Autism Research and Treatment, 2011,* Article 395190.

Silverman, W., & Albano, A. (1996). *Anxiety Disorders Interview Schedule for Children for DSM-IV: Child and Parent versions.* San Antonio, TX: Psychological Corporation/Graywind.

Silverman, W. K., Kurtines, W. M., Jaccard, J., & Pina, A. A. (2009). Directionality of change in youth anxiety treatment involving parents: An initial examination. *Journal of Consulting and Clinical Psychology, 77,* 474–485.

Simonoff, E., Pickles, A., Charman, T., Chandler, S., Loucas, T., & Baird, G. (2008). Psychiatric disorders in children with autism spectrum disorders: Prevalence, comorbidity, and associated factors in a population-derived sample. *Journal of the American Academy of Child and Adolescent Psychiatry, 47,* 921–929.

Silverman, W. K., Pina, A. A., & Viswesvaran, C. (2008). Evidence-based psychosocial treatments for anxiety disorders in children and adolescents. *Journal of Clinical Child and Adolescent Psychology, 37,* 105–130.

Skokauskas, N., & Gallagher, L. (2012). Mental health aspects of autistic spectrum disorders in children. *Journal of Intellectual Disability Research, 56*(3), 248–257.

Smith, L. E., Greenberg, J. S., Seltzer, M. M., & Hong, J. (2008). Symptoms and behavior problems of adolescents and adults with autism: Effects of mother–child relationship quality, warmth, and praise. *American Journal on Mental Retardation, 113,* 387–402.

Sofronoff, K., Attwood, T., & Hinton, S. (2005). A randomised controlled trial of a CBT intervention for anxiety in children with asperger syndrome. *Journal of Child Psychology and Psychiatry, 46,* 1152–1160.

Sung, M., Ooi, Y. P., Goh, T. J., Pathy, P., Fung, D. S. S., Ang, R. P., et al. (2011). Effects of cognitive-behavioral therapy on anxiety in children with autism spectrum disorders: A randomized controlled trial. *Child Psychiatry and Human Development, 42,* 634–649.

Tarrier, N., Barrowclough, C., Vaughn, C., Bamrah, J. S., Porceddu, K., Watts, S., et al. (1988). The community management of schizophrenia: A controlled trial of a behavioural intervention with families to reduce relapse. *British Journal of Psychiatry, 153,* 532–542.

van Steensel, F. J., Bogels, S. M., & Perrin, S. (2011). Anxiety disorders in children and adolescents with autistic spectrum disorders: A meta-analysis. *Clinical Child and Family Psychology Review, 14,* 302–317.

White, M., & Epston, D. (1990). *Narrative means to therapeutic ends.* New York: Norton.

White, S. W., Albano, A. M., Johnson, C. R., Kasari, C., Ollendick, T., Klin, A., et al. (2010). Development of a cognitive-behavioral intervention program to treat anxiety and social deficits in teens with high-functioning autism. *Clinical Child and Family Psychology Review 13,* 77–90.

White, S. W., Oswald, D., Ollendick, T., & Scahill, L. (2009). Anxiety in children and adolescents with autism spectrum disorders. *Clinical Psychology Review, 29,* 216–229.

White, S. W., Schry, A., & Maddox, B. (2012). Brief report: The assessment of anxiety in high-functioning adolescents with autism spectrum disorders. *Journal of Autism and Developmental Disorders, 42*(6), 1138–1145.

Wood, J., & McLeod, B. (2008). *Child anxiety disorders: A treatment manual for practitioners.* New York: Norton.

Wood, J. J., Drahota, A., Sze, K., Har, K., Chiu, A., & Langer, D. A. (2009). Cognitive behavioral therapy for anxiety in children with autism spectrum disorders: A randomized, controlled trial. *Journal of Child Psychology and Psychiatry, 50,* 224–234.

Wood, J. J., & Gadow, K. D. (2010). Exploring the nature and function of anxiety in youth with autism spectrum disorders. *Clinical Psychology: Science and Practice, 17,* 281–292.

6

Multimodal Treatment for Anxiety and Social Skills Difficulties in Adolescents on the Autism Spectrum

Susan Williams White, Lawrence Scahill,
and Thomas H. Ollendick

> If I say something wrong, then the other person might not want
> to talk to me anymore. I'm still learning conversation skills. . . .
> I'm not confident around other kids.
> —15-YEAR-OLD GIRL WITH HFASD,
> DESCRIBING THE SOURCE OF HER SOCIAL ANXIETY

> I want to live a happy, good life . . . to be a meteorologist . . . to
> have less worry about everything.
> —15-YEAR-OLD BOY WITH HFASD,
> WHEN ASKED, "WHAT GOALS DO YOU HAVE?"

Adolescence represents a period of increased risk for the development of secondary psychiatric problems in people with autism spectrum disorders (ASD), including the anxiety disorders. Although cognitive-behavioral therapy (CBT) has demonstrated efficacy in the treatment of anxiety disorders in adolescents (see Seligman & Ollendick, 2011, for a recent review), limited research has evaluated the feasibility and efficacy of CBT in adolescents with an ASD and co-occurring anxiety disorders. This chapter reviews research on the expression of ASD social disability and commonly co-occurring problems with anxiety in adolescents. We then describe a treatment program (Multimodal Anxiety and Social Skills Intervention

[MASSI]) developed for cognitively more able adolescents with ASD and anxiety problems. Results from a pilot, randomized clinical trial of the intervention are also provided. Finally, we discuss methodological challenges in conducting psychosocial treatment research with this population and propose specific directions for future research.

HISTORICAL BACKGROUND AND SIGNIFICANCE OF THE TREATMENT

Social Disability and ASD

Despite the heterogeneity in phenotypic expression of ASD, one defining feature of this neurodevelopmental disorder involves the presence of pervasive and severe deficits in social interaction. Regardless of the diagnosed person's global intelligence, savant-like talents, verbal ability, or mechanical giftedness, social difficulties are the primary source of impairment for most people with ASD (Carter, Davis, Klin, & Volkmar, 2005) and central to the diagnostic criteria of ASD (American Psychiatric Association, 2013). Despite changes in form and appearance over time, ASD-related social deficits rarely remit with development alone (Sigman & Ruskin, 1999). What may first emerge as a failure to respond to one's name being called or avoidance of direct eye gaze later appears as social awkwardness and immaturity in late childhood and early adolescence. In some cases, there may be complex interaction between ASD symptoms, social mistrust, hostility, or even paranoia in early adulthood. The specific deficits are diverse and include poor understanding of social interactions, failure to perceive subtle social communication signals, and absence or unusual use of nonverbal communication symbols such as hand gesture and eye gaze.

Psychosocial interventions targeting remediation of ASD-related social disability have not uniformly demonstrated efficacy across individuals or over time. Several recent, critical reviews examining the efficacy of social skills interventions have yielded inconsistent conclusions. Bellini, Peters, Benner, and Hopf (2007) concluded that school-based programs for students with ASD were only minimally efficacious, whereas Wang and Spillane (2009) found that some types of intervention (i.e., video modeling) appeared more efficacious. In contrast, Reichow and Volkmar (2010) concluded that social skills groups should be considered an established, evidence-based intervention, whereas they viewed video modeling as *promising*. There are many reasons for these seemingly disparate conclusions. In addition to different benchmarks for defining "efficacious" and "promising" interventions, replication in clinical trials evaluating the same structured interventions are few in number. Other methodological limitations include small and poorly characterized samples, inconsistent reports regarding the stability of treatment, and incomplete consensus on outcome measurement (Bellini et al., 2007; Lopata, Volker, Toomey, Chow, & Thomeer, 2008; Rao, Beidel, & Murray, 2008; White, Koenig, & Scahill, 2007). Moreover, there is great variability in the rate of positive treatment response in social skills intervention trials (e.g., White, Koenig, & Scahill, 2010). One largely unexplored but potentially important contributor to the observed variability in treatment response across participants receiving social skills interventions is within-individual characteristics.

A potential moderator that could affect the efficacy of social skills intervention is the presence of co-occurring anxiety. It is now appreciated that anxiety is common and impairing in many youth with ASD—especially among those who are not intellectually impaired (White, Oswald, Ollendick, & Scahill, 2009). Heightened anxiety and associated physiological arousal may impede social competence above and beyond the interpersonal disability conferred by the ASD diagnosis alone. Two pathways by which this effect might occur is via *avoidance* of social interactions despite the requisite knowledge of what to do, or *inability* to call upon the learned, appropriate social skills when they are needed. There are converging lines of evidence from psychophysiological, neuroimaging, and behavioral research to support a reciprocal influence between anxiety and social difficulties (e.g., Bellini, 2006; Dalton, Nacewicz, Alexander, & Davidson, 2007; Joseph, Ehrman, McNally, & Keehn, 2008; Kleinhans et al., 2010; Myles, Barnhill, Hagiwara, Griswold, & Simpson, 2001; Kyllianinen & Hietanen, 2006). Collectively, these findings suggest that when anxiety is present, the efficacy of social skills interventions in people with ASD may be enhanced by treatment that also targets anxiety.

Interventions that target social competence try to teach specific prosocial skills and to reduce socially inappropriate behaviors. Gains in these domains are believed to promote improved social functioning. Although no single theoretical orientation, conceptualization of ASD-related social deficits, or clinical approach unifies all social interventions for youth with ASD (cf. Lerner, Hileman, & Britton, in press; White & Maddox, 2011), the importance of remediating social deficits in ASD goes largely unchallenged. Indeed, *social competence,* defined by achievement and maintenance of satisfying social relationships, is essential for promoting quality of life via occupational/vocational success and satisfying interpersonal relationships (Segrin & Givertz, 2003).

Adolescents with ASD

Not all people with ASD are socially disinterested or aloof. Research and clinical experience indicate that many individuals with ASD desire interpersonal relationships and struggle with social isolation (Attwood, 2004). Anecdotally, many adolescents appear to enjoy participating in a group-delivered intervention, largely because it provides them a safe forum for talking with peers and learning new social skills. As noted by Lerner and colleagues (2011), nontargeted, positive effects (e.g., increased self-confidence, social self-efficacy, and new friendships formed in group-based programs) often result from interventions targeting social skills in adolescents with ASD. Unfortunately, in clinical trials designed to enhance social competence, many adolescents with ASD do not show significant improvement in targeted outcomes related to social functioning (Bellini et al., 2007; Rao et al., 2008). Although many adolescents verbalize a desire for friendships, recognize their interpersonal weaknesses, and take steps to improve their social behavior, they still struggle.

Adolescence may be a particularly difficult phase for people with ASD. Not only do these teens face developmentally appropriate and age-normative challenges (e.g., establishing autonomy from parents; navigating complex, sometimes volatile, and fluid peer networks), but they are also saddled with ASD-related problems such as social naiveté and misperception of social cues and "rules." Moreover, they often experience delays in the acquisition of age-appropriate adaptive skills and milestones (e.g., looking for part-time jobs, getting a driving permit). This picture may be accentuated for high-functioning adolescents with ASD (i.e., those without intellectual disability), who often have greater insight into their interpersonal differences and deficiencies (Klin & Volkmar, 2000; Myles et al., 2001; Tse, Strulovich, Tagalakis, Meng, & Fombonne, 2007). This insight may increase the risk of depression and anxiety in this subgroup (White, Oswald, et al., 2009). To date, most social skills intervention trials have focused on children 13 years of age and younger (e.g., Reichow & Volkmar, 2010; Wang & Spillane, 2009). Thus, there is a pressing need for studies targeting adolescents in the normal IQ range.

For people with HFASD, adolescence may provide the metaphorical "perfect storm" for the emergence of anxiety due to growing awareness of their social disability and emerging concept of self (which in adolescents is considerably determined by peer feedback and comments), heightened complexity in the social milieu, and decreased buffering (e.g., protection from bullying or other victimization) via parental support and structure. Although we lack longitudinal data on the ontogeny and course of anxiety in this population, emerging evidence suggests that the risk of anxiety disorders as a separate psychiatric condition is especially problematic in mid- to late-adolescence for cognitively more able people with ASD (Bellini, 2004; Kuusikko et al., 2008; White, Oswald, et al., 2009; White, Bray, & Ollendick, 2011). Although social disability is a defining feature of ASD, higher-functioning adolescents may be more aware of their deficits, which may amplify social anxiety (Klin & Volkmar, 2000; Tse, Strulovich, Tagalakis, Meng, & Fombonne, 2007; White & Roberson-Nay, 2009; Witwer & Lecavalier, 2010).

Anxiety and ASD

Among the most commonly reported co-occurring conditions in young people with ASD are anxiety (Gadow, De Vincent, Pomeroy, & Azizian, 2005; Muris, Steerneman, Merckelbach, Holdrinet, & Meesters, 1998), depression (Lainhart, 1999; Sterling, Dawson, Estes, & Greenson, 2008; Stewart et al., 2006), and attention-deficit/hyperactivity disorder (ADHD; Gadow et al., 2005; Mattila et al., 2010). Impairment due to concomitant anxiety ranges from 11 to 84% in youth with ASD (see White, Oswald, et al., 2009, for review). This wide range reflects differences in ascertainment, sample size, and assessment methods. A recent meta-analysis estimated that over 33% of children with ASD have an anxiety disorder (van Steensel, Bögels, & Perrin, 2011). Anxiety, when present, may complicate interventions designed to improve social functioning. As noted earlier, persistent social difficulties or, more specifically, the *awareness* of such difficulties, may enhance anxiety. The anxiety, in turn, may contribute to social avoidance and even greater social awkwardness, as the young person seeks refuge, for instance, in ASD-related preoccupations.

Adolescence is a developmental period of increased risk for anxiety disorders in typically developing children (Costello, Mustillo, Erkanli, Keeler, & Angold, 2003). Available evidence suggests that adolescents with ASD are at even greater risk for anxiety disorders. Onset of obsessive–compulsive disorder (separate from the preoccupations and repetitive behaviors of ASD) and social phobia (SOP) appear to be more likely to onset during adolescence. By contrast, specific phobias and separation anxiety are more likely to occur in younger children with ASD (White, Oswald, et al., 2009). SOP appears to be especially common in adolescents and adults with ASD who are not intellectually disabled (Bellini, 2004; Kuusikko et al., 2008; Simonoff et al., 2008). However, interaction of social anxiety and ASD is likely to be complex and is incompletely understood. For example, even if full diagnostic criteria for SOP are not met, higher-functioning youth with

ASD may worry about social failure and negative evaluation from peers (e.g., Kuusikko, Pollock-Warman, Jussila, Carter, Mattila, et al., 2008; White, Schry, & Maddox, 2012). The fear of rejection and social anxiety can be seen as consequences of the social disability inherent in ASD.

The relatively high prevalence of anxiety disorders in adolescents with ASD remains unexplained. It is probable that multiple pathways contribute to the onset or clinical expression of anxiety in this population. As previously discussed, anxiety may be a consequence of social problems associated with ASD (e.g., peer rejection), but other factors may also play a role. During adolescence, the age-expected physical, hormonal, and social–emotional changes likely compound preexisting challenges associated with academic, family, and social expectations (Khouzam, El-Gabalawi, Pirwani, & Priest, 2004). Structural or functional abnormalities in relevant brain regions such as the amygdala and enhanced cortisol response may also increase the likelihood of anxiety in youth with ASD (Amaral, Bauman, & Schumann, 2003; Corbett, Schupp, Simon, Ryan, & Mendoza, 2010; Juranek, Filipek, Berenji, Modahl, Osann, et al., 2006).

Many questions about the cause(s), nature, and expression of anxiety in young people with ASD remain to be answered empirically. Based on available research from our group and others, we conclude that anxiety can be reliably identified as a commonly co-occurring psychiatric condition in adolescents with ASD. We maintain that there is a reciprocal relationship between anxiety and social competence, such that severe anxiety exacerbates social impairments in youth with ASD, and poor social functioning may contribute to anxiety. Finally, adolescence may be a high-risk epoch for anxiety in youth with ASD (especially higher-functioning individuals) when social demands become more complex and their social disabilities become more salient.

PRACTICAL CONSIDERATIONS: BACKGROUND AND THEORETICAL BASIS FOR MASSI

Anxiety, if unaddressed in treatment planning, may reduce the benefits of interventions designed to target social skills deficits. Co-occurring anxiety can also contribute to the emergence of other problem behaviors (e.g., school refusal, social avoidance, poor school performance, inattention). Thus, co-occurring anxiety problems warrant consideration in treatment planning for adolescents with ASD. This consideration extends beyond the specific anxiety disorder (e.g., generalized, social, specific phobia) and may include consideration of anxiety symptoms measured dimensionally—cutting across diagnostic categories. The social deficits in early childhood, which indeed define ASD, interfere with subsequent development of peer friendships by limiting opportunities to practice age-appropriate skills. In addition to this social–developmental path, the chronically elevated physiological arousal, persistent worry, growing awareness of social deficits, and fears related to negative peer evaluation reported among young people with ASD are likely to interfere with the development and performance of age-appropriate social skills.

We began development of the MASSI treatment protocol in 2007, owing largely to the lack of treatment programs targeting the core social deficits and the added disability of anxiety in adolescents with ASD. Our early work implementing social skills training interventions in youth with ASD, based primarily on our anecdotal observations, indicated that participants with prominent anxiety symptoms did not fare well. They struggled to master and perform age-appropriate skills outside of the group context. They seemed to be less able to participate in groups and were prone to premature dropout.

A bidirectional model (Figure 6.1) of the relationship between anxiety and ASD-related social disability is the crux of the MASSI treatment program. The model holds that the core social deficit contributes to the experience of anxiety, which in turn intensifies social disability. Heightened arousal and overstimulation, especially in response to social–emotional information (Joseph et al., 2008; Kyllianinen & Hietanen, 2006), may impede accurate interpretation of social–emotional cues and appropriate response to others in the social milieu (e.g., Bal, Harden, Lamb, Van Hecke, Denver, et al., 2010). The presence of anxiety may further impair social information processing in youth with ASD (Kleinhans et al., 2010). Working in concert, social problems (e.g., awkward or unsuccessful interactions with others) may contribute to heightened anxiety (Bellini, 2006) and adversely influence functional outcomes. This bidirectional model of impairment calls for an intervention that addresses social and anxiety concerns in order to be effective in both domains.

MASSI was developed primarily as a CBT program because of the preponderance of evidence supporting CBT as an effective treatment for anxiety in children and adolescents (Seligman & Ollendick, 2011; Walkup, Albano, Piacentini, Birmaher, Compton, et al., 2008). To date, however, only a few studies have examined the efficacy of nonmedical, psychosocial treatments for anxiety in youth with ASD (Chalfant, Rapee, & Carroll, 2007; Lehmkuhl, Storch, Bodfish, & Geffken, 2008; Reaven & Hepburn, 2003; Reaven et al., 2009; Sofronoff, Attwood, & Hinton, 2005; Sze & Wood, 2007; Wood, Drahota, Sze, Chiu, & Langer, 2008; Scarpa & Reyes, 2011).

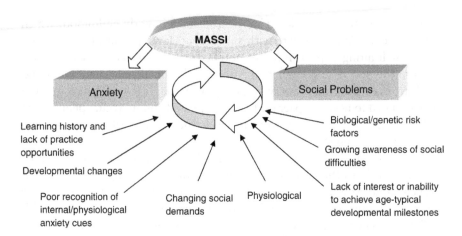

FIGURE 6.1. The MASSI model.

In most studies, adaptations to traditional CBT approaches for children with ASD have included increased structure and strategies (e.g., posted agendas) to make activities and transitions between various activities highly predictable, incorporation of visual aids, increased parental involvement, and consideration of children's special needs and interests. Treatment of social deficits included in the treatment has been secondary to the anxiety treatment (Wood et al., 2009). Most programs have been developed for school-age children up to age 14 (Reaven et al., 2009). Interventions in these studies have targeted a range of problems associated with anxiety, including co-occurring obsessive–compulsive disorder (Reaven & Hepburn, 2003; Lehmkuhl, Storch, Bodfish, & Geffken, 2008), symptoms of multiple anxiety disorders (Chalfant, Rapee, & Carroll, 2006), and symptoms of anxiety without formal diagnoses (Sofronoff et al., 2005). Although existing research indicates that CBT is a promising treatment approach for anxiety in children with ASD, few studies have targeted both social skills development and anxiety reduction or explicitly focused on treating adolescents with ASD. Also, few trials have used blinded independent evaluators in randomized trials to assess treatment outcome.

MASSI is based primarily in the principles of CBT (Ollendick & King, 1998; White et al., 2010), including functional behavior analysis, which reminds us that behaviors have antecedents and consequences (Foxx, 2008; Green, 1996; Schreibman, 2000). In the early MASSI modules, adolescents and their parents are taught how to conduct functional analysis of target behaviors. Data from these assessments are used to educate the family about the factors that serve to maintain the anxiety or social difficulty (e.g., avoidance of potential social failure experiences). These functional assessments also inform choice of specific treatment strategies, parental accommodations and needed environmental changes, and selection of effort-based reinforcers. In MASSI, the therapist tries to manipulate hypothesized triggers and consequences that likely produce or maintain target symptoms and also troubleshoots how to replace inappropriate behaviors (e.g., giving personal objects to peers as friendship bids) with more age-appropriate behaviors (e.g., verbal greetings and friendly gestures) that may serve the same social function. Although reinforcers, or rewards, are not uniformly used in the treatment, some clients enjoy having their effort and progress recognized in more tangible ways (e.g., extra time to watch a favorite television program).

OVERVIEW OF SESSIONS

Content and Delivery

MASSI was developed for adolescents (ages 12–17 years) with ASD and co-occurring problems with anxiety. It is a *multimodal* treatment that occurs simultaneously across three modalities—individual therapy, parent involvement (education, consultation, and coaching), and group therapy. The MASSI program therapist coordinates the content modules to be implemented and the sequencing of sessions based on the client's individualized treatment plan to ensure the dual focus on anxiety reduction and social skills improvement. This dual focus is integrated across treatment modalities (e.g., skills practice in group and individual sessions). MASSI was developed specifically for adolescents with HFASD and accompanying moderate to severe anxiety problems.

MASSI is designed to address the thoughts, feelings, and interpersonal interactions of adolescents with ASD and co-occurring, prominent anxiety symptoms. As with other CBT-based programs, it is an action-oriented, time-limited, intensive intervention. To promote flexibility and individualization within a structured, manual-based intervention (Chorpita, 2007), MASSI uses a modular format. There are 12 individual therapy modules to select from and seven group content modules delivered over 14 weeks (Figure 6.2). The first three modules—Orientation; Understanding Anxiety within ASD; and Thinking, Feeling, and Acting—provide for youngsters and their parents the foundational CBT skills and information on how anxiety tends to be expressed in people with ASD, and these three modules are delivered in the same sequence for all participants. Some individual therapy

---

Individual Therapy
- Orientation to MASSI and ASD Psychoeducation
- Understanding Anxiety within ASD
- Thinking, Feeling, and Acting
- Functional Assessment
- Problem Solving
- Initiating with Peers
- Coping with Worry
- Conversational Skills
- Flexibility and Recognizing the Cues of Others
- Exposure
- Handling Rejection
- Wrap-Up and Therapy Termination

Group Therapy
- Introduction
- Talking to Peers
- Following a Conversation
- Emotion Regulation 1
- Emotion Regulation 2
- Entering a Group
- Social Skills 101

FIGURE 6.2. MASSI modules.

modules may be repeated, whereas others are omitted, depending on the young person's needs. The therapist and adolescent work collaboratively to explore how cognitions contribute to anxious feelings and avoidance behaviors and, in turn, how these feelings and behaviors contribute to faulty cognitions. Exposure typically constitutes a sizable proportion of treatment time and usually focuses on developing habituation to a specific feared situation, activity, or object (e.g., exposure for fear of talking to peers).

In clinical research using MASSI to date, all participants have had Verbal IQ (VIQ) of 70 or higher. This requirement, due to the verbal and learning demands of the treatment program, ensures some similarity to peers without ASD in the group therapy component. Adolescents with multiple types of anxiety (e.g., SP, generalized anxiety) have been treated, but the MASSI protocol was not developed to target obsessive–compulsive disorder (OCD), panic disorder (PD), and posttraumatic stress disorder (PTSD); these disorders require specific forms of treatment not included in MASSI. Finally, MASSI is unlikely to be appropriate for the treatment of youth with ASD and co-occurring acute problems, such as psychosis, severe self-harming behaviors, mania or major depression, or other severe pathology that warrants more immediate treatment.

Although therapists should deliver the individual therapy modules in the sequence they deem most appropriate, the anxiety is often targeted first, prior to addressing the social deficits, because of the pervasive nature of social skills deficits in ASD, and the often more acutely distressing nature of anxiety. Specifically, improving the anxiety and distress can help build therapeutic rapport and engage the adolescent in other therapeutic tasks, such as the more long-standing problem of social disability. Of course, some adolescents need to address specific social skills problems in order to effectively address the anxiety. For instance, a teenager who struggles to initiate and carry on conversations with peers because of social difficulties (e.g., lack of appreciation for the interests of others, difficulty reading others' cues for when to speak during a conversation) may need to practice such skills before tackling exposures for anxiety about social interaction.

Because the individual adolescent's clinical presentation is essential for planning treatment in MASSI, for each subject a case conceptualization is constructed, in which the therapist formulates hypotheses about factors contributing to the anxiety and the social deficits based on all available information provided by the adolescent and his or her parents, and observations during the diagnostic assessment (see Mazefsky & White, Chapter 3, this volume). Following from the case conceptualization, a treatment plan is developed and implemented (demonstrated in the case example at end of the chapter).

Essential Elements and Unique Components

Because MASSI was developed explicitly for adolescents with ASD, we drew upon what is known about the unique strengths and challenges that often characterize this population. In doing so, we derived a set of "essential elements" (see White et al., 2010, for elaboration) that have been integrated throughout the three modalities (individual therapy, group practice, parent involvement) of the MASSI curriculum. Although these elements may be important for other psychotherapeutic programs, we view the following MASSI elements as particularly necessary for this adolescent ASD population:

• *A focus on parent and family involvement.* ASD is a chronic condition, and most people with ASD rely (to varying degrees) on parents for emotional, financial, and practical support across the lifespan. The social deficits in ASD endure into adulthood, and nonfamilial support systems (e.g., close friends, romantic partners) often do not develop as they typically would. In MASSI, adolescents are encouraged to practice new skills at home with siblings and parents, and relationships with family members are often a focus of the intervention. Thus, the individual's primary caretaker(s) are included throughout treatment.

• *Extensive practice.* The MASSI protocol involves regular practice. Repeated practice of newly learned or refined skills in contexts that approximate situations and environments in which the teen needs to use the skill is recommended (Bellini & Akullian, 2007; Bellini et al., 2007) when performing the intervention in the target environment (e.g., the classroom) is not feasible. Practice opportunities are integrated into every individual (often using role play) and group therapy session in the program. The group therapy component is especially conducive to practice within a relatively naturalistic yet highly supportive environment.

• *Immediate, direct, and specific feedback.* Youth with ASD often miss subtle cues or reminders in social discourse and have difficulty monitoring their own behavior. Many struggle with sustained attention and the ability to distinguish important from socially irrelevant stimuli (e.g., Klin, Jones, Schultz, & Volkmar, 2003). For these reasons, therapists and parents in MASSI provide feedback on performance and effort as the adolescents practice new skills and behaviors. Direct and prompt, "in the moment" feedback, as well as directive teaching, are important treatment components. Feedback is given verbally during the session. In addition, all sessions are video-recorded, so that participants can observe, critique, and learn from their own behaviors and specific feedback from the therapist during individual sessions, as well as some of the group meetings.

• *Explanation-giving.* Providing the reasons why a given behavior is appropriate (or not) in a given situation is important to the treatment. Youth with ASD are often concrete and rule-driven in their thinking, struggling with cognitive flexibility (e.g., Attwood, 2000). In some instances, a review of the rationale behind a given social skill can promote adoption of the skill.

• *Positive social learning experiences.* By adolescence, many individuals with ASD have encountered social failure and have been subjected to rejection by their peers. Group treatment in MASSI provides a positive social learning experience. Based on our pilot research with MASSI, the group is enjoyable and, for many, it is the first safe and accepting peer group experience, and an opportunity to make like-minded friends.

• *Skills modeling.* As with many social skills development programs, modeling new skills is an important part of the program. Many high-functioning individuals with ASD do not respond appropriately in social situations, because they lack knowledge of what to say or do, despite awareness of the need to do something (Loveland & Tunali-Kotoski, 2005). Modeling demonstrates what should be done in a given situation and provides an opportunity for the adolescent to learn the skill.

• *Psychoeducation.* We teach about ASD (e.g., its prevalence, course, associated problems, such as anxiety) throughout the curriculum but do so most intensively in the beginning of treatment. An adolescent with ASD, for instance, might feel excluded by peers at school. This perception, though painful and salient, may be accompanied by failure to recognize the behavior that contributed to the exclusion. Honest, candid explanation of how the teen's behavior (appearance, statements, etc.) affects how others react is designed to promote reappraisal and behavioral change. This teaching is done in individual and group therapy, and parents also are educated on relevant aspects of ASD and anxiety.

• *Structure.* Deficits in executive functioning, including the ability to plan ahead and shift between tasks effectively, have been reported in youth with ASD (Ozonoff, 1997; Ozonoff & Jensen, 1999). Although treatment modules do not use "scripts," MASSI is delivered in a structured way. Each individual and group session follows the same structured agenda to ensure that the program is delivered consistently. The same sequence of activities in each session helps participants know what to expect, which may reduce anxiety related to unpredictability in the session.

• *Therapeutic rapport.* We ask the adolescents in MASSI to face their fears and practice new social skills. These challenging and demanding tasks require active engagement on the part of the adolescents and parental support. To promote willingness to take risks and to confront anxiety-provoking situations, teens need to feel comfortable and supported. Therapeutic rapport and trust in the therapist are necessary prerequisites (e.g., Chu, Choudhury, Shortt, Pincus, Creed, et al., 2004).

• *Variety and creativity.* Finally, MASSI encourages the therapist to use creative and varied teaching strategies in treatment delivery. Visual supports, writing and drawing activities, and other approaches (e.g., drama) can be used to teach concepts and skills.

MASSI incorporates many established, evidence-based treatment strategies from CBT (e.g., psychoeducation, exposure) and applied behavior analysis (ABA; e.g., behavioral reinforcement, functional assessment). MASSI is novel in that it is designed to target anxiety and the social deficits in adolescents with ASD equally and concurrently. Other studies (e.g., Wood, Drahota, Sze, Chiu, & Langer, 2009) have included elements of social skills training in CBT treatment of anxiety. Most studies, however, have focused on change in anxiety and have not measured social disability as an outcome of interest (Chalfant, Rapee, & Carroll, 2007; Reaven et al., 2009; Sofronoff, Attwood, & Hinton, 2005; Wood et al., 2009). In addition, as noted earlier, previous studies have looked almost exclusively at younger children, with little work on CBT for adolescents with ASD. This is an important consideration, since adolescence is a period of high risk for problems with anxiety (e.g., Tse, Strulovich, Tagalakis, Meng, & Fombonne, 2007; White, Oswald, et al., 2009; Witwer & Lecavalier, 2010). Other unique elements of MASSI include integration of group and individual therapy with parental input; incorporation within individual sessions of a set of video vignettes developed for this protocol to demonstrate inappropriate–appropriate skills; and use of the client's videotaped sessions as corrective feedback on social interaction.

RESEARCH TO DATE ON THE TREATMENT

MASSI was first examined in a small ($n = 4$), open pilot study (White, Ollendick, Scahill, Oswald, & Albano, 2009). Results of this clinical series were encouraging. Three of the four adolescents showed reduced anxiety and no longer met diagnostic criteria for their primary anxiety disorder after treatment. All four participants showed improved social functioning, based on parent-reported scores. A subsequent, randomized controlled trial (RCT) with 30 adolescents, ages 12–17, compared MASSI to a wait-list control condition (White et al., 2013). The program was acceptable, and 83% of study participants completed the full program. Five different therapists implemented the curriculum with high fidelity (mean fidelity across sessions: 94%) to the manual.

Clinical outcomes of the RCT indicated a large within-group effect of treatment on social functioning, as measured by parent-report in the Social Responsiveness Scale (SRS; Constantino & Gruber, 2005) and a medium effect on symptoms of anxiety, as measured by the parent-report in the Child and Adolescent Symptom Inventory—Anxiety Scale (CASI-Anx; Sukhodolsky et al., 2008). Between-group differences on the SRS (average t-statistic = 3.433, $p = .007$) indicated that adolescents who received MASSI demonstrated greater improvement in social functioning than those who did not. Despite these social benefits, however, there was not a significant between-group difference in parent-reported anxiety symptoms over the course of treatment (average t-statistic = 1.186, $p = .22$). Overall functioning, based on Developmental Disabilities Modification of the Children's Global

Assessment Scale (DD-CGAS; Wagner, Lacavalier, Arnold, Aman, Scahill, et al., 2007) ratings clinicians blind to treatment assignment indicated that participants who received MASSI exhibited significant functional improvement (e.g., in self-care, communication, education), whereas those in the wait-list condition did not improve in overall functional outcome (average value of t-statistic = 2.280, p = .029). Six of the 15 participants assigned to MASSI were considered "treatment responders" based on blind assessments of clinical impairment (Clinical Global Impressions—Improvement Scale; Guy, 1976), while only three of the 15 wait-list participants were responders. Based on this RCT and the open trial, MASSI appears promising, though it needs additional evidentiary support.

FUTURE DIRECTIONS

The MASSI program was developed to reduce anxiety and improve social behavior and overall functioning in adolescents with HFASD. To date, it has been used only in clinical research settings. As noted, results are promising yet far from conclusive and would benefit from replication. One avenue for potential exploration with MASSI is modification for delivery in middle school and high school settings. Few manual-based programs are suitable for use in regular education settings for students with HFASD. There are challenges inherent in conducting such services in the school setting, including the brief time window for the intervention. Most class periods are 30–50 minutes long, and it may be difficult to implement programs that do not fit within these preexisting time segments. It can also be difficult to balance time needed for classroom instruction with delivery of services in a "pull-out" fashion during the school day. Another challenge is balancing the interaction with school personnel against the need to maintain confidentiality with participants. Confidentiality has several facets: the child and school personnel; the child and the parents; the parents and the school (Levitt, Saka, Romanelli, & Hoagwood, 2007).

Nonetheless, the group component of MASSI, modified for school implementation, appears to be warranted. Given the considerable body of literature indicating that behavior problems in school predict poorer academic performance (Breslau, Breslau, Miller, & Raykov, 2011; Munk & Repp, 1994), directly targeting anxiety reduction and social skills development with MASSI (School Revision) may exert positive effects on broader student outcomes, including academic performance and in-school behavior.

In addition, the effects of arousal and anxiety on functioning and development warrant further exploration given the prevalence of impairing anxiety in young people with ASD. There is still much uncertainty about how to conceptualize, diagnose, and treat anxiety in adolescents with ASD. Intervention research in this area is currently hindered by the absence of reliable and valid tools for assessing anxiety, social competence, and global outcome (e.g., functionality) in this population. Consideration on the definition of *positive treatment response* is also warranted in light of the chronicity of ASD and the associated social disability. For example, a young person completing MASSI may show a decline in anxiety symptoms after treatment but remain socially impaired. Is such a case a treatment failure? Is it reasonable or realistic to propose that the treatment goal is to achieve functioning in the "normal range" for social interaction in this population? Such questions need to be addressed in the coming years to advance this field.

CASE EXAMPLE

Maureen was a European American 13-year-old girl in the eighth grade. Presenting problems at intake, per her report and that of her mother, included feeling nervous when talking to peers—especially boys she likes—and peer pressure. Specifically, her mother was concerned that Maureen would make poor decisions in peer groups because of her impulsivity and desire to please. Maureen's mother reported that Maureen had previously received all of the following diagnoses: Asperger syndrome, ADHD, OCD, sensory integration disorder, adjustment disorder, and central auditory processing disorder. In the past, she had also received occupational and speech therapy, individual counseling and pet-assisted therapy, as well as family counseling. Although she had been tried on multiple medications in the past, at intake the only medication prescribed was Abilify, which, her mother said, seemed to help calm her down.

Maureen's stated goals for treatment were simply "to be able to go to the eighth grade dance." Her mother stated that she wanted Maureen to have more self-direction, to be able to work through her anxiety and frustration, and to work on improving her impulse control (e.g., not touching undergarments or private parts in public), and to further develop age-appropriate social skills. During the diagnostic assessment, Maureen was found to meet criteria for SP on a diagnostic interview, the Anxiety Disorders Interview Schedule for Children (ADIS-C; Silverman & Albano, 1996); she obtained a Clinician Severity Rating [CSR] of 5. Some of the specific problems endorsed included anxiety about working in groups at school or having to read aloud; fear of joining conversations or calling peers on the telephone; and intense fear of attending social functions, such as school dances or friends' parties, although she desperately wanted to be invited to such functions. No other disorder was above threshold, although she was subthreshold, or just below the diagnostic cutoff (CSR of 3 on the ADIS-C) for separation anxiety disorder, generalized anxiety disorder, and specific phobia—fear of the dark. Maureen's Autism Diagnostic Interview—Revised [ADI-R]; Lord, Rutter, & LeCouteur, 1994) score was above the diagnostic threshold, but her Autism Diagnostic Observation Schedule (ADOS; Lord, Rutter, DiLavore, & Risi, 2002) score was not. Based on all available information, including clinical judgment and ADOS and ADI-R scores, Maureen was judged to meet criteria for a mild ASD. In the prior DSM, she would be diagnosed with Asperger syndrome (per DSM-IV-TR; American Psychiatric Association, 2000). Based on recent psychoeducational assessment, she was functioning in the average range cognitively.

Maureen was conceptualized clinically as facing several age-appropriate and normative developmental changes (e.g., developing interest in the opposite sex), but her social immaturity, interpersonal difficulties, information-processing biases (e.g., assuming she would fail if she tried to interact with peers), and social anxiety prevented her from mastering such challenges. She was bright, motivated to improve her social functioning, and had supportive parents—all assets to her in treatment. Because many of her social difficulties made her appear awkward or unusual to peers (e.g., asking people if she looked okay, interjecting random comments into conversations), these behaviors were targeted prior to conducting in-session exposures or community-based practices and were revisited throughout the intervention. In the MASSI program, the specific treatment goals identified that guided Maureen's treatment plan were to talk to others more often, to act like herself (or to feel more at ease around others), and to stay on topic in conversations with others.

She spent much of the individual session practicing how to cope with anxiety and what to do and say in anticipated social situations (e.g., talking to a new boy in class). A considerable amount of thought challenging addressed some of Maureen's "thinking errors," which she identified as magnification ("I made a huge, unforgiveable mistake"), jumping to conclusions (assuming the worst outcome will come true, catastrophizing), and labeling ("I am a loser because I didn't say anything to him"). Exposure exercises included having Maureen read something she wrote first to the therapist, then to an unfamiliar male.

Following treatment, Maureen was determined to be a treatment responder based on her CGI-I score of 2 (much improved), as rated by a clinician blind to her treatment assignment. Her scores on various indices of anxiety, social functioning, and overall functioning were somewhat inconsistent, however. Her self-reported anxiety symptoms on the Multidimensional Anxiety Scale for Children (MASC; March, 1997) did not show improvement (baseline Total T-score = 54, endpoint = 52). She demonstrated considerable improvement in ASD-related social disability as measured by the SRS; her total score based on parent report was 88 at baseline and dropped 30 points to 58 at endpoint. Parent-reported MASC scores also showed considerable decline, from a raw score of 70 at baseline to 46 at endpoint. Finally, in terms of her global functioning rated by a clinician blind to her treatment assignment, Maureen's baseline score of 57 (moderate impairment in functioning in most domains) rose to 77 (slight impairment in functioning) at endpoint.

CONCLUSION

Anxiety is a common problem in youth with ASD and may be particularly important during adolescence. When present, anxiety likely has reciprocal effects with the social disability in ASD. For example, anxiety may exacerbate social avoidance and amplify self-awareness of social disability. MASSI is a manualized program developed specifically for adolescents with ASD who do not have cognitive impairment. The program targets social skills and anxiety concurrently, with group and individual CBT, as well as parent involvement. Research conducted to date indicates that the program is feasible, and preliminary results suggest that it may also be efficacious. Larger randomized clinical trials are needed to demonstrate efficacy.

REFERENCES

Amaral, D. G., Bauman, M. D., & Schumann, C. M. (2003). The amygdala and autism: Implications from nonhuman primate studies. *Genes, Brain, and Behavior, 2*, 295–302.

American Psychiatric Association. (2000). *Diagnostic and statistical manual of mental disorders* (4th ed., text rev.). Washington, DC: Author.

American Psychiatric Association. (2013). *Diagnostic and statistical manual of mental disorders* (5th ed.). Arlington, VA: Author.

Attwood, T. (2000). Cognitive behavior therapy for children and adults with Asperger's syndrome. *Behaviour Change, 21*(3), 147–161.

Bal, E., Harden, E., Lamb, D., Van Hecke, A. V., Denver, J. W., & Forges, S. W. (2010). Emotion recognition in children with autism spectrum disorders: Relations to eye gaze and autonomic state. *Journal of Autism and Developmental Disorders, 40*, 358–370.

Bellini, S. (2004). Social skill deficits and anxiety in high-functioning adolescents with autism spectrum disorders. *Focus on Autism and Other Developmental Disabilities, 19*(2), 78–86.

Bellini, S. (2006). The development of social anxiety in adolescents with autism spectrum disorders. *Focus on Autism and Other Developmental Disabilities, 21*, 138–145.

Bellini, S., & Akullian, J. (2007). A meta-analysis of video modeling and video self-modeling interventions for children and adolescents with autism spectrum disorders. *Exceptional Children, 73*(3), 264–287.

Bellini, S., Peters, J. K., Benner, L., & Hopf, A. (2007). A meta-analysis of school-based social skills interventions for children with autism spectrum disorders. *Remedial and Special Education, 28*(3), 153–162.

Breslau, N., Breslau, J., Miller, E., & Raykov, T. (2011). Behavior problems at ages 6 and 11 and high school academic achievement: Longitudinal latent variable modeling. *Psychiatry Research, 185*, 433–437.

Carter, A., Davis, N., Klin, A., & Volkmar, F. (2005). Social development in autism. In F. R. Volkmar, R. Paul, A. Klin, & D. Cohen (Eds.), *Handbook of autism and pervasive developmental disorders* (3rd ed., pp. 312–334). Hoboken, NJ: Wiley.

Chalfant, A., Rapee, R., & Carroll, L. (2007). Treating anxiety disorders in children with high functioning autism spectrum disorders: A controlled trial. *Journal of Autism and Developmental Disorders, 37*, 1842–1857.

Chorpita, B. F. (2007). Modular cognitive-behavioral therapy for childhood and anxiety disorders. In J. B. Persons (Ed.), *Guides to individualized evidence-based treatment*. New York: Guilford Press.

Chu, B. C., Choudhury, M. S., Shortt, A. L., Pincus, D. B., Creed, T. A., & Kendall, P. C. (2004). Alliance, technology, and outcome in the treatment of anxious youth. *Cognitive and Behavioral Practice, 11*, 44–55.

Constantino, J. N., & Gruber, C. P. (2005). *Social Responsiveness Scale (SRS)*. Los Angeles: Western Psychological Services.

Corbett, B. A., Schupp, C. W., Simon, D., Ryan, N., & Mendoza, S. (2010). Elevated cortisol during play is associated with age and social engagement in children with autism. *Molecular Autism, 1*(13), 1–12.

Costello, E. J., Mustillo, S., Erkanli, A., Keeler, G., & Angold, A. (2003). Prevalence and development of psychiatric disorders in childhood and adolescence. *Archives of General Psychiatry, 60*, 837–844.

Dalton, K. M., Nacewicz, B. M., Alexander, A. L., & Davidson, R. J. (2007). Gaze-fixation, brain activation, and amygdala volume in unaffected siblings of individuals with autism. *Biological Psychiatry 61*, 512–520.

Foxx, R. M. (2008). Applied behavior analysis treatment of autism: The state of the art. *Child and Adolescent Psychiatric Clinics of North America, 17*, 821–834.

Gadow, K. D., DeVincent, C. J., Pomeroy, J., & Azizian, A. (2005). Comparison of DSM-IV symptoms in elementary school-age children with FDD versus clinic and community samples. *Autism, 9*(4), 392–415.

Green, G. (1996). Early behavioral intervention for autism: What does research tell us? In C. Maurice, G. Green, & S. C. Luce (Eds.), *Behavioral intervention for young children with autism: A manual for parents and professionals.* Austin, TX: PRO-ED.

Guy, W. (1976). ECDEU assessment manual for psychopharmacology. *U.S. Department of Health, Education, and Welfare Publication,* ADM No. 76-338, pp. 218–222.

Joseph, R. M., Ehrman, K., McNally, R., & Keehn, B. (2008). Affective response to eye contact and face recognition ability in children with ASD. *Journal of the International Neuropsychological Society, 14,* 947–955.

Juranek, J., Filipek, P. A., Berenji, G. H., Modahl, C., Osann, K., & Spence, M. A. (2006). Association between amygdala volume and anxiety level: Magnetic resonance imaging (MRI) study in autistic children. *Journal of Child Neurology, 21,* 1051–1058.

Khouzam, H., El-Gabalawi, F., Pirwani, N., & Priest, F. (2004). Asperger's disorder: A review of its diagnosis and treatment. *Comprehensive Psychiatry, 45,* 184–191.

Kleinhans, N. M., Richards, T., Weaver, K., Johnson, L. C., Greenson, J., Dawson, G., et al. (2010). Association between amygdala response to emotional faces and social anxiety in autism spectrum disorders. *Neuropsychologia, 48*(12), 3665–3670.

Klin, A., Jones, W., Schultz, R., & Volkmar, F. (2003). The enactive mind—from actions to cognition: Lessons from autism. In D. J. Cohen & F. R. Volkmar (Eds.), *Handbook of autism and pervasive developmental disorders* (2nd ed., pp. 682–704). New York: Wiley.

Klin, A., & Volkmar, F. R. (2000). Treatment and intervention guidelines for individuals with Asperger syndrome. In A. Klin, F. R. Volkmar, & S. S. Sparrow (Eds.), *Asperger syndrome* (pp. 340–366). New York: Guilford Press.

Kuusikko, S., Pollock-Wurman, R., Jussila, K., Carter, A. S., Mattila, M., Ebeling, H., et al. (2008). Social anxiety in high-functioning children and adolescents with autism and Asperger syndrome. *Journal of Autism and Developmental Disorders, 38,* 1697–1709.

Kyllianinen, A., & Hietanen, J. (2006). Skin conductance responses to another person's gaze in children with autism. *Journal of Autism and Developmental Disorders, 36*(4), 517–525.

Lainhart, J. E. (1999). Psychiatric problems in individuals with autism, their parents and siblings. *International Review of Psychiatry, 11,* 278–298.

Lehmkuhl, H. D., Storch, E. A., Bodfish, J. W., & Geffken, G. R. (2008). Brief report: Exposure and response prevention for obsessive–compulsive disorder in a 12-year-old with autism. *Journal of Autism and Developmental Disorders, 38,* 977–981.

Lerner, M. D., Hileman, C. M., & Britton, N. (in press). Promoting the social and emotional development of adolescents with autism spectrum disorder. In T. Guillotts, & C. Leukefeld (Eds.), *Encyclopedia of primary prevention and health promotion: adolescence* (Vol. 3, 2nd ed.). New York: Springer.

Levitt, J. M., Saka, N., Romanelli, L. H., & Hoagwood, K. (2007). Early identification of mental health problems in schools: The status of instrumentation. *Journal of School Psychology, 45,* 163–191.

Lopata, C., Volker, M. A., Toomey, J. A., Chow, S., & Thomeer, M. L. (2008). Asperger's and other high functioning autism spectrum disorders: A review of group-based social enhancement research and a model for school-based social intervention. In D. H. Molina (Ed.), *School psychology: 21st century issues and challenges* (pp. 299–325). Hauppauge, NY: Nova Science.

Lord, C., Rutter, M., DiLavore, P. C., & Risi, S. (2002). *Autism Diagnostic Observation Schedule*. Los Angeles: Western Psychological Services.

Lord, C., Rutter, M., & LeCouteur, A. (1994). Autism Diagnostic Interview— Revised: A revised version of a diagnostic interview for caregivers of individuals with possible pervasive developmental disorders. *Journal of Autism and Developmental Disorders, 24,* 659–685.

Loveland, K. A., & Tunali-Kotoski, B. (2005). The school-age child with an autistic spectrum disorder. In F. R. Volkmar, R. Paul, A. Klin, & D. Cohen (Eds.), *Handbook of autism and pervasive developmental disorders* (3rd ed., pp. 247–287). New York: Wiley.

March, J. S. (1997). *Multidimensional Anxiety Scale for Children manual*. North Tonawanda, NY: Multi-Health Systems.

Mattila, M., Hurtig, T., Haapsamo, H., Jussila, K., Kuusikko-Gauffin, S., Kielinen, M., et al. (2010). Comorbid psychiatric disorders associated with Asperger syndrome/high-functioning autism: A community- and clinic-based study. *Journal of Autism and Developmental Disorders, 40,* 1080–1093.

Mimk, D. D., & Repp, A. C. (1994). The relationship between instructional variables and problem behavior: A review. *Exceptional Children, 60*(5), 390–401.

Munk, D. D., & Repp, A. C. (1994). The relationship between instructional variables and problem behavior: A Review. *Exceptional Children, 60*(5), 390–401.

Muris, P., Steerneman, P., Merckelbach, H., Holdrinet, I., & Meesters, C. (1998). Comorbid anxiety symptoms in children with pervasive developmental disorders. *Journal of Anxiety Disorders, 12*(4), 387–393.

Myles, B., Barnhill, G., Hagiwara, T., Griswold, D., & Simpson, R. (2001). A synthesis of studies on the intellectual, academic, social/emotional and sensory characteristics of children with asperger syndrome. *Education and Training in Mental Retardation and Developmental Disabilities, 36,* 304–311.

Ollendick, T. H., & King, N. J. (1998). Empirically supported treatments for children with phobic and anxious disorders: Current status. *Journal of Clinical Child Psychology, 27,* 156–167.

Ozonoff, S. (1997). Causal mechanisms of autism: Unifying perspectives from an information-processing framework. In D. J. Cohen & F. R. Volkmar (Eds.), *Handbook of autism and pervasive developmental disorders* (2nd ed., pp. 868–879). New York: Wiley.

Ozonoff, S., & Jensen, J. (1999). Brief report: Specific executive function profiles in three neurodevelopmental disorders. *Journal of Autism and Developmental Disorders, 29,* 171–177.

Rao, P. A., Beidel, D. C., & Murray, M. J. (2008). Social skills interventions for children with Asperger's syndrome or high-functioning autism: A review and recommendations. *Journal of Autism and Developmental Disorders, 38,* 353–361.

Reaven, J., & Hepburn, S. (2003) Cognitive-behavioral treatment of obsessive-compulsive disorder in a child with Asperger syndrome. *Autism, 7*(2), 145–164.

Reaven, J. A., Blakeley-Smith, A., Nichols, S., Dasari, M., Flanigan, E., & Hepburn, S. (2009). Cognitive-behavioral group treatment for anxiety symptoms in children with high-functioning autism spectrum disorders: A pilot study. *Focus on Autism and Other Developmental Disabilities, 24*(1), 27–37.

Reichow, B., & Volkmar, F. R. (2010). Social skills interventions for individuals with autism: Evaluation for evidence-based practices within a best evidence synthesis framework. *Journal of Autism and Developmental Disorders, 40,* 149–166.

Scarpa, A., & Reyes, N. M. (2011). Improving emotion regulation with CBT in young children with high functioning autism spectrum disorders: A pilot study. *Behavioural and Cognitive Psychotherapy, 39,* 495–500.

Schreibman, L. (2000). Intensive behavioral/psychoeducational treatments for autism: Research needs and future directions. *Journal of Autism and Developmental Disorders, 30,* 373–378.

Segrin, C., & Givertz, M. (2003). Methods of social skills training and development. In J. O. Greene & B. R. Burleson (Eds.), *Handbook of communication and social interaction skills* (pp. 135–178). Mahwah, NJ: Erlbaum.

Seligman, L. D., & Ollendick, T. H. (2011). Cognitive behavior therapy for anxiety disorders in children and adolescents. *Psychiatric Clinics of North America, 20,* 217–238.

Sigman, M., & Ruskin, E. (1999). Continuity and change in the social competence of children with autism, Down syndrome, and developmental delays: With commentary by Carolyn B. Mervis and Byron F. Robinson. *Monographs of the Society for Research in Child Development, 61,* v–139.

Silverman, W. K., & Albano, A. M. (1996). *The anxiety disorders interview schedule for DSM-IV—Child and Parent versions.* San Antonio, TX: Graywind.

Simonoff, E., Pickles, A., Charman, T., Chandler, S., Loucas, T., & Baird, G. (2008). Psychiatric disorders in children with autism spectrum disorders: Prevalence, comorbidity, and associated factors in a population-derived sample. *Journal of the American Academy of Child and Adolescent Psychiatry, 47*(8), 921–929.

Sofronoff, K., Attwood, T., & Hinton, S. (2005). A randomized controlled trial of a CBT intervention for anxiety in children with Asperger syndrome. *Journal of Child Psychology and Psychiatry, 46*(11), 1152–1160.

Steensel, F. J. A., Bögels, S. M., & Perrin, S. (2011). Anxiety disorders in children and adolescents with autistic spectrum disorders: A meta-analysis. *Clinical Child and Family Psychology Review, 14*(3), 303–317.

Sterling, L., Dawson, G., Estes, A., & Greenson, J. (2008). Characteristics associated with presence of depressive symptoms in adults with autism spectrum disorder. *Journal of Autism and Developmental Disorders, 38,* 1011–1018.

Stewart, M. E., Barnard, L., Pearson, J., Hasan, R., & O'Brien, G. (2006). Presentation of depression in autism and Asperger syndrome. *Autism, 10*(1), 103–116.

Sukhodolsky, D. G., Scahill, L., Gadow, K. D., Arnold, E., Aman, M. G., McDougle, C. J., et al. (2008). Parent-rated anxiety symptoms in children with pervasive developmental disorders: Frequency and association with core autism symptoms and cognitive functioning. *Journal of Abnormal Child Psychology, 36*, 117–128.

Tse, J., Strulovich, J., Tagalakis, V., Meng, L., & Fombonne, E. (2007). Social skills training for adolescents with Asperger syndrome and high-functioning autism. *Journal of Autism and Developmental Disorders, 37*, 1960–1968.

Wagner, A., Lecavalier, L., Arnold, L. E., Aman, M. G., Scahill, L., Stigler, K. A., et al. (2007). Developmental disabilities modification of Children's Global Assessment Scale (DDCGAS). *Biological Psychiatry, 61*, 504–511.

Walkup, J. T., Albano, A. M., Piacentini, J. C., Birmaher, B., Compton, S. N., Sherrill, J. T., et al. (2008). Cognitive behavioral therapy, Sertraline, or a combination in childhood anxiety. *New England Journal of Medicine, 359*, 2753–2766.

Wang, P., & Spillane, A. (2009). Evidence-based social skills interventions for children with autism: A meta-analysis. *Education and Training in Developmental Disabilities, 44*, 318–342.

White, S. W., Albano, A., Johnson, C., Kasari, C., Ollendick, T., Klin, A., et al. (2010). Development of a cognitive-behavioral intervention program to treat anxiety and social deficits in teens with high-functioning autism. *Clinical Child and Family Psychology Review, 13*(1), 77–90.

White, S. W., Bray, B. C., & Ollendick, T. H. (2012). Examining shared and unique aspects of social anxiety disorder and autism spectrum disorder using factor analysis. *Journal of Autism and Developmental Disorders, 42*(5), 874–884.

White, S. W., Koenig, K., & Scahill, L. (2007). Social skills development in children with autism spectrum disorders: A review of the intervention research. *Journal of Autism and Developmental Disorders, 37*, 1858–1868.

White, S. W., Koenig, K., & Scahill, L. (2010). Group social skills instruction for adolescents with high-functioning autism spectrum disorders. *Focus on Autism and Other Developmental Disabilities, 25*, 209–219.

White, S. W., & Maddox. (in press). Solid interventions. In R. F. Volkmar (Ed.), *Encyclopedia of autism spectrum disorders* (Vol. 3). New York: Springer.

White, S. W., Ollendick, T., Albano, A., Oswald, D., Johnson, C., Southam-Gerow, M. A., et al. (2013). Randomized controlled trial: Multimodal anxiety and social skill intervention for adolescents with autism spectrum disorder. *Journal of Autism and Developmental Disorders, 43*(2), 382–394.

White, S. W., Ollendick, T., Scahill, L., Oswald, D., & Albano, A. (2009). Preliminary efficacy of a cognitive-behavioral treatment program for anxious youth with autism spectrum disorders. *Journal of Autism and Developmental Disorders, 39*, 1652–1662.

White, S. W., Oswald, D., Ollendick, T., & Scahill, L. (2009). Anxiety in children and adolescents with autism spectrum disorders. *Clinical Psychology Review, 29*(3), 216–229.

White, S. W., & Roberson-Nay, R. (2009). Anxiety, social deficits, and loneliness in youth with autism spectrum disorders. *Journal of Autism and Developmental Disorders, 39*(7), 1006–1013.

White, S. W., Schry, A. R., & Maddox, B. M. (2012). Brief report: The assessment of anxiety in high-functioning adolescents with autism spectrum disorder. *Journal of Autism and Developmental Disorders, 42*, 1138–1145.

Witwer, A. N., & Lecavalier, L. (2010). Validity of comorbid psychiatric disorders in youngsters with autism spectrum disorders. *Journal of Developmental and Physical Disabilities, 22*, 367–380.

Wood, J. J., Drahota, A., Sze, K., Har, K., Chiu, A., & Langer, D. A. (2009). Cognitive behavioral therapy for anxiety in children with autism spectrum disorders: A randomized, controlled trial. *Journal of Child Psychology and Psychiatry, 50*(3), 224–234.

7

Cognitive-Behavioral Therapy for Stress and Anger Management in Young Children with ASD

The Exploring Feelings Program

ANGELA SCARPA, NURI REYES,
AND TONY ATTWOOD

The cognitive-behavioral therapy (CBT) program *Exploring Feelings* teaches children how thoughts, feelings, and behaviors interact, with the goal of providing skills to monitor and control anger and anxiety. This intervention program has been found to be an efficacious treatment for older children (ages 9–12) with high-functioning autism spectrum disorders (ASD) and comorbid anger or anxiety problems (Sofronoff, Attwood, & Hinton, 2005; Sofronoff, Attwood, Hinton, & Levin, 2007). Pilot testing of the intervention, called the *Stress and Anger Management Program* (STAMP; Scarpa, Wells, & Attwood, 2013), in young children (ages 5–7) with ASD also shows promising results. In general, STAMP has been shown to increase knowledge of emotion regulation skills and to decrease emotional outbursts in young children with ASD. This chapter reviews components of the *Exploring Feelings* program, necessary developmental modifications for younger children, and supporting research.

HISTORICAL BACKGROUND
AND SIGNIFICANCE OF THE TREATMENT

Emotional competence generally involves the ability to identify one's own and others' emotional states (e.g., appraisal), to display appropriate affect, and to regulate those emotional states (Saarni, 1999, 2000). Significant changes in emotional competence are observed in early childhood (Wellman, Phillips, & Rodriguez, 2000; Widen & Russell, 2003). Gradually, children become skilled at appraising, expressing, and managing basic emotions such as fear, anger, sadness, and happiness, and later more complex emotions such as shame, jealousy, pride, and guilt. Thus, in addition to recognizing and knowing the appropriate display of emotional experiences, developing an optimal ability to regulate emotions is an important component of emotional competence. Emotion regulation capacity, an advanced skill, is the most complex component of emotion competence (Saarni, 1999).

Emotion regulation has been by some researchers defined as voluntary management and modulation of emotional responses (e.g., occurrence, form, duration, and intensity) by engaging in cognitive processes to regulate continuous affective states to achieve one's goal (Eisenberg & Spinrad, 2004; Gross & Thompson, 2007; Stringaris & Goodman, 2009; Zelazo & Cunningham, 2007). Others note that emotion regulation involves both extrinsic and intrinsic regulatory processes that facilitate the monitoring, evaluation, and modification of emotional reactivity to facilitate the attainment of a goal and to make social adaptations (Calkins, 1994; Fox, 1994; Kopp, Neufeld, Davidson, Scherer, & Goldsmith, 2003; Thompson, 1994).

Such emotional development in children appears to transition from extrinsic to intrinsic regulators of emotional states; that is, infants need to rely on others to help regulate their emotional states (e.g., a mother soothing her crying child); as children mature, however, they tend to become more independent in their ability to self-regulate their emotions (Calkins, 1994). Less is known, however, about the developmental trajectory in atypical populations, such as children with autism. It has been proposed that the emotional development deficits that are primary to autism in turn generate other social and cognitive difficulties (e.g., Hobson, 1993; Sigman, Kasari, Kwon, & Yirmiya, 1992).

Emotion Regulation Abilities and Emotionality in ASD[1]

Children with ASD have difficulty comprehending the significance of, interpreting, and reacting to others' emotional states (Kasari, Sigman, Yirmiya,

---

[1]This section refers to research on ASD that includes autistic disorder, as well as other ASD, such as Asperger syndrome and pervasive developmental disorders.

& Mundy, 1993; Sigman et al., 1992). These deficits may in turn affect the way children understand, interpret, and deal with both their own emotions and the emotions of others. Sofronoff et al. (2007) suggest that children with HFASD might not be able to distinguish physiological signals that accompany emotional experiences, such as anger. In fact, Shalom, Mostofsky, Hazlett, Goldberg, Landa, et al. (2006) did not find differences in physiological responses (i.e., skin conductance) between typically developing children and children with high-functioning autism, but they did find that children with ASD had difficulty reporting their emotion states. Thus, children with ASD might not appreciate physiological cues associated with emotional states that might facilitate their regulation of emotion.

Emotional competence, therefore, involves several components, such as regulation, recognition, understanding, and display of emotions, and multiple studies have noted difficulties with emotional competence in children with ASD. Downs and Smith (2004), for example, found that children with autism show more deficits in emotion recognition than typically developing peers and children with other mental health disorders, such as attention-deficit/hyperactivity disorder and oppositional defiant disorder. Children with autism also appear to have more difficulties expressing their emotions than do their same-age peers (Shalom, 2006), and they are described as having difficulty identifying and conceptualizing thoughts and feelings of others and themselves (Baron-Cohen, 1995; Sofronoff et al., 2007).

While multiple studies have examined deficits in emotion recognition and emotion understanding in children with ASD, less has been reported about the appropriate display of emotions and emotion regulation abilities, the other two components of emotional competence (Bauminger, 2002; Konstantareas & Stewart, 2006). Some initial reports suggest that children with autism demonstrate less effective and less mature emotion regulation abilities compared to typically developing children (Begeer, Koot, Rieffe, Meerum Terwogt, & Stegge, 2008; Konstantareas & Stewart, 2006).

Negative emotionality has been described as an inclination to generate an intense negative emotional response to affective provoking stimuli (Eisenberg, Fabes, Murphy, et al., 1996). Similarly, *emotional lability* is described as irritability, hot temper, low frustration tolerance, and abrupt volatile shifts toward negative emotions such as anger, dysphoria, and sadness (Sobanski et al., 2010). Previous research in children without autism indicates a link between emotionality and emotion regulation, whereby negative emotionality is related to poorer adjustment in children who are less able to regulate emotions (Caspi, 1998; Caspi, Henry, McGee, Moffitt, & Silva, 1995; Colder & Chassin, 1997); however, research studies on the emotionality of children with autism have been limited. In one study, Kasari and Sigman (1997) found that parents described children with ASD as more emotionally and temperamentally difficult than typically developing children. Thus, it is possible that children with autism show elevated negative emotionality and may be at risk for excessive mood changes or outbursts because of delays in emotion regulation.

Internalizing and Externalizing Difficulties in ASD

Current research indicates that children with high-functioning autism experience elevated internalizing (i.e., depressed mood, anxiety) and externalizing (i.e., aggression, disruptive behaviors) problems. According to Eisenberg and Fabes (1992), children who tend to experience intense negative emotions and show less ability to regulate their emotions are more likely to experience elevated externalizing problems. Although children may be prone to experiencing elevated levels of emotionality, this tendency might not interfere with their social functioning if they have appropriate repertoires of emotion regulation abilities (Eisenberg, Fabes, Guthrie, & Reiser, 2000). Children with ASD who lack emotion regulation skills and have increased emotionality (as noted earlier) may be at increased risk for externalizing behavior problems.

Parents of children with ASD report that their children experience more anxiety-related difficulties than do parents of children diagnosed with anxiety disorders and typically developing children (Evans, Canavera, Kleinpeter, Maccubbin, & Taga, 2005; Russell & Sofronoff, 2005). The presence of comorbid anxiety disorders ranges from 47.0 to 84.1% in children with autism and may change with age (Chalfant, Rapee, & Carroll, 2007; Evans et al., 2005). Specifically, younger children with Asperger syndrome have been found to experience general anxiety (13.6%), separation anxiety (8.5%), situational phobias, and medical phobias (Evans et al., 2005; Sofronoff et al., 2005). Moreover, Evans et al. (2005) report a link between anxiety symptoms and behavioral problems in children with ASD. Children with Asperger syndrome also tend to experience mood disorders (16.9%), are described as more aggressive and demanding of parents than typically developing children (Sofronoff et al., 2005), and are more likely to show anger-related difficulties (Sofronoff et al., 2007).

Significance of Emotion Regulation Intervention in ASD

The high rates of internalizing and externalizing problems in children with ASD may cause significant distress and daily life interference (Farrugia & Hudson, 2006). Although no longitudinal studies of individuals with ASD have examined the trajectory of emotional development and its possible link to internalizing and externalizing problems, it is possible that these problems may persist into adolescence and adulthood, and cause further difficulties with employment, social relationships, and overall quality of life (Simonoff et al., 2008).

Emotional competence is also associated with social competence (Denham et al., 2003; Izard et al., 2001; Mostow, Izard, Fine, & Trentacosta, 2002). Thus, emotion understanding and emotion regulation abilities are considered important skills, because they are likely to be used in everyday interactions and are needed for successful social interchanges (Gross, Richards, & John, 2006).Whereas social competence and emotion regulation abilities have been found to be positively related (Eisenberg et al., 1991), social competence and emotional intensity are inversely related (Eisenberg et al., 1993). Negative emotional intensity predicts aggression and reduced peer status and prosocial behavior (Eisenberg, Fabes, Guthrie, et al., 1996; Eisenberg et al., 2000).

Taken together, previous research provides supportive evidence for the interface between emotional and social competence in childhood. However, these associations have not been fully examined in children with autism. We can hypothesize that utilization of ineffective emotion regulation strategies (e.g., avoidance, aggression, self-injury) might result in elevated displays of negative emotionality that in turn affect successful social interactions in young children with autism. As such, developing evidence-based interventions to improve emotion regulation abilities in children with ASD could ultimately decrease internalizing–externalizing problems and improve the quality of their social relations and overall well-being.

THE EXPLORING FEELINGS INTERVENTION FOR EMOTION REGULATION IN CHILDREN WITH HIGH-FUNCTIONING ASD

Because of the need to address emotion regulation issues in high-functioning youth with ASD, Attwood (2004a, 2004b) developed the treatment program Exploring Feelings, based on cognitive-behavioral principles. The program is highly structured and interesting, with the goal of encouraging the cognitive control of emotions. It is manualized and designed to be implemented by psychologists, speech pathologists, teachers, occupational therapists, parents, and any other person who has experience with ASD.

The original program designed for youth 9–12 years of age was implemented in groups, although it may be adapted for work with a single client.

Its six 2-hour sessions include activities and information meant to teach children how to understand and to manage emotions. There are two Exploring Feelings programs—one designed to address anxiety and another to address anger. Every child in the group is provided a workbook to record comments and questions during each of the six sessions. At the end of each session, the child is provided a project to complete before the next session; this project is discussed at the beginning of the next session.

The Exploring Feelings program includes two primary stages that are meant to address the difficulties with emotion understanding and regulation inherent in ASD. The first stage, *affective education*, includes discussion and activities to teach the connection among thoughts, feelings, and behaviors. Affective education teaches children the range of both positive and negative emotions and the vocabulary to express their emotions. The children are also taught about the bodily sensations, thoughts, and behaviors that function as early warning signs of emotional escalation.

The second stage, *cognitive restructuring*, includes the practice of new cognitive skills to correct distorted conceptualizations and dysfunctional beliefs. Cognitive restructuring teaches the children to identify thoughts that may increase their anxiety–anger (e.g., "They will laugh at me"), then replace those thoughts with antidotes (e.g., "I can stay calm"). This challenges distorted/biased thoughts or misinterpretations that may arise out of delayed theory of mind abilities, literal or concrete thinking, or poor *pragmatics* (both understanding the meaning of a situation and seeking to clarify the comments of others). For example, the therapist sometimes uses pictures of scenes with thought bubbles to identify what people might be thinking in situations (e.g., Gray, 1998); this strategy can help the child identify the thoughts of other people rather than assume that the other person is thinking the same thing the child is thinking or take the other person's comments too literally and not consider the context.

Children also explore appropriate and inappropriate responses to situations that elicit anxiety or anger, and they review the consequences for each option. With the help of the therapist, the child determines the best response for the long-term. It is often difficult, however, for the child with ASD to formulate a variety of appropriate responses to help manage these emotional experiences. Attwood developed the Emotional Toolbox, a strategy for cognitive restructuring that is one of the main components of the Exploring Feelings program. The metaphor of a toolbox enlists different types of "tools" to help "repair" the problems related to feeling anxiety, anger, or sadness. The tools comprise different strategies that help to release (e.g., a physical tool such as exercise) or to soothe (e.g., a relaxation tool such as deep breathing) emotional arousal. Other aids include social, cognitive, and special interest tools to increase help-seeking behaviors and thoughts, and pleasurable activities.

STAMP for Young Children with ASD

Based on the Exploring Feelings program, Scarpa et al. (2013) modified the program to suit young, high-functioning children (ages 5–7 years) with ASD. The new program, called the Stress and Anger Management Program (STAMP) is for young children with ASD. The following sections on practical considerations and session overviews draw heavily from the manual, which was recently published (Scarpa et al., 2013). The reader is referred to the manual for more details on the intervention and specific outlines of each session, which include timing of activities, description of tasks, and materials/supplies needed.

STAMP uses a skill-building cognitive-behavioral approach to educate young children with ASD about emotions and the various relaxation, physical, social, and cognitive tools they can use to calm themselves when distressed. The treatment is designed to teach children how thoughts, feelings, and behaviors interact in relation to anger and anxiety; how to recognize these components in themselves; and how to use a toolbox of skills to control these strong emotions (i.e., emotion regulation skills). The goal of STAMP is that the child should be able to list/recite specific strategies for managing anxiety and/or anger, and be able to implement these strategies in natural situations. For example, a child who initially responds with intense anger would instead ask for help when feeling frustrated with a task; or a child who initially exhibits anxiety and avoidance prior to a school recital would use deep breathing to self-soothe. It is expected that such skills serve to decrease overall levels of anxiety and anger, and will lead to improvements in social behavior.

Although CBT was originally developed for adults suffering from depression and anxiety (Albert & Beck, 1975), it has successfully been extended downward for children as young as 3 years old (Ollendick & Cerny, 1981). This is important given the consistent agreement among professionals that early intervention provides the best prognosis for children with ASD (Bryson, Rogers, & Fombonne, 2003). Even though some have questioned the appropriateness of CBT at young ages given children's immature level of cognitive understanding, there is growing empirical support for the benefits of CBT in treating young children, if developmental issues are carefully considered (Choate-Summers et al., 2008; Grave & Blissett, 2004; Ollendick, Grills, & King, 2001; Southam-Gerow & Kendall, 2000). The CBT approach can be modified, for example, to incorporate

concrete and tangible examples, to use methods that match the child's cog
nitive abilities, to incorporate lessons into developmentally appropriate
play routines, and to include parents or other key caregivers in the treatment process.

Specific adaptations to the Exploring Feelings program made STAMP
developmentally appropriate for 5- to 7-year-old children. These adaptations include shorter sessions (i.e., 60 minutes), longer program duration (i.e., 9 weeks), inclusion of parents, and games/activities designed
for young children (e.g., duck–duck–goose, musical chairs). In addition,
the CBT approach was adapted for verbally limited children and those
with different learning styles to include pictures and visual supports, such
that every concept in the intervention is accompanied by a visual aid. For
example, the relaxation tools are depicted on a poster with picture of a
person taking deep breaths, a child swinging on a hammock, and other
examples of relaxing activities. Children in STAMP meet once a week,
for 1 hour, in groups of two to six children over 9 weeks. Note that this
program is shorter than typical CBT treatments, some of which last as
long as 90 minutes each over 12–16 weeks. This program, however, was
adapted from the Exploring Feelings intervention, which was implemented
for 90-minute sessions over only 6 weeks. In our initial feasibility work,
we determined that this framework was not tolerable for many younger
children with ASD; therefore, we shortened each session, simplified content, and extended the time frame to 9 weeks. We found this protocol to be
feasible and suitable in our pilot work (Scarpa & Reyes, 2011), although it
may certainly be lengthened for slower learners. As in the Exploring Feelings program, practice assignments (called "home projects") are provided
each week and discussed at the beginning of the following session. The
inclusion of parents is viewed as critical for this developmental modification, because parents are considered to be primary in getting children
to complete the practice assignments. In addition, parents are taught the
therapeutic strategies, so they can encourage their use in settings outside
the clinic, thereby promoting consistency and generalizability of the intervention.

PRACTICAL CONSIDERATIONS FOR EXPLORING FEELINGS AS ADAPTED IN STAMP

Therapist Qualifications and Number

STAMP was originally tested using therapists that were advanced,
post-master's degree students in clinical psychology or master's level

occupational therapists. Therapists participated in a 2-day STAMP training session, and were supervised and assessed weekly to maintain fidelity throughout the efficacy test. Based on this initial work, a comprehensive manual was developed, so that anyone can implement the program; however, it is recommended that the person implementing the program have a good working knowledge about how to work with children and the characteristics of ASD.

The program is designed so that two adults are in the room with the children, although it can be adapted to work with a single child client and adult teacher. In group settings, one adult serves as the primary therapist, and the other serves as an assistant to keep children engaged or to troubleshoot individual issues that may arise during the session.

Child Eligibility

The program was designed for children with a diagnosis of ASD, however, it can be adapted for any child with anger–anxiety difficulties who meets all other eligibility criteria. The activities in STAMP (e.g., singing, crafts, stories) are best suited for children who have developmental levels similar to those in preschool or kindergarten. Although visuals are used throughout to help explain concepts and strategies, the program still requires that children have functional verbal communication and be able to understand basic verbal directions (e.g., look and listen, sit in a circle) and young children's stories. They should be able to engage in preschool-level games (e.g., duck–duck–goose, musical chairs) and to tolerate singing and the group setting.

Parent Psychoeducational Groups

Parents meet simultaneously with a separate therapist who reviews the skills, troubleshoots, and describes practice assignments the parents are to do with their children during the following week. This parental psychoeducational component provides parents with support and access to STAMP personnel, trains parents to use the therapeutic skills, and encourages practice at home, thereby promoting parental self-efficacy and generalization of skills to other settings and people.

Room Setup

The room should be arranged so as to include plenty of space for games. It is preferable to have a table on one side of the room for craft activities and snacks, and an open space on the other for games, stories, and discussion. Children should be seated in chairs or in some other assigned space (e.g., a carpet square), in which they have a visual guide for seating. Children should be seated in a semicircle in front of the lead therapist.

Schedule

Each session follows the same schedule—cool down, welcome, singing, story/discussion, activity, snack/stickers, and good-byes. The schedule is provided to give the children a sense of predictability and to help with transitions between activities. The schedule is reviewed in Session 1 and is posted on the wall during each session.

Home Projects

Every session ends with a review of a homework assignment that the children are to complete with their parent before the next session, with the purpose of practicing or reminding the child of the main lesson learned. For example, in Session 1, parents are asked to help their children cut out different expressions of happy feelings from magazines or books. Children and parents are to identify the intensity of the happy feeling, from a *little bit happy* to *very very happy*. The purpose of this project is to practice identification and labeling of varying degrees of happy feelings during affective education. Project assignments are reviewed with parents and children at the beginning of the next session.

Visual Aids

In order to accommodate children who may be less verbal or have a visual learning style, it is important to accompany all concepts in STAMP with a visual supplement, pictures, or illustrations (suggestions and printables are included in the manual; Scarpa et al., 2013). Visuals should be posted on the wall or where they may be easily seen by the group. Rules and the schedule should be written on a poster board on the wall every session. The schedule can have a movable arrow attached to show children the part of the session in which they are involved. A visual timer can be included to show the length of each part of the schedule. The room should be equipped with a whiteboard or easel, so that the therapist can write comments or important concepts for the children to see. Less verbal children can be encouraged to draw their comments or responses as pictures. Finally, therapists should use gestures, as well as words, when describing things (e.g., cup a hand around one's ear when saying "Listen," place hand on chest when describing the heart racing).

Behavioral Management

As in all good behavioral programs, the primary mode of behavior management is through reinforcement of desired behaviors. In STAMP, therapists are encouraged to use lots of praise, to be specific (e.g., "I like how you're sitting and waiting"), consistent, and immediate with their praise. Both verbal and nonverbal (e.g., high fives, pats on the back) praise are recommended. Therapists are also encouraged to maintain a positive atmosphere, to use an enthusiastic tone of voice and smile often. Finally, stickers are provided for the children as a tangible reinforcer for any demonstration of appropriate behavior (following the rules, completing homework, making an on-topic comment, etc.). The program can be adapted so that stickers are provided immediately after each behavior and placed on a chart, or praise may be provided immediately, with stickers distributed during review at the end of the session. We have seen both styles work in this program. Either way, we recommend that stickers be distributed liberally to encourage and maintain desired behavior. Each session ends with a snack time, during which the therapist reviews the sticker chart for that day. Children are told that if they earn enough stickers, they can have a group party at the end of the program; thus, obtaining stickers has the potential to benefit both the group and the individual.

In some cases, an additional behavior plan is needed to maintain a child in the group. If a child is aggressive, then he or she must be removed for the safety of the group. However, therapists should attempt to create a behavior plan in advance to prevent such escalation of undesirable behavior. For example, the therapist could put in place a reward system, so that the child could earn a "break" or some preferred activity (e.g., jumping on a trampoline) after earning rewards for appropriate behavior in group. Another option is to teach the child to ask for help or request a break when feeling agitated. It helps to have an assistant in the room who can redirect the child to appropriate behavior. Sometimes, the child simply needs to be kept engaged and active in the session. Some ways to do this include having the child move the arrow on the schedule, asking the child to write on the whiteboard or erase the board, questioning a specific child by name, and having the child jump, stretch, or illustrate an answer.

OVERVIEW OF STAMP SESSIONS

Session 1: Exploring Positive Feelings (Happiness)

The primary goal for the first few sessions is to introduce different feelings as part of the affective education stage. In the first two sessions, STAMP emphasizes positive feelings. Session 1 explores the feeling of happiness, through understanding of its experience, expression, and varying levels of intensity. Since this is the first session, it begins with introductions and an exercise for the children to get to know one another. Singing and story time activities prime the children for thinking about happy feelings as they sing "If You're Happy and You Know It" and read a story about being happy. The ruler game, designed to explore degrees of happiness, is conducted while playing musical chairs. Each child has a turn during the game to choose a card with varying levels of happiness and place the card on the ruler (or thermometer). Finally, each session ends with a snack and good-byes for a brief review of the session, to count stickers, and to say good-bye to each other. During the parent session, parents are introduced and provide brief descriptions of their children. The parent therapist reviews the session and allows parents to view the session, while discussing the therapeutic strategies. Finally, parents are given home projects at the end of each session, which are always reviewed at the beginning of remaining sessions.

Session 2: Exploring Positive Feelings (Relaxation) and Anger–Anxiety, Emotional Toolbox Introduction

This session focuses not only on being relaxed but it also introduces anger and anxiety. The children are taught a welcome song to welcome them to each of the remaining sessions, and in each remaining session they then review homework assignments. The singing and story activities help children start to think about relaxation. The activity involves tracing each child's body on paper and helping the children see how parts of the body feel when they are relaxed. Then this is contrasted with how the body feels when they are angry or anxious. Finally, the emotional toolbox of options to use when feeling angry or anxious is introduced. These tools include some of the following:

- Take a break.
- Sit by yourself.
- Talk to someone.
- Stretch.
- Take deep breaths.

- Count.
- Ask for help.

For Session 2, the parent session focuses primarily on education about reasons that children with ASD may have difficulties with emotion management, and on review of the emotional toolbox. Since the emotional toolbox forms the crux of this intervention, it is emphasized to the parents. In the home project, a shoebox or other container is used to design the child's own "toolbox" to bring to each session and fill with tools to repair angry and anxious feelings.

Session 3: Exploring Anxiety–Anger, Physical and Relaxation Tools

This session continues the focus on anger, anxiety, and emotional toolbox options for cooling down when children feel angry or anxious. The children are taught the "If I'm Angry and I Know It" song, which they sing in all remaining sessions as an additional method to help them remember each of the tools they learn. The story activity permits discussion about a child who gets angry in a typical scenario where children might lose their temper (e.g., losing a cherished toy or being denied a desired food), and the tools the child might use to feel better. The ruler game, introduced in Session 1, is designed to explore varying degrees of anger–anxiety, and the children are taught that it is easier to use these tools at lower levels of emotion, before the feeling gets too strong. Finally, the children practice using physical tools that energize the body and release energy (e.g., jumping, dancing, exercise), and relaxation tools that calm the body (e.g., deep breathing, counting, meditation). Parents are also taught about the physical and relaxation tools.
Physical tools may include the following:

- Physical exercise (e.g., walking, running, jumping on a trampoline)
- Sports
- Creative destruction (e.g., recycling)
- Dance

Relaxation tools may include the following:

- Music
- Drawing
- Solitude
- Massage

- Reading
- Repetitive action (e.g., swinging)
- Sleep
- Deep breathing

The home projects emphasize the child's practice of the skills by singing the "If I'm Angry" song, identifying degrees of anger or anxiety at home, and using physical and relaxation tools when the child is calm.

Session 4: Social Tools

This session explores social tools to cool down. In this session, children discuss how people and other living beings (e.g., pets) help them when they feel anxious or angry. To introduce this topic, the story is about a character who is lonely and feels better after he finds a friend. The children are then taught a script that demonstrates how to ask friends or others for help ("I have a problem. Can you help me?"). The activity uses puppet shows to illustrate situations that can lead to anger–anxiety, and how others may help in these situations. Parents are also taught the script so that they may practice with their child; they are reminded that it may be difficult for children with ASD to ask for help, because they do not always think of others as social agents. Also, parents may naturally want to soothe their children with physical affection (e.g., hugging, holding their hand), but this may bother some children with ASD who have sensory issues. Therefore, the parent is instructed to ask the child for permission before providing physical affection. Finally, the home projects additionally include an interview between the parent and child to learn how they can help each other when they feel upset.

Session 5: Thinking Tools

This session explores how thoughts can help us feel better when we become anxious or angry. This is one of the more difficult sessions to teach, because it directly targets the ability to identify thoughts in ourselves and other people. This ability, often referred to as "theory of mind," tends to be impaired or delayed in children with ASD, and young children vary in their cognitive maturity to grasp these concepts. The concept of "thoughts" is first introduced through a story in which the character thinks about good things to help him fall asleep. The pictures, coupled with thought bubbles over the character's head, help to make the abstract concept more concrete. The children then discuss how they might change their thoughts to feel better. The identification of thoughts is further practiced in two games. First, each child has a turn to identify whether a given thought (e.g., "I'm a loser") would make him or her feel better or worse, then is taught an opposing thought that might help (e.g., "I'm a winner"). Children also play a card game in which they are taught that positive thoughts need to be bigger than negative thoughts to "win." Finally, in the head trace activity, children trace their heads on paper and write words or strategies to say to themselves in times of anger–anxiety to feel better. They are provided an index card with the thought written on it, and take this home to practice with their parent. The parent session emphasizes teaching parents how to use drawings (e.g., Gray, 1998) to illustrate a situation in which their child became upset, then together fill thought bubbles first with words/thoughts that made the child upset, then with new words/thoughts the child can use to feel better in that situation.

Session 6: Special Interest Tools

This session explores how children have their own special way to make themselves feel better when they become anxious or angry. This skill capitalizes on children's special interests but uses that behavior as an intentional tool to manage intense feelings. Through the story and discussion, the children discuss different activities or interests that make some children happy and lessen anxiety or anger (e.g., singing, blowing bubbles, playing with trains). The children discuss and create a collage of their own special ways/interests to make them feel better in situations that may make them angry or anxious. Parents are asked to post the collage somewhere visible in the home and use it as a prompt to remind the child of activities to use at home. Parents are encouraged to place a time limit on these activities if the child tends to perseverate and overfocus on the activity. Once the child is calm, they can move on. Prior to this session, practice was primarily encouraged while children were still calm, in order to firmly establish the skills. In this session, parents can begin to practice the skills with their child at low levels of distress.

Session 7: Appropriate and Inappropriate Tools

Session 7 begins the final one-third of the group program. In the final three sessions, including Session 7, children and parents review all the skills and concepts learned in STAMP. In Session 7, the children engage in activities and discuss tools that are appropriate ("right tools") or inappropriate ("wrong tools"). The story primes them with ideas of things that make some people "feel good," and things that make some people "feel bad." Through a game, they review all the tools in their emotional toolbox (e.g., take a break, ask for help, think of something happy), as well as other tools that might not be so helpful (hit, cry, scream). They then create a chart to use with their parents to track the tools they use during the week and identify them as "right" or "wrong" based on whether the tools helped them to feel better or made things worse. Parents are asked to help complete this chart with their child and identify which kind of tool it was (i.e., physical, relaxation, social, cognitive, special). In this way, parent and child can begin to identify specific tools that might be most beneficial for each child and tailor the program accordingly.

Session 8: Review (Group Story and Create a Commercial)

This session is dedicated to reviewing all the tools learned in STAMP. For the story, the therapist creates a personalized story that uses children in the group as characters who need to use their various STAMP tools to deal with some crisis. Photos of each child are used as illustrations in the story to make it more likely that the children will identify with the main characters/models. With parental permission, each child is given a copy of the illustrated book to take home and use as a reminder of the skills learned in the program. Names of the children can be changed to protect confidentiality. Puppets are then used in another review activity. Finally, the children create their own commercial to demonstrate each of the skills they learned. The therapist can video-record each child using his or her favorite tool, then splice the scenes into one commercial. Each child is provided with a copy of the video commercial at the final session as another means to promote maintenance of skills. At this time, it is recommended that clinicians obtain permission from parents to distribute this commercial to the other families in the group, as confidentiality can be a concern. If any parent declines permission, we recommend making individual commercials, with only one child per video, with the child receiving only his or her video to take home after the final session. Parents are asked to review the toolbox with their child over the next week, to personalize the toolbox by adding any other tools the child may find helpful, and to continue to practice the skills.

Session 9: Group Reward/Celebration

This session focuses on review, assessments, and celebration after completing the group. Instead of a story, the children view the video commercial they created and discuss the various skills they have learned. They then have the opportunity to complete posttreatment assessments to evaluate treatment gains. Finally, they end with a party they have earned by obtaining stickers for their good work. During the party, the children show the video commercial to their parents and have snacks. The therapists then distribute the gift of the video commercial to each family, and each child is presented with a certificate of completion. Parents and children are thanked and reminded to watch their video and read their group story when they want to "remember the things they learned in group."

RESEARCH SUPPORT FOR THE TREATMENT

Three research studies evaluated the efficacy of the *Exploring Feelings* program and STAMP for managing anxiety and anger in high functioning children with ASD using a randomized controlled design (Scarpa & Reyes, 2011; Sofronoff et al., 2005, 2007). Sofronoff et al. (2005) examined the Exploring Feelings program specific to anxiety management, and also examined whether intensive parental involvement would increase a child's ability to manage anxiety outside of the clinic. Seventy-one children ages 10–12 with Asperger syndrome, whose parents were concerned about problems with high anxiety, participated in the study. The children were randomly assigned to one of three groups: (1) an intervention group in which the child was treated in a group without parents, (2) an intervention group with parental involvement, or (3) a wait-list control group. Five children did not complete the study, one from each intervention type and three from the wait-list. Relative to the control group, children in both intervention groups showed overall improvement from pre- to posttreatment in terms of parent-reported anxiety (including obsessive–compulsive tendencies, generalized anxiety tendencies, and social phobic tendencies) and strategies generated by the child to manage anxiety, with greater improvement in the intervention with added parental involvement.

Sofronoff et al. (2007) examined the efficacy of the Exploring Feelings program for anger management. Forty-five children ages 9–13 diagnosed with Asperger syndrome and anger problems participated in the study. The children were randomly assigned to an intervention group or to a wait-list control group. All parents engaged in a separate psychoeducational parent group. Parent reports indicated reduced anger episodes and improvement in the areas of frustration, peer relationships, and authority relationships. Parents and children also reported increased confidence with managing the child's anger. In a teacher survey, 88% reported a positive change in the children, and 12% reported no change in behavior following the intervention.

Scarpa and Reyes (2011) examined the efficacy of STAMP as a developmental adaptation of the Exploring Feelings program for 5- to 7-year-old children with high-functioning ASD. In this study, 11 children (two girls, nine boys) were assigned randomly to treatment ($n = 5$) or to a wait-list ($n = 6$) condition. All children met research criteria for autism or the autism spectrum, using the Autism Diagnostic Observation Schedule (ADOS; Lord et al., 2000; Lord, Rutter, DiLavore, & Risi, 1999). The manualized treatment was delivered by master's-level clinicians to groups of two to four children. At the same time, parents met with another clinician, reviewed the child sessions on a video monitor, and learned the components of each session, so they could practice with their child at home and other settings. Outcome measures were taken pre- and immediately postintervention for both conditions, then again for the wait-list group after receiving treatment. Initial comparison of pre- to posttreatment means indicated significantly decreased negative affect and a trend toward increased emotion regulation after treatment as reported by parents. Children also showed decreases from pre- to posttreatment in the duration of emotional outbursts, and increases in the number of emotion regulatory strategies they named in response to vignettes. Parental self-confidence in managing children's anger and anxiety, and confidence in the child's ability to self-soothe anger and anxiety also increased following treatment. In expanded analyses that compared posttreatment data on the treatment group and the wait-list control group, children in the treatment group showed fewer and shorter outbursts, and generated more emotion-regulatory strategies in response to the vignettes than children in the wait-list group. Parents of children in the treatment versus those in the wait-list condition also reported greater self-confidence in their ability to manage their children's anger–anxiety and greater confidence in their children's ability to manage their own emotions. More details of the results can be found in Scarpa and Reyes (2011).

FUTURE DIRECTIONS

Taken together, these three studies provide encouraging support for the use of CBT to treat anger and anxiety in high-functioning children with ASD, and suggest that it can be developmentally modified for use with younger children (PreK and kindergarten), as well as school-age children. Advantages of the studies included random assignment to treatment or control conditions and multiple informants to assess children's behavior. Limitations included reliance on parent report and small sample sizes. As such, these studies need replication with larger samples and objective assessments, though they now provide encouraging support in three studies across two research teams.

For future studies, parental involvement, delivery of treatment to other age groups, the role of treatment gains in other areas of development, and individual differences should be addressed. These initial studies suggest that the parental role in treatment may be important. Sofronoff et al. (2005), in particular, found that treatment gains occurred in conditions with and without parental involvement, although some effects were greater in the group with parent involvement. As such, the finding by Sofronoff et al. requires replication, and further research is needed to clarify whether the CBT program has equally beneficial effects with or without parental involvement, and whether the role of parental involvement changes with child age.

To date, the Exploring Feelings program and STAMP have focused on preschool to school-age children. As the field moves toward understanding the lifelong challenges of people with ASD, it would be worthwhile to expand the treatments to different developmental stages, including adolescence and young adulthood (e.g., college settings). Although some studies address anxiety in adolescents with ASD, to our knowledge, currently no evidence-based CBT programs address both anxiety and anger or deal with general emotion regulation in older individuals with ASD.

As noted earlier, previous research on typically developing children showed some initial evidence of the link between emotion regulation and psychological adjustment. Thus, it is reasonable to expect that improvement in stress and anger management in children with ASD would also extend to improvements in other areas, such as positive well-being, peer acceptance, improved social abilities, and decreased parent stress. Future research should examine these widespread outcomes subsequent to improved emotion regulation.

Finally, as with any psychosocial and biomedical intervention, it would be helpful to be able to tailor the treatment to specific child characteristics and to identify subgroups that may be most responsive to this intervention. It possible that individual differences, such as emotionality, sensory difficulty, or cognitive maturity, might also affect treatment gains; that is, children with certain characteristics, such as higher levels of emotionality, might be more likely to benefit.

The interventions discussed in this chapter are based primarily on the notion that individuals with ASD show poor self-awareness, self-regulation, and less mature perspective-taking abilities that underlie the cognitive difficulties associated with negative emotions and emotion dysregulation in ASD. Therefore, affective education and cognitive restructuring are emphasized in the treatments. It should be noted, however, that the specific mechanisms of change in Exploring Feelings or STAMP have not yet been studied and would be a fruitful area of future work.

In conclusion, children with autism experience severe social–emotional difficulties in their daily lives that can have long-lasting effects. By intervening early and developing interventions designed to improve their emotional awareness, knowledge, and management, it may be possible to prevent the cascade of adjustment problems that can develop in later years. CBT for emotion regulation skills has been shown to be a promising intervention to ameliorate some of these early difficulties in children with ASD.

REFERENCES

Albert, N., & Beck, A. T. (1975). Incidence of depression in early adolescence: A preliminary study. *Journal of Youth and Adolescence, 4*(4), 301–307.

Attwood, T. (2004a). *Exploring feelings: Cognitive behaviour therapy to manage anger.* Arlington, TX: Future Horizons.

Attwood, T. (2004b). *Exploring feelings: Cognitive behaviour therapy to manage anxiety.* Arlington, TX: Future Horizons.

Baron-Cohen, S. (1995). *Mindblindness: An essay on autism and theory of mind.* Boston: MIT Press/Bradford Books.

Bauminger, N. (2002). The facilitation of social–emotional understanding and social interaction in high-functioning children with autism: Intervention outcomes. *Journal of Autism and Developmental Disorders, 32*(4), 283–298.

Begeer, S., Koot, H. M., Rieffe, C., Meerum Terwogt, M., & Stegge, H. (2008). Emotional competence in children with autism: Diagnostic criteria and empirical evidence. *Developmental Review, 28*(3), 342–369.

Bryson, S. E., Rogers, S. J., & Fombonne, E. (2003). Autism spectrum disorders: Early detection and intervention, education and psychopharmacological treatment. *Canadian Journal of Psychiatry, 48*, 506–516.

Calkins, S. D. (1994). Origins and outcomes of individual differences in emotion regulation. *Monographs of the Society for Research in Child Development, 59*(2–3), 53–72.

Caspi, A. (1998). Personality development across the life course. In W. E. Damon & N. Eisenberg (Eds.), *Handbook of child psychology* (pp. 311–388). Hoboken, NJ: Wiley.

Caspi, A., Henry, B., McGee, R. O., Moffitt, T. E., & Silva, P. A. (1995). Temperamental origins of child and adolescent behavior problems: From age three to age fifteen. *Child Development, 66*(1), 55–68.

Chalfant, A. M., Rapee, R., & Carroll, L. (2007). Treating anxiety disorders in children with high functioning autism spectrum disorders: A controlled trial. *Journal of Autism and Developmental Disorders, 37*(10), 1842–1857.

Choate-Summers, M. L., Freeman, J. B., Garcia, A. M., Coyne, L., Przeworski,

A., & Leonard, H. L. (2008). Clinical considerations when tailoring cognitive behavioral treatment for young children with obsessive compulsive disorder. *Education and Treatment of Children, 31*(3), 395–416.

Colder, C. R., & Chassin, L. (1997). Affectivity and impulsivity: Temperament risk for adolescent alcohol involvement. *Psychology of Addictive Behaviors, 11*(2), 83–97.

Denham, S. A., Blair, K. A., DeMulder, E., Levitas, J., Sawyer, K., Auerbach-Major, S., et al. (2003). Preschool emotional competence: Pathway to social competence? *Child Development, 74*(1), 238–256.

Downs, A., & Smith, T. (2004). Emotional understanding, cooperation, and social behavior in high-functioning children with autism. *Journal of Autism and Developmental Disorders, 34*(6), 625–635.

Eisenberg, N., & Fabes, R. A. (1992). Emotion, regulation, and the development of social competence. In M. S. Clark (Ed.), *Emotion and social behavior: Review of personality and social psychology* (Vol. 14, pp. 119–150). Thousand Oaks, CA: Sage.

Eisenberg, N., Fabes, R. A., Bernzweig, J., Karbon, M., Poulin, R., & Hanish, L. (1993). The relations of emotionality and regulation to preschoolers' social skills and sociometric status. *Child Development, 64*(5), 1418–1438.

Eisenberg, N., Fabes, R. A., Guthrie, I. K., Murphy, B. C., Maszk, P., Holmgren, R., et al. (1996). The relations of regulation and emotionality to problem behavior in elementary school children. *Development and Psychopathology, 8*, 141–162.

Eisenberg, N., Fabes, R. A., Guthrie, I. K., & Reiser, M. (2000). Dispositional emotionality and regulation: Their role in predicting quality of social functioning. *Journal of Personality and Social Psychology, 78*(1), 136–157.

Eisenberg, N., Fabes, R. A., Murphy, B., Karbon, M., Smith, M., & Maszk, P. (1996). The relations of children's dispositional empathy-related responding to their emotionality, regulation, and social functioning. *Developmental Psychology, 32*(2), 195–209.

Eisenberg, N., Fabes, R. A., Schaller, M., Miller, P., Carlo, G., Poulin, R., et al. (1991). Personality and socialization correlates of vicarious emotional responding. *Journal of Personality and Social Psychology, 61*(3), 459–470.

Eisenberg, N., & Spinrad, T. L. (2004). Emotion related regulation: Sharpening the definition. *Child Development, 75*(2), 334–339.

Evans, D. W., Canavera, K., Kleinpeter, F. L., Maccubbin, E., & Taga, K. (2005). The fears, phobias and anxieties of children with autism spectrum disorders and Down syndrome: Comparisons with developmentally and chronologically age matched children. *Child Psychiatry and Human Development, 36*(1), 3–26.

Farrugia, S., & Hudson, J. (2006). Anxiety in adolescents with Asperger syndrome: Negative thoughts, behavioral problems, and life interference. *Focus on Autism and Other Developmental Disabilities, 21*(1), 25–35.

Fox, N. A. (1994). Dynamic cerebral processes underlying emotion regulation. *Monographs of the Society for Research in Child Development, 59*(2–3), 152–166.

Grave, J., & Blissett, J. (2004). Is cognitive behavior therapy developmentally appropriate for young children?: A critical review of the evidence. *Clinical Psychology Review, 24*(4), 399–420.

Gray, C.A. (1998). Social Stories™ and Comic Strip Conversations with students with Asperger syndrome and high-functioning autism. In E. Schopler, G. Mesibov, & L. J. Kunce (Eds.), *Asperger's syndrome or high-functioning autism* (pp. 167–198). New York: Plenum Press.

Gross, J. J., Richards, J. M., & John, O. P. (2006). Emotion regulation in everyday life. In J. J. Gross (Ed.), *Emotion regulation in couples and families: Pathways to dysfunction and health.* Washington, DC: American Psychological Association.

Gross, J. J., & Thompson, R. A. (2007). Emotion regulation: Conceptual foundations. In J. J. Gross (Ed.), *Handbook of emotion regulation* (Vol. 3, pp. 3–26). New York, NY: Guilford Press.

Hobson, R. P. (1993). The emotional origins of social understanding. *Philosophical Psychology, 6*(3), 227–249.

Izard, C., Fine, S., Schultz, D., Mostow, A., Ackerman, B., & Youngstrom, E. (2001). Emotion knowledge as a predictor of social behavior and academic competence in children at risk. *Psychological Science, 12*(1), 18–23.

Kasari, C., & Sigman, M. (1997). Linking parental perceptions to interactions in young children with autism. *Journal of Autism and Developmental Disorders, 27*(1), 39–57.

Kasari, C., Sigman, M., Yirmiya, N., & Mundy, P. (1993). Affective development and communication in young children with autism. In A. P. Kaiser & D. B. Gray (Eds.), *Enhancing children's communication: Research foundations for intervention* (Communication and language intervention series) (Vol. 2, pp. 201–222). Baltimore: Brookes.

Konstantareas, M. M., & Stewart, K. (2006). Affect regulation and temperament in children with autism spectrum disorder. *Journal of Autism and Developmental Disorders, 36*(2), 143–154.

Kopp, C., Neufeld, S., Davidson, R., Scherer, K., & Goldsmith, H. (2003). Emotional development during infancy. *Handbook of Affective Sciences*, 347–374.

Lord, C., Risi, S., Lambrecht, L., Cook, E. H., Leventhal, B. L., DiLavore, P. C., et al. (2000). The Autism Diagnostic Observation Schedule—Generic: A standard measure of social and communication deficits associated with the spectrum of autism. *Journal of Autism and Developmental Disorders, 30*(3), 205–223.

Lord, C., Rutter, M., DiLavore, P. C., & Risi, S. (1999). Autism Diagnostic Observation Schedule—WPS (ADOS-WPS). Los Angeles: Western Psychological Services.

Mostow, A. J., Izard, C. E., Fine, S., & Trentacosta, C. J. (2002). Modeling emotional, cognitive, and behavioral predictors of peer acceptance. *Child Development, 73*(6), 1775–1787.

Ollendick, T. H., & Cerny, J. A. (1981). *Clinical behavior therapy with children.* New York: Plenum Press.

Ollendick, T. H., Grills, A. E., & King, N. J. (2001). Applying developmental theory to the assessment and treatment of childhood disorders: Does it make a difference? *Clinical Psychology and Psychotherapy, 8*(5), 304–314.

Russell, E., & Sofronoff, K. (2005). Anxiety and social worries in children with Asperger syndrome. *Australian and New Zealand Journal of Psychiatry, 39*(7), 633–638.

Saarni, C. (1999). *The development of emotional competence.* New York: Guilford Press.

Saarni, C. (2000). Emotional competence: A developmental perspective. In R. P. Bar-On & D. A. James (Ed.), *The handbook of emotional intelligence: Theory, development, assessment, and application at home, school, and in the workplace* (pp. 68–91). San Francisco: Jossey-Bass.

Scarpa, A., & Reyes, N. M. (2011). Improving emotion regulation with CBT in young children with high functioning autism spectrum disorders: A pilot study. *Behavioural and Cognitive Psychotherapy, 39*(4), 495–500.

Scarpa, A., Wells, A. O., & Attwood, T. (2013). *Exploring Feelings for young children with high-functioning autism or Asperger's disorder: The STAMP treatment manual.* London: Jessica Kingsley.

Shalom, B., Mostofsky, S. H., Hazlett, R. L., Goldberg, M. C., Landa, R. J., Faran, Y., et al. (2006). Normal physiological emotions but differences in expression of conscious feelings in children with high-functioning autism. *Journal of Autism and Developmental Disorders, 4*(36), 395–400.

Sigman, M., Kasari, C., Kwon, J., & Yirmiya, N. (1992). Responses to the negative emotions of others by autistic, mentally retarded, and normal children. *Child Development, 63*(4), 796–807.

Simonoff, E., Pickles, A., Charman, T., Chandler, S., Loucas, T., & Baird, G. (2008). Psychiatric disorders in children with autism spectrum disorders: Prevalence, comorbidity, and associated factors in a population-derived sample. *Journal of the American Academy of Child and Adolescent Psychiatry, 47*(8), 921–929.

Sobanski, E., Banaschewski, T., Asherson, P., Buitelaar, J., Chen, W., Franke, B., et al. (2010). Emotional lability in children and adolescents with attention deficit/hyperactivity disorder (ADHD): Clinical correlates and familial prevalence. *Journal of Child Psychology and Psychiatry, 51*(8), 915–923.

Sofronoff, K., Attwood, T., & Hinton, S. (2005). A randomised controlled trial of a CBT intervention for anxiety in children with Asperger syndrome. *Journal of Child Psychology and Psychiatry, 46*(11), 1152–1160.

Sofronoff, K., Attwood, T., Hinton, S., & Levin, I. (2007). A randomized controlled trial of a cognitive behavioural intervention for anger management in children diagnosed with Asperger syndrome. *Journal of Autism and Developmental Disorders, 37*(7), 1203–1214.

Southam-Gerow, M. A., & Kendall, P. C. (2000). A preliminary study of the emotion understanding of youths referred for treatment of anxiety disorders. *Journal of Clinical Child Psychology, 29*(3), 319–327.

Stringaris, A., & Goodman, R. (2009). Mood lability and psychopathology in youth. *Psychological Medicine, 39*(8), 1237–1245.

Thompson, R. (1994). Emotion regulation: A theme in search of definition. *Monographs of the Society for Research in Child Development, 59*(2), 25–52.

Wellman, H. M., Phillips, A. T., & Rodriguez, T. (2000). Young children's understanding of perception, desire, and emotion. *Child Development, 71*(4), 895–912.

Widen, S. C., & Russell, J. A. (2003). A closer look at preschoolers' freely produced labels for facial expressions. *Developmental Psychology, 39*(1), 114–128.

Zelazo, P. D., & Cunningham, W. A. (2007). Executive function: Mechanisms underlying emotion regulation. In J. J. Gross (Ed.), *Handbook of emotion regulation* (pp. 135–158). New York: Guilford Press.

PART III

SOCIAL COMPETENCE

Multimodal Intervention for Social Skills Training in Students with High-Functioning ASD

The Secret Agent Society

RENAE BEAUMONT AND KATE SOFRONOFF

HISTORICAL BACKGROUND AND SIGNIFICANCE OF THE TREATMENT

The diagnosis of autism became known in the 1940s through the work of Leo Kanner (1943), but it was not included in the American Psychiatric Association's *Diagnostic and Statistical Manual of Mental Disorders* (DSM) in either 1952 (DSM-I) or 1968 (DSM-II). In 1980, "infantile autism" was included in DSM-III, with the description amended to autistic disorder in 1987. Although Hans Asperger described children with similar characteristics in 1944, the diagnosis of Asperger syndrome was not recognized until 1981, when Lorna Wing characterized it. In 1994 both autistic disorder and asperger's disorder (Asperger syndrome) were included in DSM-IV (American Psychiatric Association, 1994) within the category of pervasive developmental disorders. Most recently, in 2013, the DSM-5 grouped these syndromes into a single, unified diagnosis of Autism Spectrum Disorder (American Psychiatric Association, 2013).

Early interventions for autism were developed in the area of behaviorism, and this was very much in line with the theoretical perspective of the time. Professor Ivar Lovaas evaluated the first randomized controlled trial of the behavioral approach that came to be known as the "Lovaas method," based in the theoretical approach of applied behavior analysis. The first trial of intensive behavior therapy with children with autism (Lovaas, 1987) demonstrated significant improvements in child skills and raised the hope of "recovery" from core deficits. The intervention was replicated (McEachin, Smith, & Lovaas, 1993), and the principles of applied behavior analysis are considered to be well established and are included in many current programs supported by research.

Since this time there have been numerous interventions that purport to demonstrate significant improvements in children with a diagnosis of an autism spectrum disorder (ASD). A number of review papers have evaluated the evidence base of interventions offered (e.g., Rogers & Vismara, 2008), and the authors of these papers have made useful suggestions with respect to the components considered to be important. Many of the components were outlined in the National Research Council (2001) report and in an article by McConnell (2002). Rogers and Vismara (2008) also provided a brief overview of core components in their paper, including the use of positive behavior supports, functional analysis, and a positive teaching approach to encourage appropriate skills and behaviors to replace unwanted or dysfunctional behaviors. There is an emphasis on teaching in a naturalistic environment and using child interests to enhance motivation. It is also stressed that children with ASD need encouragement and support in peer interactions, and that parents are included in an intervention.

The development and evaluation of interventions for children diagnosed with high-functioning autism or Asperger syndrome (HFASD) start somewhat later than the intensive behavioral interventions. It is in this area that we first see the use of cognitive-behavioral interventions to regulate emotion and assist with the development of social skills and social understanding. The first randomized controlled trial of a cognitive-behavioral intervention was reported by Sofronoff, Attwood, and Hinton (2005) for an anxiety program for children with Asperger syndrome. The results of the trial demonstrated that the program was successful in reducing child anxiety based on parent report and increasing child knowledge of strategies to use in anxiety-provoking situations based on child generation of strategies for a hypothetical scenario. The results of this trial also demonstrated a significant additional benefit of direct parent involvement in the program.

Following this trial, an increasing number of trials have used cognitive-behavioral strategies for anxiety (Chalfant, Rapee, & Carroll, 2007; Wood et al., 2009), anger management (Sofronoff, Attwood, Hinton, & Levin, 2007), and to increase understanding of affectionate behavior (Sofronoff,

Eloff, Sheffield, & Attwood, 2011). Each of these programs has modified cognitive-behavioral strategies to make the content accessible to children with ASD: The programs take a strengths-based approach and use the interests of the child to increase motivation; parents are always included as an integral and essential part of the program; concepts are made concrete; and rehearsal or role play is central.

Following the start of an evidence base for the efficacy of cognitive-behavioral strategies for children with high-functioning ASD, research efforts turned to tackling social interactions. Two review papers (Reichow & Volkmar, 2010; White, Koenig, & Scahill, 2007) provided outlines of the strength of evidence for social skills interventions for children with ASD. Reichow and Volkmar (2010) accessed publications between 2001 and mid-2008, and found that despite an increased focus on social interaction, only a few studies reported significant effects from social skills groups or programs, and the findings with respect to the approach used are inconsistent. Kroeger, Schultz, and Newsom (2007) reported outcomes from a comparison of direct instruction in social interaction and a playgroup, with each intervention running for 5 weeks. The groups were similar in structure, beginning with a "hello" circle and ending with a "good-bye" circle, and the children were ages 4–6 years. The active component of the direct teaching group was video modeling, followed by prompts to use the play skills modeled. The program used video clips of same-age peers separated by short bursts of a popular cartoon. While both groups showed improvement from pre- to postintervention, the direct instruction group made greater gains.

Owens, Granader, Humphrey, and Baron-Cohen (2008) compared LEGO therapy (LeGoff, 2004), the Social Use of Language Programme (SULP; Rinaldi, 2004) and a no-intervention control group. The high-functioning children were ages 6 to 11 years. The LEGO method used a more naturalistic and collaborative approach, while SULP used direct teaching. LEGO therapy relies on the reinforcing nature of play with LEGO to encourage collaborative interactions among children. A typical "project" might involve a small group of children building with a LEGO set, with each child given a designated role and requirements for social interaction to achieve the desired end result. The results suggested that LEGO therapy produces a reduction in autism-specific social difficulties, while SULP does not, and observational data suggest that children in the LEGO group engaged in social interaction for longer periods of time than those in the SULP group. The SULP approach uses a curriculum and a hierarchical approach to teach skills (Owens et al., 2008). Both interventions did result in reduced maladaptive child behaviors. The authors suggest further investigation isolate the active ingredients in these interventions. These approaches are behavioral rather than cognitive and based on structured modeling processes.

A number of recent programs reported after the previous reviews have looked at ameliorating social deficits in children with ASD. The social skills group intervention (S.S.GRIN; DeRosier, 2002) developed for typical children ages 6–12 years has been evaluated with children with high-functioning ASD (DeRosier, Swick, Davis, McMillen, & Matthews, 2011). The program has 15 sessions and uses a small-group format, with four to five children and two group leaders. Parents are encouraged to participate actively in four of the groups and to encourage generalization of learned skills to other settings. Parents reported a significant effect of intervention for both child social skills and parent self-efficacy, with a moderate to large effect size. The study was not able to capture changes on child reports of self-efficacy or feelings of loneliness, and the authors reflect that this may emerge over time as the children have more opportunities to use the skills learned.

The Secret Agent Society (SAS) social–emotional skills program (Beaumont, 2010) was developed specifically for children ages 8–12 years with HFASD. The program includes an interactive computer game to teach emotion recognition and regulation in the context of social situations, weekly small-group sessions, parent sessions, and teacher tip sheets. The program draws on the appeal of being a cadet attending a Secret Agent Society academy to learn the detective skills needed to identify and manage emotions, and to engage effectively in social situations. Results from a randomized controlled trial demonstrated significant gains in social skills and emotion regulation, as reported by parents postintervention and at 5-month follow-up (Beaumont & Sofronoff, 2008). This program takes advantage of a likely interest in computers and games in this population of children, and incorporates all of the components outlined in the National Research Council (2001) report as best practice in working with children diagnosed with an ASD.

The SAS program is based within the theoretical frameworks of applied behavior analysis and cognitive-behavioral therapy (CBT). Practitioners are trained in the program and follow a manual to ensure fidelity to the treatment framework. A profile of skills is developed for each child is monitored, so that the program can be tailored to suit the needs of each individual, and data are collected and analysed throughout the program to evaluate progress. The program employs a hierarchical approach to skills development, with each social skill broken down into its component steps, and skills taught later in the program build on those introduced, practiced, and mastered earlier in the program. The SAS computer game is also structured in this hierarchical manner.

Specific components built into the program maximize the likelihood of skills generalization and include the use of weekly "home missions" to facilitate skills practice in home and school settings. The home–school diary monitors a child's use of individual skills and is linked to a reward system. Weekly parent information sessions and a parent workbook allow parents to learn how to support their child in generalizing skills at home. Weekly teacher tip sheets and intermittent contact help teachers to support skills use in the school setting. The program also uses many visual supports to help children use their skills in real-world contexts.

The SAS program takes a strengths-based approach and engages children via common areas of special interest. There are a wide variety of immediate and intermittent reinforcement schedules used both within and outside of sessions. The program uses both a direct instruction approach and a naturalistic approach as skills are shaped within and across sessions. Prompts that are used throughout the program to promote errorless learning are gradually faded as skills are mastered. Modeling is a central component of the program (i.e., each strategy is demonstrated by the therapist prior to a child trying it), and task analysis and chaining are also central (i.e., each task is broken into small, manageable steps and tried consecutively). Every effort is made to ensure that an individual child is supported and has a positive experience throughout the program.

OVERVIEW OF SESSIONS

Program Synopsis

The SAS program is a multimodal social skills intervention for 8- to 12-year-old children with high-functioning ASD (HFASD). Children are initially taught core emotion recognition, emotion regulation, and social problem-solving skills by a four-level, animated computer game played at home or at school with adult support. The computer game format optimizes child engagement (technology is a common special interest for children with HFASD and caters to all learning styles—visual, verbal and kinesthetic), reduces social anxiety associated with therapist and peer interactions during initial learning, and allows for self-paced instruction and repetition. Once children have developed a basic understanding of core emotional and social concepts by playing assigned sections of the game, they attend weekly group sessions to practice these skills in therapist-facilitated activities with peers. Information sessions and resources are also provided to help parents and school staff support children's use of social skills at home and at school, and to create ASD-friendly environments. A home–school diary and weekly home practice tasks ("home missions") also help children, parents, and school staff to monitor children's skill usage on an ongoing basis.

Program Structure and Content

SAS Computer Game

In the SAS Computer Game (Beaumont, 2009), the user assumes the role of a Junior Detective training to be a mind-reading specialist at the International Secret Agent Society Headquarters. To graduate from the academy, the user is required to complete a four-level training program.

In Level 1, children learn how to detect suspects' feelings from face, body and voice clues. In Level 2, they calibrate body clue and thought scales to detect emotions in themselves, and piece together clues to detect how others are feeling in a series of animated vignettes. In Level 3, skills from Levels 1 and 2 are applied to four virtual reality missions. In these missions, the user decides how his or her character will manage emotions and respond to social challenges, such as trying a new activity, engaging in group work, losing a game, and bullying. These virtual reality missions adopt a similar format to choose-your-own-adventure-style storybooks, whereby the outcome of the mission is dependent on the response chosen. To successfully complete Level 3 of the game, the user is required to attempt each mission at least twice, choosing a different course of action on each attempt. This encourages users to view and consider different ways of solving social problems instead of fixating on only one possible solution—a common challenge for children with HFASD. After successfully completing Levels 1–3 of the game, the player graduates from the academy as a Special Agent in Level 4. For screen shots from the game, see Figures 8.1–8.3. To view footage from the game, go to the Social Skills Training Institute website *www.sst-institute.net*.

Research suggests that many children with HFASDs have the same intact understanding of simple emotions (e.g., happy, sad, angry, and afraid) as same-age peers (Capps, Yirmiya, & Sigman, 1992). The SAS Computer Game consolidates and extends this knowledge to teach children how to recognize and manage complex emotions that have important implications for their social development and peer acceptance (e.g., boredom, confusion, embarrassment, and sarcasm). A range of real-life and computer-animated male and female characters of different ages and ethnicities display these emotions throughout the game.

The game features a mentor special agent who praises the player for

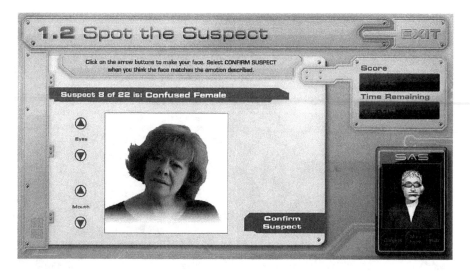

FIGURE 8.1. Screen shot from the Spot the Suspect activity in Level 1 of the SAS Computer Game—Detecting emotions from other people's facial expressions. From Beaumont (2009). Reprinted with permission from the Social Skills Training Institute, a subdivision of Triple P International Pty. Ltd.

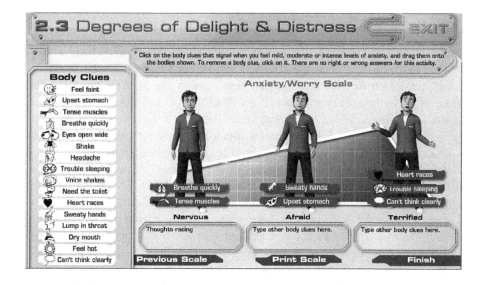

FIGURE 8.2. Screen shot from the Degrees of Delight and Distress activity in Level 2 of the SAS Computer Game—Recognizing the intensity of your own emotions from body clues. Reprinted with permission from the Social Skills Training Institute, a subdivision of Triple P International Pty. Ltd.

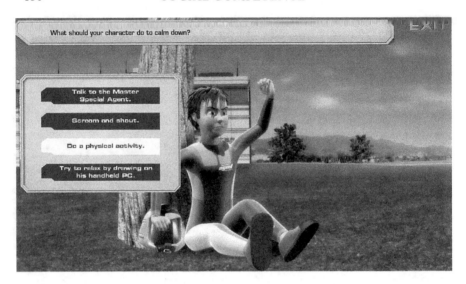

FIGURE 8.3. Screen shot from the Detective Flight Challenge Virtual Reality Mission in Level 3 of the SAS Computer Game—Coping with anger. Reprinted with permission from the Social Skills Training Institute, a subdivision of Triple P International Pty. Ltd.

good performance, gives hints, and explains correct answers when needed. Detective gadgets (e.g., an invisible ink reader, night vision contact lenses) are also awarded when the user reaches the target score for an activity, or attempts it on two occasions. These devices are used to complete the Level 3 virtual reality missions successfully. Short quizzes are included at the beginning and end of each game level to track the user's learning outcomes. To facilitate skills generalization, a Secret Agent Journal containing weekly "home missions" is integrated into the computer game. Children are asked to complete these weekly home missions to give them real-life practice in using the skills they have learned in the computer game. Within the journal, users can describe how they have used a skill by typing their response and/or creating pictures with a Scene Generator. The Scene Generator is similar to a computerized Comic Strip Conversation (Gray, 1994) creation device, whereby speech and thought bubbles can be added, and the emotion(s) that people were feeling can be displayed in full-color images (see Figure 8.4). Children are encouraged to print out their journal entries and bring them to weekly child group meetings to discuss with their facilitator(s) and peers.

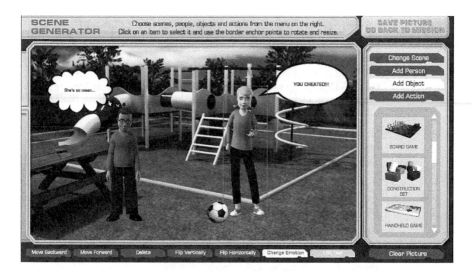

FIGURE 8.4. Screen shot of a picture created using the Scene Generator in the SAS Computer Game Journal. Reprinted with permission from the Social Skills Training Institute, a subdivision of Triple P International Pty. Ltd.

Child Group Meetings and Resources

In its standard format, the SAS program is delivered as a series of nine weekly, 2-hour, small-group child therapy sessions ("child group meetings"), with 3- and 6-month booster sessions. The program is ideally co-facilitated by two trained practitioners with a group of four to six children, but may be delivered to a group of three children by a sole facilitator. The first 90 minutes of child group meetings involve games and activities to practice and extend the skills introduced in the SAS Computer Game. Table 8.1 provides a summary of the activities scheduled for the weekly child group meetings.

To optimize group members' enjoyment and learning, the child group meeting activities are visually engaging, physically active, and relate to common special interests for children with HFASD (including science, transport, weaponry, collectibles, and technology). A selection of resources used by a facilitator to deliver the child group meetings is shown in Figure 8.5. These include walkie-talkies, a foam "helpful thought missile" game in which a player shoots down enemy thought targets with "helpful thought missiles," collectible pocket-size "code cards" featuring full-color character illustrations of the social skills steps, and a

TABLE 8.1. Summary of Weekly Child Group Meeting Content

Session	Content
1	Introduction Code—Steps for introducing yourself to others. Group rules and discussion of session rewards. Detection of the Expression Game—Detecting emotions from facial expressions. Secret Message Transmission Device Game—Detecting how people feel from their voice tone using walkie-talkies.
2	Secret Agent Body Signals and Body Clues Freeze Game—Identifying body clues that signal how people are feeling. Emotionometer Device Activity—Creating individualized pocket-sized devices to measure degrees of anxiety and anger, and affixing stickers showing the body clues and situations in which these emotions are felt. Movie Mania—Acting out scenes that show different degrees of emotions in different situations.
3	Detective Gadgets to Help You Feel Better—Reviewing relaxation strategies to help you feel happier, calmer, and braver and to make smart choices. Thought Missile Game—Shooting down unhelpful enemy thoughts with foam helpful thought missiles.
4	Detective Gadgets to Help You Feel Better—Reviewing additional relaxation strategies. SAS Friendship Force Game—Investigating the qualities that make good and not-so-good friends or allies. Helping Others Code—Steps for being helpful to others. D.E.C.O.D.E.R. formula for solving social problems.
5	Conversation Code—Steps for starting, continuing, and ending conversations. Secret Agent Fact File Cards—Conversation topics for making new friends, or becoming closer friends with others. Dialogue Duel—Practicing conversation skills with others.
6	Play Code—Steps for playing with others in a friendly way. Damage Control Code—Steps for coping with mistakes. Introduction to the Secret Agent Society Challenger Board Game—Group members practice their social skills through role plays and physical challenges included in the board game.
7	Continue playing the Secret Agent Society Challenger Board Game to practice social skills. Clues for detecting the difference between accidents, jokes, and intentional nasty deeds.
8	Bully-Guard Body Armor—Strategies for preventing and managing bullying and teasing. Continue playing the Secret Agent Society Challenger Board Game.
9	Confusion Code—Steps for coping with feelings of confusion and uncertainty. SAS Review Game. Try to finish the Secret Agent Society Challenger Board Game. Future planning. Program evaluation.
3 month follow-up	Progress update. Review games. Self-esteem activity. Future planning. Program evaluation. Party.
6-month follow-up	Progress update. Finish the Secret Agent Society Challenger Board Game (if children haven't done so already). Future planning. Program evaluation. Presentation of graduation certificates and medals.

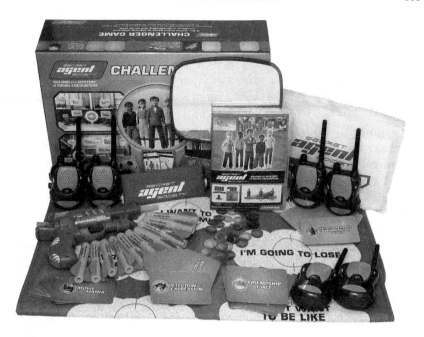

FIGURE 8.5. A selection of practitioner resources used to deliver SAS child group meetings. Reprinted with permission from the Social Skills Training Institute, a subdivision of Triple P International Pty. Ltd.

role-play-based board game (SAS Challenger Board Game) that includes fun physical challenges.

Each child group meeting is structured in a similar way to ensure consistency and predictability for group members. Session structure includes a review of group members' home missions and what they learned in the previous group meeting, scheduled activities for the session (which consolidate and build on previously taught skills), home mission planning for the current week, and a final session activity. The final 30 minutes of weekly child group meetings is typically an informal play and skills generalization period. While one facilitator helps group members to use their SAS skills while they play games (e.g., board games and card games), the other delivers a structured parent information session (see below).

Parent Group Meetings and Resources

The SAS program commences with a 2-hour parent information session that introduces parents to the aims and content of the program, and advises them of the important role they play in helping children to generalize their

social skills to home and school environments. In addition to learning how
to help their child play the SAS Computer Game and complete the weekly
"home missions," parents are provided with a home–school diary to monitor their child's SAS skills usage (see Figure 8.6).

At the top left of the diary, parents and/or teachers write down the
target skill or behavior on which a child will focus for a given week (this
typically aligns with a skill learned in their SAS child group meeting). Children are awarded diary points at home and at school when they display
the target behavior. These points are then tallied at a standard daily "tally
time" at home and exchanged for either daily and/or longer-term rewards.
Completion of this exercise typically requires about 5 minutes of a parent's
time. Parents and children collaboratively create a rewards menu featuring
practical and desirable daily and/or longer-term rewards from which the
child can choose. Alternatively, they can make a "lucky dip bag" containing a selection of daily rewards from which the child randomly selects.
Parents set a daily points target for the child that takes into account his or
her current skills level in performing the target behavior.

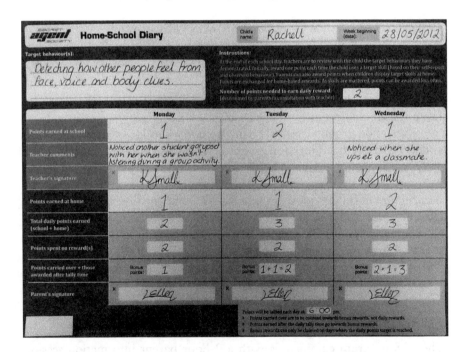

FIGURE 8.6. SAS home–school diary. Reprinted with permission from the Social
Skills Training Institute, a subdivision of Triple P International Pty. Ltd.

After the 2-hour introductory meeting, caregivers are asked to attend a weekly, 30-minute group meeting during the last half-hour of weekly child group meetings. During this time, a facilitator discusses with parents how they have done using the home–school diary and helping their child to do home missions for the week, briefly summarizes the child group meeting session activities, and informs caregivers how they can provide support for their children's home missions in the coming week. During the 90-minute child group meetings (which immediately precede the structured parent group meetings), caregivers are encouraged to discuss among themselves the successes and challenges they have faced in helping their children use their social skills. This informal discussion can take place at the SAS program venue or at a nearby park or coffee shop.

School Resources and Support

Weekly teacher tip sheets and home–school diaries included in the SAS program materials provide for school staff members a summary of what children learn in the program and tips on how they can help students use these skills in the classroom and on the playground. Recommendations are also provided for establishing school-based policies and procedures that promote friendly and compassionate behavior among all members of the school community, and prevent and manage bullying and teasing. These include strategies such as providing psychoeducation about ASD to members of the school community, creating a "class code" of friendly behaviors that are reinforced with a class-based reward system, and establishing a peer mentor system for students with ASD. Teacher tip sheets are typically distributed to a child's classroom teacher, teacher aide, behavior support personnel, school guidance officer/counselor, special education teacher, and/or the head of special education services. An optional 2-hour school seminar summarizing the core principles of the intervention is included in the program materials that trained facilitators deliver to key members of the school community when possible and appropriate (including the deputy/assistant principal or principal). Facilitators also phone or e-mail the most appropriate contact at a child's school to check on his or her progress throughout the program.

Clinic versus School Delivery

To optimize the flexibility with which the SAS program can be delivered in different settings (e.g., private practice, community clinic, hospital or school), a variety of program modifications are possible. These include

replacing the weekly parent group meetings with four 2-hour parent semi-
nars timed at strategic points throughout the intervention, omitting the
informal child play periods, and/or delivering the program as weekly or
twice weekly sessions that are half the usual session length (i.e. 45 minute
child session + 15 minute parent session). Guidelines on how to make these
modifications without compromising the integrity of the program are provided in the SAS facilitator manual (Beaumont, 2010).

PRACTICAL CONSIDERATIONS

Selection Criteria

In some of the efficacy trials reported earlier in this chapter, necessary
constraints were placed on recruitment of child participants. For example,
some of the programs required that the child have a basic cognitive and verbal ability such that he or she could understand the content of the program
(Beaumont & Sofronoff, 2008; DeRosier et al., 2011). Interestingly, results
from the initial randomized controlled trial (Beaumont & Sofronoff, 2008)
showed that the SAS program was equally effective regardless of child IQ
(within the normal range); ASD symptom severity; age (between 7.5 and
11.0 years at program entry); number of comorbid diagnoses; medication
usage; and level of parental ASD symptomatology, depression, anxiety, and
stress. The only significant predictor of treatment outcome was the number
of home missions completed by children. These findings suggest that the
program is generally effective for children ages 7½ to 11 years with an
Asperger-type ASD and language, intellectual, and reading skills within
the normal range. However, clinical experience, anecdotal evidence, and
practitioner feedback suggest some important indicators of limited treatment engagement or responsiveness, as summarized below. Current and
future research aims to evaluate empirically the effects of these factors on
treatment outcome.

Caregiver Skills, Confidence and Well-Being

Some programs also require the child to have a level of behavioral control
that will not be problematic when working in a group with other children (e.g., DeRosier et al., 2011). The SAS program requires parents to
implement a variety of parenting strategies to support children's application of SAS skills to real-world social interactions. Such strategies include
a monitoring and rewards system, prompting their children to use relaxation gadgets or strategies, disengaging when they or their children are

very distressed, and using visual resources and formulas to review social problems when both they and their children are calm. Because SAS parent group sessions are of a standard length, there is limited opportunity to provide individualized support to families struggling with basic parenting skills or other concerns (e.g., child behavior management, grief reactions to a recent ASD diagnosis, financial stressors, partner relationship issues). Because these issues can significantly impair caregivers' abilities to support their children in practicing their SAS skills, it is important that these issues be adequately assessed prior to a family participating in the program (typically through intake interviews and psychometric measures) and treated if required. If caregivers wish to proceed with the SAS program in the face of identified risk factors, their progress should be closely monitored and their decision to participate revisited in the face of poor treatment engagement or responsiveness. A case can certainly be made for a stepped intervention approach for children with HFASD, which ideally would begin with some work with parents around teaching new skills and behavior management. The issue may often be one of child readiness for a specific program.

Child Depression, Anxiety and Anger

In looking at a program that addresses social interaction skills it is also important to consider emotion regulation. Some programs already have this as a central component (e.g., Beaumont & Sofronoff, 2008; White et al., 2010), but children suffering from high levels of depression, social anxiety, and/or aggressive outbursts are likely to benefit from individual therapy that teaches them how to recognize and manage their feelings more effectively before participating in an SAS group therapy program. This approach is not only in the best interests of the child, but it also enhances the enjoyment and learning outcomes for other group members, who are likely to become distressed by frequent meltdowns or aggressive outbursts. Commencing with individual therapy (ideally with the same practitioner who delivers the SAS group intervention) also allows the child to become familiar with the therapeutic environment and the rules for participating in therapy, increasing the likelihood that he or she will be able to participate actively and have fun in the group intervention.

Group Composition and Physical Space

To improve group cohesiveness and to optimize time efficiency for program delivery, it is recommended that all children within a group be at a similar functional level with regard to intellectual ability, expressive and receptive language skills (especially verbal comprehension), and reading level. It may also be preferable (but not essential) for group members to be of a similar age, the same gender, and to have similar interests and hobbies. For girls-only groups, often more attention is focused on understanding popularity hierarchies and cliques, tailoring social exchanges based on closeness of friendship (e.g., conversation topics with an acquaintance vs. best friend), and detecting the more subtle nuances of nonverbal communication and unfriendly behavior (e.g., eye rolling, smirking, whispering). Where group members vary in their level of intellectual functioning and/or expressive and receptive language skills, it is often helpful to subdivide the group into smaller groups for therapy activities and to enlist the help of an additional staff member for behavior management support.

Because the SAS program involves physical games and activities to engage children, practitioners require a room with a minimum 11.5 feet × 18 feet to deliver child group sessions, and a separate area with access to a computer, data projector, and seating for parent sessions.

Optimizing Skills Generalization

One of the greatest challenges in conducting social skills training groups for children with HFASD is supporting skills generalization. Several features of the SAS program have been designed to optimize children's application of skills to the real world. These include prompting skills usage with pocket-size collectable "Code Cards," providing information to parents and teachers on how to support children's use of their SAS skills at home and at school, assigning children weekly "home missions" that involve practicing and reviewing skills in their Secret Agent Journal, and the home–school diary monitoring and rewards system (see Figure 8.6).

An important consideration for facilitators and families using these generalization enhancement tools is the need to tailor them to the needs of an individual child, family, and/or school support team. Children learn the skills taught in the SAS program at different rates, so it is important for parents and facilitators to tailor home missions and target behaviors for the home–school diary accordingly. For example, if a child is struggling to use relaxation gadgets when prompted to do so by a caregiver(s) or teacher, the "Relaxation Gadgetry" home mission may be repeated over multiple weeks, until the child's competence at this skill improves. Then, the child may be encouraged to move on to later home missions that involve applying this skill during peer or sibling interactions. Similarly, if caregivers or teachers find it too difficult to use the home–school diary in the recommended manner, they are encouraged to adapt it to make it more manageable (e.g., using the diary every second day instead of daily, or enlisting the help of another staff member to complete the diary with the child). Before the end of each parent group meeting, caregivers are asked to state what they will do during the coming week to help their children to use their SAS skills, and how this relates to their goals for program attendance. The underlying philosophy of the intervention is to set up every child, family, and school support team for success.

Preventing and Managing Meltdowns in Child Group Meetings

Some of the common causes of distress in child group meetings and appropriate strategies for preventing and managing these are summarized in Table 8.2. Further details about each of these prevention and management strategies are described below.

TABLE 8.2. Summary of Common Causes of Distress in Child Group Meetings and Possible Prevention and Management Strategies

Cause of distress	Prevention and management strategies
Not knowing what to do	Set clear ground rules in the first child group meeting (and review these as necessary); review the agenda at the beginning of each group meeting; provide specific instructions and time limits for activities.
Restlessness, inattentiveness or boredom	Provide a clear rationale for why each skill is taught; use a token reward system to encourage participation; ensure that children are actively engaged; modify activities; provide sensory tools or strategies; program delivery as 45-minute child group meetings, if needed.
Sensory understimulation or overstimulation	Provide appropriate sensory tools or adaptations to the sensory environment; request occupational therapist recommendations.
Perfectionism or competitiveness	Activity modifications; review relaxation gadgets before competitive activities; reward children for staying calm when they make a mistake or lose a game with praise, tokens and/or a friendship award.
Task too difficult	Activity modifications; reward effort with tokens.
Cognitive rigidity	Provide a clear rationale for why each skill is taught; avoid arguing with children (engage the child as a "consultant" to adapt program materials as needed).
Difficulties recognizing and managing anxiety and anger	Prompt the use of relaxation gadgets when early signs of distress are detected; set up a chill-out zone; reward children for using their relaxation gadgets and/or going to the chill-out zone to calm down with praise and tokens.

Ground Rules

At the beginning of the first child group meeting, program facilitators help children to create an SAS group rules poster, which summarizes the rules that group members are to follow to help them have fun and learn at SAS group meetings. These rules typically include having one person speak at a time; listening to other group members; using a friendly face, voice, and words; and keeping one's hands and feet to oneself. The group rules poster is displayed and reviewed at the beginning of each child group meeting to remind children what is expected.

Specific Instructions and Time Limits for Session Activities

To reduce children's anxiety about participating in unfamiliar activities, each SAS child group meeting begins with an overview of the session activities that will be completed (this agenda is also shown in children's SAS Cadet Handbooks). To set up group members for success with session activities, they are initially also taught core skills and concepts through the SAS Computer Game before coming to their weekly child group meeting, and are given a clear explanation of the procedure and duration of each session activity. It is recommended that facilitators give children a warning (e.g., 2 minutes) before transitioning to a new activity.

Clear Rationale for Why Each Skill Is Taught

As children with HFASD typically lack awareness and understanding of the implicit rules for human social interaction, each skill taught in the SAS program is introduced with a clear explanation of why it is important, and how it will help children to achieve their own goals and objectives (e.g., making friends and keeping them; feeling happier, calmer and/or braver; making smart choices). Providing a clear rationale for program activities and skills appeals to the hunger for knowledge and wisdom that characterizes many children with HFASD, increasing their motivation to use the skills they learn in the program.

Token Reward System

To encourage participation in session activities and to prevent behavioral difficulties, a token reward system is established in the first child group meeting. This involves each child nominating small rewards they would like to receive over the course of the program for trying hard and following the group rules. These individualized rewards typically include items such as mini LEGO men, candy, stationery, collector cards, and character figurines. A token target is set at the beginning of each child group meeting, and group members are awarded tokens throughout the session for trying hard and following the group rules. As facilitators develop a better understanding of the unique behavioral challenges faced by group members, specific behavioral goals can be set for each child to earn tokens. For example, quieter group members may be awarded tokens for trying to answer questions, whereas overtalkative children may be given tokens for keeping comments brief and listening to others. A child who reaches the token target by the end of the group meeting is given one of the rewards. As the program progresses and children's social skills improve, the token targets for each session gradually increase.

Ensuring That Children Are Actively Engaged

Children are likely to become bored if they are required to do the same thing for too long in session, or to sit and listen to others for an extended period of time. To prevent boredom, the SAS program has been designed to include short, fun, physical activities and visual resources related to common special interest areas of children with HFASD. Facilitators can create additional opportunities for active involvement by asking children to draw or write down their own ideas for an activity before sharing them with the group; encouraging them to draw or write down other group members' ideas to promote active listening; splitting larger groups (e.g., six children) into smaller groups (e.g., two groups of three), so that each child gets more turns at activities; and involving all children in some capacity (e.g., becoming the movie director who yells out "Action" and "Cut" for a role play if a child is initially too anxious to participate).

Activity Modifications

Although the SAS program is a manualized intervention, practitioners are encouraged to adapt child session activities to children's interests, ability levels, and learning style(s). For example, if a child is too anxious to role-play a skill, the facilitator may encourage them to discuss or draw what they might say or do in the situation, ask other group members to act out the solution, then encourage the anxious child to imitate what others said and did. For a group of young children, initial program activities may focus on simple emotions (e.g., happy, sad, angry, and afraid), introducing more complex emotions (e.g., embarrassment, teasing) later as group members' knowledge and understanding of emotions improves. Task demands are gradually increased as children's skills and confidence improve, and they are rewarded for their efforts with praise and tokens.

Sensory Items and Activity Adaptations

Sensory processing difficulties of some children with HFASD may present in many different ways. For example, some children (including those with comorbid features of attention-deficit/hyperactivity disorder, ADHD) find it difficult to concentrate unless they have a sensory item to fidget with (e.g., a stretchy rubber animal, a stress ball, a piece of rope) or something active they can do while listening (e.g., drawing). Facilitators may also prompt children to use these relaxation gadgets to calm down when they first notice their distress levels rising, then reward their efforts with praise and tokens. Children should be encouraged to use these items as inconspicuously as possible to minimize distraction for other group members.

Some of the children's activities in the SAS program (e.g., physical challenges in the SAS Challenger Board Game) involve coming in close physical contact with each other, or using items that may cause distress because of sensory sensitivities (e.g., the sound of walkie-talkie static). Facilitators are encouraged to adapt these activities as needed to prevent certain children becoming distressed, while gently encouraging and rewarding them for gradually facing their fears as they learn skills to manage their anxiety more effectively.

Program Delivery as 45-Minute Child Group Meetings

If child group members still find it difficult to stay focused in group meetings after facilitators have implemented the previous recommendations, it may be advisable to deliver the program as 45- to 60-minute sessions (instead of 90- to 120-minute sessions). This program format works particularly well for younger children and those with ADHD features.

Relaxation Gadget Review before Competitive Activities

The SAS program includes several games and activities with an optional winner. Because losing games is a common trigger of distress for children with HFASD, before starting a game, facilitators are encouraged to discuss with group members the relaxation gadgets and helpful thought missiles to use if they lose, and remind them of these as the activity progresses. Children are rewarded with praise and tokens for staying calm if they are not winning, and SAS Friendship Awards may also be used to reward children for playing session games in a kind and friendly way. This helps to refocus their attention on the rules for friendly talk and play, and to enjoy the process of socializing with others rather than fixating on winning a game or activity.

Avoiding Arguing with Children

Children can be resistant to certain concepts and skills steps featured in the SAS curriculum. For example, a child may claim that certain relaxation gadgets "don't work" for them. Rather than arguing or reasoning with the child, facilitators are encouraged to ask the child why the strategy does not work and to provide an example of it not working. From the example provided, the facilitator may be able to explain why the strategy did not work (e.g., the child may have tried to use a calming relaxation gadget instead of a physical one when he or she was very upset), or encourage the child to try alternative strategies that may be more appropriate.

Children can also be pedantic or critical about the terminology or specific examples provided in their SAS Cadet Handbook. For example, one child insisted that someone who was being truly friendly would offer you a turn on his or her computer game, before he or she had a turn, not afterwards, as described in the example in the book. In such instances, it is often helpful to engage the child as a "consultant" to provide feedback on the written materials, changing words and examples as he or she sees fit. This approach also works well when delivering the program to young teenagers, who may find some of the terminology immature. For example, a group of teens preferred to rename "Play Code" the "Hang Out Code."

Setting Up a Chill-Out Zone

If a child becomes visibly distressed in session, it is valuable to have a chill-out zone where he or she can go to relax, then return to the group when calmer. The chill-out zone can be a corner of the room, separated by a partition, that contains a variety of relaxation gadgets and sensory items. The chill-out zone is typically introduced to group members in the third child group meeting as a place to calm down if they are feeling moderately to very anxious or angry in session. Children are rewarded with praise and tokens for going to the chill-out zone when needed (prompted or unprompted) and for returning to the task at hand. To prevent use of the chill-out zone as an avoidance strategy, token reinforcement is typically withheld until a child returns to the session activity after visiting the chill-out zone. If a child refuses to move to the chill-out zone when prompted, it is recommended that the facilitator move the other group members away from him or her. When the child is calm (at the end of the session or at the beginning of the next session), the facilitator can take the child aside to review what upset him or her and develop a coping plan for next time, using the skills learned in the program.

Preventing and Managing Resistance in Parent Group Meetings

Caregiver resistance to recommendations presented in the parent group meetings typically arises from one or more of the following: (1) The program content is not aligned with the caregiver's current goals or priorities; (2) the parent has unrealistic expectations about the speed and manner in which his or her child should be developing their social skills; (3) the parent is having difficulties understanding the concepts and content discussed in the parent group meetings; and (4) the parent lacks confidence in his or her ability to implement the recommendations.

Providing a clear explanation of the objectives, content, and structure of the program, highlighting in the initial intake assessment the importance of caregiver support as a major predictor of program effectiveness, and emphasizing that SAS is not a "cure" for ASD can help caregivers to set realistic expectations for treatment outcome. Assessing and discussing the impact of risk factors on program effectiveness can also help caregivers to make an informed decision about whether SAS is the best service for their family at the present time, or whether alternative supports are more appropriate. Setting ground rules and an agenda for parent group meetings; providing clear, step-by-step explanations for skills and concepts; acknowledging parents' concerns; asking for clarifying information; and using strategic questioning to help parents see distinctions between how they've tried a strategy in the past and the recommended implementation protocol can help parents to develop more positive attitudes toward program content. It can also be helpful to encourage other caregivers in the group to share their successes in trying a strategy or to suggest appropriate alternatives.

If a caregiver expresses persistent concerns about the program, if child home missions are rarely completed, and/or if minimal improvements in a child's social skills are observed or reported, then it is recommended that an individual consultation be scheduled with the caregiver to discuss obstacles preventing his or her family from engaging in and benefiting from the program, and how these can be overcome. This might involve the family withdrawing from the program to participate in therapy addressing other issues, or accessing concurrent additional support to learn and apply the SAS skills and concepts.

RESEARCH TO DATE ON THE TREATMENT

A randomized controlled efficacy trial showed that children with Asperger syndrome who participated in the SAS program (formerly the Junior Detective Training Program) showed greater improvements in social and emotion management skills based on parent-report measures than did children who received treatment as usual during the intervention period (Beaumont & Sofronoff, 2008). Teacher-report data suggested that treatment gains generalized to the school environment, and improvements in children's social skills at school during the intervention period were greater than those made during a baseline period of similar length. Treatment group participants, compared to controls, were better able to suggest appropriate strategies for how story characters could manage feelings of anxiety and anger at postintervention than at preintervention.

Analyses showed that the program was equally effective irrespective of children's age (between 7½ and 11 years at program entry), IQ (all participants had a prorated Wechsler Intelligence Scale for Children [WISC] Full-Scale IQ score of 85 or above), severity of ASD symptoms, level of comorbidity, use of psychotropic medication, and primary caregiver psychopathology (depression, anxiety, stress and Asperger syndrome symptomatology). The only significant predictor of treatment outcome was the number of home missions completed by children.

Follow-up parent-report data indicated that treatment gains were maintained at 5-month follow-up, with 76% of children who displayed clinically significant social impairments at pretreatment improving to within the normal range by the end of the program and/or 5-month follow-up (Beaumont & Sofronoff, 2008). On parent report measures, there was continued improvement in children's social skills from posttreatment to 5-month follow-up. Due to the intensive, time-limited nature of the SAS intervention, children sometimes develop only a basic understanding of some of the social concepts taught during the program, and require ongoing prompting, practice, feedback, and reinforcement to continue using and developing these skills over the weeks, months, and years ahead.

An effectiveness trial of the SAS program is currently underway in Autism Spectrum Australia satellite classes in New South Wales. This trial is evaluating the effectiveness of the intervention when delivered by school staff to students attending specialist ASD satellite classes (typically six students with ASD, a teacher, and teacher-aide) affiliated with mainstream schools. Treatment outcome is evaluated at baseline, intervention, and 1-year follow-up phases using parent, child, program-facilitator, and teacher/teacher-aide-report measures and observational assessments. Children participating in this trial were age 7 to 14 years at the time of program entry, and were not excluded based on comorbidity, symptom severity, IQ, or verbal comprehension deficits. Analyses will be conducted to determine the impact of sociodemographic factors on treatment outcome in this school-based evaluation. A pilot evaluation of the SAS program for children without an ASD diagnosis who have social skill difficulties is also currently underway. This trial includes children who meet diagnostic criteria for other psychological disorders (e.g., ADHD, anxiety disorders), and those who do not meet formal criteria for any diagnosis but report peer interaction difficulties. Parent- and child-report data are being collected at pretreatment, posttreatment, and 6-week follow-up to explore the effectiveness of the program in improving children's social skills and reducing their anxiety levels.

FUTURE DIRECTIONS

Future research aims to answer several outstanding questions about the SAS program. Firstly, the relative contribution of the different program components (i.e., computer game, child group meetings, parent group meetings, teacher information and support) to treatment outcome needs to be evaluated. It is important to examine the risk factors for limited treatment response proposed in this chapter, to clarify how these may be addressed to optimize treatment gains. Trials of the program with rural and remote families are scheduled to elucidate further the core program ingredients and to determine whether a self-directed variant of the program can be successfully delivered with therapist support provided via telephone or Skype.

Planned research also aims to examine how the intervention may be supplemented with further technological innovations to help children review, apply, and monitor their use of emotion regulation and social skills. There is some early evidence to suggest that programs incorporating technology such as computers and computer games result in better social skills outcomes (Wainer & Ingersoll, 2011). Perhaps the next stage is the use of virtual environments and virtual peers, as piloted by Mitchell, Parsons, and Leonard (2007). This emerging development may offer further advances in assisting the social skills of young people with ASD.

Cross-cultural trials of the SAS intervention, a classroom-based adaptation of the program, and upward extensions of the content for teenagers and young adults are being explored. The impact of improved social and emotional functioning on children's relationships with others, their academic and vocational outcomes, and their overall happiness and well-being across the lifespan also needs to be evaluated empirically.

REFERENCES

American Psychiatric Association. (1994). *Diagnostic and statistical manual of mental disorders* (4th ed.). Washington, DC: Author.

American Psychiatric Association. (2013). *Diagnostic and statistical manual of mental disorders* (5th ed.). Arlington, VA: Author.

Beaumont, R. (2009). *Secret Agent Society: Solving the mystery of social encounters—computer game.* Queensland, Australia: The Social Skills Training Institute, a subdivision of Triple P International Pty. Ltd.

Beaumont, R. (2010). *Secret Agent Society: Solving the mystery of social encounters—facilitator manual.* Queensland, Australia: Social Skills Training Institute, a subdivision of Triple P International Pty. Ltd.

Beaumont, R., & Sofronoff, K. (2008). A multi-component social skills intervention for children with Asperger syndrome: The Junior Detective Training Program. *Journal of Child Psychology and Psychiatry, 49*(7), 743–753.

Capps, L., Yirmiya, N., & Sigman, M. (1992). Understanding of simple and complex emotions in non-retarded children with autism. *Journal of Child Psychology and Psychiatry, 33*(7), 1169–1182.

Chalfant, A., Rapee, R., & Carroll, L. (2007). Treating anxiety disorders in children with high-functioning autism spectrum disorders: A controlled trial. *Journal of Autism and Developmental Disorders, 37,* 1842–1857.

De Rosier, M. E. (2002). *Group interventions and exercises for enhancing children's communication, cooperation, and confidence.* Sarasota, FL: Professional Resources Press.

De Rosier, M. E., Swick, D. C., Davis, N. O., McMillen, J. S., & Matthews, R. (2011). The efficacy of a social skills group intervention for improving social behaviors in children with high functioning autism spectrum disorders. *Journal of Autism and Developmental Disorders, 41,* 1033–1043.

Gray, C. (1994). *Comic strip conversations.* Arlington, TX: Future Horizons.

Kanner, L. (1943). Autistic disturbances of affective contact. *Nervous Child, 2,* 217–250.

Kroeger, K. A., Schultz, J. R., & Newsom, C. (2007). A comparison of two group-delivered social skills programs for young children with autism. *Journal of Autism and Developmental Disorders, 37,* 808–817.

LeGoff, D. B. (2004). Use of LEGO as a therapeutic medium for improving social competence. *Journal of Autism and Developmental Disorders, 34*(5), 557–571.

Lovaas, O. I. (1987). Behavioral treatment and normal educational and intellectual functioning in young autistic children. *Journal of Consulting and Clinical Psychology, 55,* 3–9.

McConnell, S. R. (2002). Interventions to facilitate social interaction for young children with autism: Review of available research and recommendations for educational intervention and future research. *Journal of Autism and Developmental Disorders, 32,* 351–372.

McEachin, J. J., Smith, T., & Lovaas, O. I. (1993). Long-term outcome for children with autism who received early intensive behavioral treatment. *American Journal on Mental Retardation, 97*(4), 385–391.

Mitchell, P., Parsons, S., & Leonard, A. (2007). Using virtual environments for teaching social understanding to 6 adolescents with autistic spectrum disorders. *Journal of Autism and Developmental Disorders, 37,* 589–600.

National Research Council. (2001). *Educating children with autism.* Washington, DC: National Academic Press.

Owens, G., Granader, Y., Humphrey, A., & Baron-Cohen, S. (2008). LEGO therapy and the Social Use of Language Programme: An evaluation of two social skills interventions for children with high functioning autism and Asperger syndrome. *Journal of Autism and Developmental Disorders, 38,* 1944–1957.

Reichow, B., & Volkmar, F. R. (2010). Social skills interventions for individuals with autism: Evaluation for evidence based practices within a best evidence synthesis framework. *Journal of Autism and Developmental Disorders, 40,* 149–166.

Rinaldi, W. (2004). *Social use of Language Programme: Infant and primary school teaching pack.* Cranleigh, Surrey, UK: Author.

Rogers, S., & Vismara, L. (2008). Evidence-based comprehensive treatments for early autism. *Journal of Clinical Child and Adolescent Psychology, 37,* 8–38.

Sofronoff, K., Attwood, T., & Hinton, S. (2005). A randomized controlled trial of a CBT intervention for anxiety in children with Asperger syndrome. *Journal of Child Psychology and Psychiatry, 46,* 1152–1160.

Sofronoff, K., Attwood, T., Hinton, S., & Levin, I. (2007). A randomized controlled trial of a cognitive behavioural intervention for anger management in children diagnosed with Asperger syndrome. *Journal of Autism and Developmental Disorders, 37,* 1203–1214.

Sofronoff, K., Eloff, J., Sheffield, J., & Attwood, T. (2011). Increasing the understanding and demonstration of appropriate affection in children with Asperger syndrome: A pilot trial. *Autism Research and Treatment, 2011,* Article 214317.

Wainer, A. L., & Ingersoll, B. R. (2011). The use of innovative technology for teaching social communication to individuals with autism spectrum disorders. *Research in Autism Spectrum Disorders, 5,* 96–107.

White, S. W., Albano, A. M., Johnson, C. R., Kasari, C., Ollendick, T., Klin, A., et al. (2010). Development of a cognitive-behavioral intervention program to treat anxiety and social deficits in teens with high-functioning autism. *Clinical Child and Family Psychology Review, 13,* 77–90.

White, S. W., Koenig, K., & Scahill, L. (2007). Social skills development in children with autism spectrum disorders: A review of the intervention research. *Journal of Autism and Developmental Disorders, 37,* 1858–1868.

Wood, J. J., Drahota, A., Sze, K., Har, K., Chui, A., & Langer, D. A. (2009). Cognitive behavioural therapy for anxiety in children with autism spectrum disorders: A randomized controlled trial. *Journal of Child Psychology and Psychiatry, 50*(3), 224–234.

9

A Manualized Summer Program for Social Skills in Children with High-Functioning ASD

CHRISTOPHER LOPATA, MARCUS L. THOMEER,
MARTIN A. VOLKER, AND GLORIA K. LEE

HISTORICAL BACKGROUND AND SIGNIFICANCE OF THE TREATMENT

The autism spectrum is characterized by significant variability in the manifestation and severity of social and communicative impairments, and circumscribed behaviors and interests (American Psychiatric Association, 2013). The relative strengths in cognitive and formal language abilities exhibited by children with ASD without accompanying intellectual impairment can mask their significant needs and hinder access to services and treatment (Klin & Volkmar, 2000; Marans, Rubin, & Laurent, 2005). Lack of access to appropriate treatment is especially problematic for children with HFASD as their pervasive and chronic impairments have been associated with long-term negative outcomes including limited ability to secure and maintain employment, social isolation, and prolonged dependence on family members for financial and interpersonal support (Portway & Johnson, 2005; Shattuck, Wagner, Narendorf, Sterzing, & Hensley, 2011), highlighting the need for effective treatments for these children.

Significant heterogeneity across the autism spectrum poses a significant treatment challenge as subgroups, including children with HFASD, often require distinct interventions (Rao, Beidel, & Murray, 2008). This chapter presents an intensive comprehensive psychosocial treatment for children with HFASD that is administered in a summer program format. The treatment was developed to target the unique features of children with HFASD, and its efficacy has been supported in a number of increasingly rigorous uncontrolled and controlled trials. As we describe later, the trials were conducted following National Institute of Mental Health (NIMH) working-group guidelines for evaluating and validating psychosocial interventions for ASD (Smith et al., 2007). Because the comprehensive treatment protocol was developed specifically to target the features of children with HFASD, it is appropriate to begin with a review of the areas affected in HFASD and research related to the active treatment components in the program. This provides a clear rationale and framework for the treatment model, therapeutic targets, and manualized protocol.

Consistent with the new nosology in the DSM-5 (American Psychiatric Association, 2013), children with former diagnoses of Asperger syndrome, autistic disorder (high-functioning), and PDD-NOS are characterized as having HFASD in this chapter. There is ongoing disagreement about whether the disorders that make up HFASD are distinct or better characterized along a continuum (see Klin, McPartland, & Volkmar, 2005). Shared relative strengths in cognitive and language abilities, along with studies that have failed to find differences between the groups (e.g., Macintosh & Dissanayake, 2006) have supported the inclusion of children with Asperger syndrome, high-functioning autism, and PDD-NOS under the broader grouping of HFASD.

Overview of Clinical and Associated Features of HFASD

Social Interaction Impairments

A central feature of HFASD is a significant and pervasive deficit in social interaction skills. This characteristic is often regarded as the most handicapping and it is featured prominently in the diagnostic criteria for the disorders that comprise ASD (American Psychiatric Association, 2013). Diagnostic criteria involving marked social dysfunction include impairments in nonverbal behaviors used to regulate social interactions (eye-to-eye gaze, body posture); failure to establish developmentally appropriate relationships; failure to seek spontaneously to share enjoyment, interest, or activities; and lack of emotional or social reciprocity (American Psychiatric Association, 2013). For individuals with ASD, social impairments range from deficits in rudimentary social skills (McConnell, 2002) to more complex social-cognitive processing (e.g., interpreting the intentions of others; Carothers & Taylor, 2004). The social deficits of children with HFASD have been documented in a number of studies (e.g., Macintosh & Dissanayake, 2006; Volker et al., 2010) and they most often extend into adolescence and adulthood (Church, Alisanski, & Amanullah, 2000; Portway & Johnson, 2005). Despite these impairments, individuals with HFASD generally exhibit greater social awareness and social interest than their lower-functioning peers with autism (Church et al., 2000; Portway & Johnson, 2005).

Circumscribed Behaviors, Interests, and Activities

The second core feature involves restricted, repetitive, and stereotyped behaviors, interests, and activities. These can be observed in preoccupations or narrow and intense interests, inflexible adherence to nonfunctional routines or rituals, repetitive and stereotyped motor mannerisms, and/or significant preoccupation with parts of objects (American Psychiatric Association, 2000). For children with HFASD, their intense and narrow focus on an area of interest and their inability to inhibit preoccupations can have cognitive and behavioral ramifications; such perseverative tendencies often interfere with their ability to attend to important environmental content and can disrupt daily functioning (e.g., poor retention of academic material; Safran, Safran, & Ellis, 2003). While circumscribed behaviors, interests, and activities constitute distinct clinical features of HFASD (American Psychiatric Association, 2013), they can also impede social performance and exacerbate social difficulties. To illustrate, rigidly focusing on a narrow area of interest restricts children's interests, range of responses to others, and social learning opportunities (Klin, Sparrow, Marans, Carter, & Volkmar, 2000; McConnell, 2002). This has been observed in the children's propensity for sustained one-sided conversations on a restricted topic of interest (Klin et al., 2000). Additionally, children with HFASD have been found to restrict their conceptualizations of *friends* to others who share their interests (Carrington, Templeton, & Papinczak, 2003). Given these findings, a reduction in circumscribed behaviors, interests, and activities would appear to have collateral social benefits for children with HFASD.

Associated Features

Several associated features also affect daily functioning and social performance of this population. While children with HFASD are generally characterized by relative strength in formal language/vocabulary, pragmatic communication (i.e., social communication) deficits commonly contribute to social interaction breakdowns. In this way, children with HFASD also exhibit communicative deficits, although their deficits are qualitatively different from those of lower-functioning children with autism. Pragmatic communication problems for children with HFASD can include impaired understanding of nonliteral language, abstract language, and abstract concepts (Klin et al., 2005; Safran et al., 2003). Deficits in accurate comprehension (decoding) of affective information in facial expression have also been noted (Lindner & Rosén, 2006). Problems with decoding can exacerbate social-communicative problems, because facial expressions allow communicative recipients to make important inferences about the internal/emotional experience of the sender (Baron-Cohen, Jolliffe, Mortimore, & Robertson, 1997; Cohn & Ekman, 2005). Studies have documented a range of decoding difficulties for children with HFASD, including impairments in recognizing basic and/or complex emotions in facial expressions (Downs & Smith, 2004; Lindner & Rosén, 2006).

Last, children with HFASD can exhibit a range of behavioral difficulties. Evidence has indicated elevated externalizing symptoms in children with HFASD (Volker et al., 2010) including behaviors such as interrupting, noncompliance, verbal aggression, and instigating others (Klin & Volkmar, 2000). Internalizing problems, including elevated symptoms of depression and anxiety, have also been reported in children with HFASD (Lopata, Toomey, et al., 2010) and may further contribute to social withdrawal and isolation. Laurent and Rubin (2004) noted that emotion regulation and behavioral responses are influenced by the ability to communicate effectively, understand emotions, contemplate another's perspective, and determine salient information in the presence of environmental and social stimuli, all of which may be compromised in HFASD.

The broad range of areas affected in HFASD warrants a comprehensive treatment approach. The following section summarizes recent reviews of psychosocial intervention studies for ASD/HFASD. These papers provide a basis for understanding the current state of psychosocial treatment research and the techniques commonly employed in this research.

Intervention Research for HFASD

Despite their pervasive and significant impairments, children with HFASD have received less treatment research attention than their peers with classic autism (Lord et al., 2005). Reviews of social skills and psychosocial interventions have generally not differentiated between studies involving HFASD samples and samples from the broad ASD population (e.g., Bellini, Peters, Benner, & Hopf, 2007; Reichow & Volkmar, 2010; White, Koenig, & Scahill, 2007). Given the variable composition of the study samples and treatment settings in these reviews, it is perhaps not surprising that the authors have arrived at different conclusions. For example, the Bellini et al. (2007) review of single-subject, school-based social skills intervention studies for children and adolescents with ASD concluded that social skills interventions had low-to-questionable treatment effects. In contrast, White et al. (2007) examined the state of social intervention research studies in ASD and concluded that evidence for social skills interventions was emerging and that a number of treatment techniques were *promising*. In their review, Reichow and Volkmar (2010) determined that social skills interventions had adequate support to be considered an evidence-based practice for school-age children with ASD.

While most of the previous reviews included intervention studies from the broad population of ASD, two evaluated the evidence for social interventions specifically for children and adolescents with HFASD. Rao et al. (2008) evaluated the outcomes of 10 social intervention studies for children and adolescents with HFASD. Of the 10 studies, seven found positive outcomes associated with treatment, though some of the positive findings were limited to a portion of participants or subset of the measures. Significant methodological weaknesses in the studies led Rao et al. to conclude that some support was emerging for social interventions, but that more rigorously controlled studies were needed. In the other review, Lopata, Volker, Toomey, Chow, and Thomeer (2008) evaluated 17 group-based social intervention studies for children and adolescents with HFASD. All 17 studies reported some type of social improvement resulting from treatment. Nine of the studies used standardized measures and conducted statistical analyses, with eight studies yielding significant improvements on one or more measures. Similar to Rao et al. (2008), Lopata, Volker, et al. (2008) noted significant methodological limitations in the studies. Nonetheless, they concluded that group-administered social interventions for HFASD had some preliminary support and held promise.

While these reviews clearly point to methodological limitations in many earlier social intervention studies for ASD/HFASD, the following techniques have been identified as particularly promising for HFASD/ASD social interventions (cf. Koenig et al., 2010; Lopata, Volker, et al., 2008; White et al., 2007):

- Clear and concrete rules
- Structured environments
- Direct and explicit instruction
- Modeling
- Role playing/rehearsal

- Repeated practice
- Performance feedback/reinforcement
- Parent training

These techniques allow task analysis of complex skills and teaching in a part-to-whole sequence, using reinforcement to increase acquisition and maintenance (Howlin, Baron-Cohen, & Hadwin, 1999). In fact, recent randomized clinical trials (RCTs) of social interventions for children with HFASD have yielded findings that support these techniques (e.g., Koenig et al., 2010). Though not always explicitly stated, the techniques used in many social interventions for HFASD are generally consistent with a cognitive-behavioral orientation. This orientation exploits the relative cognitive and language strengths of these children and allows a greater focus on social impairments unique to them, including understanding of social conventions and social problem solving, along with development of basic social skills (Volker & Lopata, 2008; see also Attwood & Scarpa, Chapter 2, this volume).

One additional point that is relevant to the discussion of psychosocial interventions for HFASD/ASD involves the breadth of the interventions and primary treatment target(s). The previously noted reviews made no distinction between *focused* and *comprehensive* interventions. Focused interventions are designed to produce a specific and narrowly defined outcome, whereas comprehensive treatment models (CTMs) are designed to affect core ASD features and broader learning/development (Odom, Boyd, Hall, & Hume, 2010). CTMs comprise multiple treatment components that target multiple domains and are typically applied intensively for an extended period of time and/or at a specified level of engagement (Odom et al., 2010; Smith et al., 2007). The distinction between focused interventions and CTMs is noteworthy; the manualized summer program described in this chapter is a CTM.

It is clear from this review that development of effective social interventions is a challenge for treatment researchers, requiring a systematic approach to development and evaluation. The following section details some of the practical considerations in the creation and study of comprehensive social interventions for children with HFASD.

PRACTICAL CONSIDERATIONS

While diagnostic criteria and research examining features of HFASD have defined a set of deficits to be targeted and social intervention studies have identified some effective treatment techniques, development of effective psychosocial treatments poses a significant challenge due to the multiple areas affected by the disorder. This requires a comprehensive model that addresses critical skills areas and core features of the syndrome, and that is manualized to foster replication and dissemination (Lord et al., 2005; Odom et al., 2010; Smith et al., 2007). An additional challenge involves the need for manualized protocols that address common features of HFASD and the unique needs of an individual child (i.e., manualized and individualized; Smith et al., 2007). Given these challenges, the following are practical considerations for researchers and clinicians seeking to develop and evaluate social interventions for children with HFASD.

A basic but critical consideration is the need to ensure that "treatment targets are derived from a clearly identified source or sources (e.g., theory, diagnostic criteria, etc.) and operationally defined" (Lopata, Volker, et al., 2008, p. 318). Poorly defined treatment targets make assessment of outcomes impossible. Once treatment targets are identified, specific elements of the treatment must be codified in the manual. Such elements include *dosage* (e.g., number and length of sessions), *what to teach* (content), and *how to teach it* (administration procedures; Lord et al., 2005; Odom et al., 2010; Smith et al., 2007). Also important is a clear rationale for how the active components in the model foster symptom reduction, skills development, or management of problem behaviors. Development of a model with these factors in mind allows treatment researchers and providers to understand better how the content and treatment procedures operate to produce the desired effect. A treatment manual also allows development of fidelity measures and assessment of fidelity during implementation (White et al., 2007). In the absence of fidelity data, it is not possible to determine whether observed changes are attributable to the treatment (Bellini et al., 2007).

Another practical consideration is the procedures used for staff training. Some studies of manualized psychosocial treatments have used professional clinicians (e.g., Koenig et al., 2010) while others have used undergraduate and graduate students to administer the treatment protocol (Lopata, Thomeer, et al., 2010). Regardless of the individuals chosen, it is essential that staff members be rigorously trained in the protocol and proficient in its administration (Rao et al., 2008). Manualization of the protocol allows researchers and clinical supervisors to assess staff competency and fidelity with the protocol prior to and throughout protocol delivery.

One final consideration involves the considerable time, attention, infrastructure, resources, and expertise required to develop and systematically evaluate CTMs for HFASD (Lord et al., 2005; Rao et al., 2008). Researchers working to develop and test such treatments may benefit from the structure and systematic progression outlined in the NIMH working-group guidelines for developing and evaluating psychosocial interventions for ASD (Smith et al., 2007; an overview is described in the "Research to Date on the Manualized Summer Program for Children with HFASD" section). Once a treatment is manualized and validated, however, it may be more feasibly implemented by trained individuals. For example, the manualized program described in this chapter was implemented by under-graduate and graduate students as part of clinical internships and practica. Under the supervision of a trained clinician, it is possible that manualized protocols can be administered in a cost-effective manner in community settings.

OVERVIEW OF THE MANUALIZED SUMMER PROGRAM FOR CHILDREN WITH HFASD

As noted, the complexity of HFASD requires a comprehensive treatment model that addresses the core features of ASD and development of adaptive skills. In addition, the model must not only be manualized but also respon-sive to the unique needs of individual children (Lord et al., 2005; Smith et al., 2007). The comprehensive summer protocol described in this sec-tion was developed to address the core and associated features of HFASD. Shared diagnostic and associated features allowed for development of a protocol that is administered to all of the child participants. Whereas the core treatment curriculum is administered to all the child participants, an additional component allows for the targeting of skills/behaviors unique to the individual child. This individualized component is a small part of the overall treatment model, yet it allows for some individualization in an otherwise highly manualized protocol. As we describe later in the chapter, the efficacy of the comprehensive summer program has been supported in a series of treatment trials, including a recent RCT. This line of research has produced a fully developed and operationalized manual that delineates the curriculum *(what to teach)*, treatment procedures *(how to administer it)*, and staff training protocol *(knowledge and competence),* as well as fully developed behavioral tracking forms, fidelity forms with psychometric data, and outcome measures that have shown treatment sensitivity (ele-ments considered essential for comprehensive treatment models; Lord et al., 2005; Odom et al., 2010; Smith et al., 2007).

The treatment program is administered 5 days per week over 5 weeks during the summer to children ages 7–12 years with HFASD. Treatment groups comprise six children (mixed gender) with HFASD and three staff members. Each treatment day is highly structured and comprises five 70-minute treatment cycles. Every 70-minute treatment cycle includes 20 minutes of intensive skills instruction, followed by a 50-minute therapeutic activity. The skills instruction and therapeutic activities target social and social-communicative skills, face–emotion recognition (decoding) skills, and interpretation of nonliteral language skills, and the therapeutic activities also target interest expansion. Each skills group and therapeutic activity is aligned with a specific deficit area associated with HFASD (see Table 9.1). The manualized curriculum is administered using direct instruction, modeling, role playing/rehearsal, performance feedback/reinforcement, homework, and repeated practice. A behavioral reinforcement system also fosters skills development and reduces ASD symptoms and problem behaviors, and parent training is provided. During each of the skills groups and therapeutic activities, one staff member facilitates group activities, while a second staff member serves in a support role and provides performance feedback/reinforcement to the children. A third staff member records response–cost and individual daily note (IDN) data on standardized tracking sheets, in addition to serving in a support role and providing feedback/reinforcement. The three staff members within each group who alternate roles throughout the treatment day, however, remain with the same group of six children during the 5-week program. The following describes the areas targeted by the specific skills groups and therapeutic activities.

Skills Groups

Social Skills Groups

The social and social-communicative skills targeted in these groups were selected from the Skillstreaming curriculum, which is a structured program for teaching interpersonal skills to children with social skills deficits (McGinnis & Goldstein, 1997). Each of the selected skills is aligned with and directly addresses a specific diagnostic feature of children with HFASD (American Psychiatric Association, 2000). The manual includes a table delineating each skill and its associated target clinical feature. The skills in the curriculum have been task-analyzed, and each skill's component steps are taught in correct sequence. Participants are taught the most basic skills first (e.g., listening, having a conversation) and progress to more complex social and social-communicative skills (e.g., negotiating, understanding another's feelings). The conduct of the groups is by direct instruction, modeling, role playing/rehearsal, performance feedback/reinforcement,

TABLE 9.1. Linkage between Treatment Components and Targeted Clinical Features

Treatment component	Targeted clinical feature
Social skills instruction	Social impairment
Face–emotion recognition instruction	Social impairment (decoding)
Nonliteral language instruction	Pragmatic communication
Therapeutic activities	Social impairment Pragmatic communication Restricted/repetitive interests and activities
Response–cost behavioral system	Social impairment Pragmatic communication Restricted/repetitive interests and activities
Individual daily note	Behavior problems Social impairment Restricted/repetitive interests and activities
Parent training	Parent understanding of HFASDs Development of parent strategies for promoting skills/generalization

and transfer of learning. The staff member conducting the group follows a manualized, nine-step procedure as follows: (1) Define the skill; (2) model the skill; (3) establish trainee skill need; (4) select a role player; (5) set up the role play; (6) conduct the role play; (7) provide performance feedback; (8) assign skill homework; and (9) select the next role player (Goldstein, McGinnis, Sprafkin, Gershaw, & Klein, 1997, p. 37). Each child is a primary treatment recipient at least once every two social skills groups, in addition to being an active participant in other children's role plays and providing performance feedback to peers.

Face–Emotion Recognition (Decoding) Skills Groups

Six skills groups specifically target face–emotion decoding skills. Each lesson delineates the target decoding element, the link to the specific HFASD deficit, and procedures for conducting the group. These skills groups involve identification of facial features and positions that characterize different emotions, and recognition of physiological reactions related to emotions. Children's recognition of their own physiological reactions (i.e., emotions) fosters understanding of the emotional state conveyed in the facial expressions of others. Each child is a primary treatment recipient in every face–emotion decoding group, in addition to being an active co-participant in decoding exercises with peers and staff.

Nonliteral Language Skills Groups

Six skills groups specifically target interpretation of nonliteral language skills. Each lesson plan delineates the target nonliteral language skill, link to the specific HFASD deficit, and procedures for conducting the group. Nonliteral language instruction promotes understanding that language can have multiple meanings. Practice activities that involve decoding of idioms and other nonliteral elements of language are conducted during each group. Each child is a primary treatment recipient in every nonliteral language skills group, in addition to being actively involved in practice exercises.

Therapeutic Activities

The last 50 minutes of each treatment cycle are devoted to a therapeutic activity. As previously noted, these activities have been designed to practice and reinforce social and social-communicative skills, face–emotion recognition skills, and nonliteral language skills, and expand the children's interests and behaviors. The activities were developed to be fun and engaging, so that children perceive the program as a *summer camp* (not a treatment program). Each activity lesson plan delineates the target skill(s), link(s) to the specific HFASD deficit, and procedures for conducting the activity.

All activities are cooperative in nature and require interpersonal interaction and collaborative problem solving among the children to complete the activity successfully. As such, each therapeutic activity either directly or indirectly involves practice of social and social-communicative skills. Other activities target development and practice of face–emotion decoding skills in a group format. Face–emotion recognition activities begin with tasks involving children's identification of basic facial expressions in pictures and progress to more naturalistic activities involving the examination of their own and other children's expressions during activities. The children also learn and practice identification of physiological reactions associated with different facial expressions, and discuss how facial expressions convey meaning and how to decode and use facial expressions in social situations. Therapeutic activities targeting interpretation of nonliteral language involve practice in decoding non-literal expressions. These activities build on the nonliteral language skills group lessons and generally require that children initially determine whether a statement is meant to be interpreted literally and, if not, what are potential alternative interpretations based on other contextual clues. The children then determine the best interpretation and receive performance feedback.

The final area targeted in the therapeutic activities is interest expansion activities, developed to increase children's engagement in topics and activities beyond their own circumscribed interests. This may allow them to interact more effectively without dominating social exchanges, perseverating on a narrow topic, or precluding social interactions with others who do not share their target area of interest. Interest expansion activities require active engagement in activities and tasks outside their narrow areas of interest. The children work together on non-self-selected topics and share their newly learned information with their peers. An example involves having children, working in pairs, randomly select a topic from a *grab bag* of topics. Together, members of a pair conduct a computer search on the selected topic and develop a book on the novel topic. At the end of the activity each pair presents the book and new information they discovered, discusses possible social scenarios when the newly discovered information might be useful, and describes the social skills used to complete the project. Each child is a primary treatment recipient in every therapeutic activity, engages in multiple practice trials, and receives high rates of performance feedback.

Behavioral Reinforcement System

Children with HFASD have significant difficulty acquiring and maintaining new social and social-communicative skills, and decreasing their repetitive and restricted interests and behaviors. Two behavioral procedures address shared clinical features of HFASD, as well as the needs of individual children (manualized and individualized; Smith et al., 2007). The two behavioral procedures are applied across the treatment day, and feedback is provided to parents at the end of each treatment day by a designated staff member from each group.

Response–Cost Behavioral System

The response–cost system comprises operationally defined skills and problem behaviors that characterize children with HFASD. Because these skills and behaviors are derived from diagnostic criteria and research characterizing common clinical features of children with HFASD, they are universally applied with all the participants. Each operationally defined category carries a designated point value, and points are verbally awarded or withdrawn immediately following the occurrence of a target skill/behavior. Children earn points for following operationally defined rules and using any previously taught social skill (positive categories), and lose points for not following instructions, for violating a group rule, or engaging in operationally defined negative social behavior (ASD-related behaviors that include violating another's personal space, sharing irrelevant information, poor eye contact, etc.). Children also earn a point bonus during any interval for exhibiting any three or more social/social-communicative skills previously taught and not losing any points for a negative social behavior. Points are verbally awarded or withdrawn by any of the group's three staff members; however, one staff member each treatment cycle is designated to record the points on a standardized point sheet. When withdrawing points, the staff member quickly identifies in a calm tone the operationally defined negative behavior and the specific point loss associated with that negative behavior, then continues with the lesson/activity; this approach to point withdrawal has been highly effective in prior treatment studies of the summer program and generally has not elicited negative reactions from children with HFASD. Children receive brief (< 1 minute) point-based feedback every 20 minutes (on their performance during that interval) throughout the treatment day from the staff member recording points for that interval. Points earned in the response–cost system (and on the IDN; see below) are used to earn an end-of-week outing as a reinforcer. The outings are also used for practice and generalization of skills beyond the treatment setting (Rao et al., 2008). Every week, each child's target points are increased 10% above the prior week's point total. One staff member from each group provides a summary of each child's point-based performance to parents at the end of every treatment day. Notably, fidelity of program implementation (including point allocation or withdrawal) is monitored regularly to ensure proper use of procedures.

Individual Daily Note

Each child also has an IDN targeting two to three skills/behaviors unique to the child. This component integrates targets that may not be covered in the standard protocol and allows for some degree of individualization (e.g., teasing peers). IDN targets and baseline rates are derived from observations and behavioral tracking during the first week of the program. Each IDN is created using a standardized template that includes the child's unique skills/behavioral targets and target performance levels. Verbal feedback on IDN performance is provided to children by all the staff members during the treatment day. Each child receives brief (< 1 minute) IDN feedback every 20 minutes (on his or her performance during that interval) throughout the treatment day from the staff member recording IDN performance for that interval. IDN feedback is provided at the same time the response–cost feedback is given. A small reward (i.e., reinforcer) is provided onsite at the end of each treatment day to each child who reaches his or her IDN target level.

Parents also provide a daily reward at home (typically a preferred activity) for reaching the IDN target level. The home-based reward is determined collaboratively with parents during parent training (Smith et al., 2007). In addition to the daily IDN reinforcers, the overall weekly IDN performance (along with the response–cost point target previously described) is used to earn an end-of-week outing. Each week the child is required to have earned ≥ 75% overall on his or her IDNs (along with the target level of response–cost points) to earn the end-of-week outing. One staff member from each group provides a summary of each child's IDN performance to parents at the end of every treatment day (the same staff member who provides the response–cost performance to parents).

Parent Training

Parents participate each week in one 90-minute onsite parent training session conducted by one of the program directors. Content and instructional procedures for parent training are manualized to ensure delivery of consistent content. The sessions are conducted to educate parents on features of HFASD, components of the program, and effective use of behavioral strategies. Parents also learn about and develop strategies for skills growth and generalization beyond the treatment site. As previously noted, parents and the parent-training facilitator work collaboratively to develop a home-based reinforcement system for the children's performance at the summer program. This increases parent participation in the treatment, focuses parents on critical treatment targets, and fosters children's skills acquisition and reduces ASD symptoms and problem behaviors.

Staff Training

To ensure that all staff members are competent in delivering the treatment (Rao et al., 2008; Smith et al., 2007) a structured staff training protocol is instituted. This protocol assesses mastery of the treatment manual (i.e., knowledge) and proficiency in treatment delivery (i.e., competence). All staff complete a rigorous, 5-day (40-hour) training that has been manualized to ensure that all staff members receive the same content and skills development exercises and demonstrate competence. The treatment manual is distributed 1 month prior to training. At the beginning of the training week, each staff member is required to pass a written exam that assesses mastery of the manual, with a score of 100%. Among other knowledge items, each staff member must precisely write out the operational definitions for each of the skills/behaviors in the response–cost system and identify its corresponding point value. Staff then complete 5 days of intensive classroom and applied practice training. Competence is assessed by clinical supervisors during applied practice exercises toward the end of the training week. Using standardized fidelity forms (the same forms used to assess fidelity during treatment), each staff member is required to demonstrate ≥ 90% fidelity administering the treatment protocol.

Fidelity Monitoring during Implementation

Because the protocol is manualized, implementation is assessed using standardized fidelity forms. The forms indicate dose (i.e., number and duration of session) and adherence (i.e., percentage of specific elements accurately administered per component). These forms have been found to yield high levels of interobserver agreement (i.e., average per session interobserver agreement across individual intervention elements was 97.2%; Lopata, Thomeer, et al., 2010).

RESEARCH TO DATE ON THE MANUALIZED SUMMER PROGRAM FOR CHILDREN WITH HFASD

To address the significant complexities in developing and evaluating psychosocial interventions for ASD, a NIMH working group has proposed a set of guidelines for systematically developing, studying, validating, and disseminating psychosocial interventions for this population (Smith et al., 2007). Although the authors noted that studies often deviate from this linear progression, studies in the model generally progress in a four-phase, stepwise manner from Phase 1—development, systematic implementation, and assessment of a new technique(s), to Phase 2—creation of an intervention manual and plan of evaluation (including fidelity measures) and pilot testing, to Phase 3—RCTs, and finally Phase 4—community effectiveness studies. This model is noted here because the summer program has been systematically evaluated in a series of increasingly rigorous studies that have largely paralleled the NIMH guidelines, including a Phase 3 RCT. The RCT was also executed according to Consolidated Standards of Reporting Trials (CONSORT) guidelines. Interested readers are encouraged to consult both the NIMH working group (Smith et al., 2007) and CONSORT guidelines for conducting treatment trials.

One additional point that deserves mention involves the measurement challenges faced by treatment researchers. While there is a recognized need to assess the core features of ASD and broader adaptive skills, there is a significant lack of treatment-sensitive measures (Lord et al., 2005; Smith et al., 2007). Suggestions to improve the accuracy of outcome assessments have included use of scales that assess ASD features, skills directly targeted by the treatment, and broader adaptive functioning, as well as the inclusion of ratings by multiple informants (Lord et al., 2005; Odom et al., 2010; Smith et al., 2007; White et al., 2007). The need to assess such a broad range of variables is confounded, however, by problems with statistical power and the need to control error associated with multiple comparisons. To address these challenges, researchers have been encouraged to utilize a limited number of primary measures/analyses and a small number of secondary measures (Smith et al., 2007). This approach to measure selection, hypothesis testing, and data analysis is reflected in the progression described in Table 9.2.

To date, four published studies have evaluated and supported the efficacy of the summer program for children with HFASD. Although these four studies are summarized in Table 9.2, interested readers are referred to the original published papers for more details. The following brief, narrative descriptions are presented in the following order to illustrate the general progression through the NIMH working-group phases. It is important to note that the manualized program evaluated in the following studies involved the same treatment protocol; however, the program was initially delivered during a 6-week summer format (four treatment cycles per day). This was changed to a 5-week format (five cycles per day) in the Phase 3— RCT to accommodate the wait-list children in the same summer. Based on the strength of the design and findings resulting from the RCT, the 5-week format (described in the previous section) is now considered the final version.

Phase 1–Phase 2: Case Study ($n = 1$)

Although not published until after two of the group studies, the case study (Toomey, Lopata, Volker, & Thomeer, 2009) was based on data collected during the initial development and assessment of the protocol. The study included elements from Phase 1– and Phase 2–type studies. Phase 1 elements included use of a case study design to gather initial evidence that the intervention may be beneficial for an individual with an HFASD. In addition, it utilized observational data collected across the intervention period, as well as the tracking of behavioral data specific to the target child. Because the study involved implementation of a multicomponent, manualized protocol, it also had elements of a Phase 2 trial (Smith et al., 2007). The participant was a 9-year-old male with an HFASD, participating in the 6-week summer

TABLE 9.2. Summary of Comprehensive Summer Program Treatment Studies and Outcomes for Children with HFASD

Study	N (ages)	Comprehensive treatment program	Study design	Results
Toomey, Lopata, Volker, & Thomeer (2009)	1 (9)	6-week treatment program, 5 days per week, four treatment cycles per day. Targets included social skills, face–emotion recognition, interest expansion, and interpretation of nonliteral language. High rates of verbal (noncategorical) feedback and parent training provided.	Case study	Observational data collected on five operationally-defined behaviors during game sessions (four times per week; 20-minute observation periods). A significant increase was found in on-task participation in social activities and significant decreases in problem behaviors (i.e., whining and verbal aggression and verbal defiance). Data on conversational behaviors (i.e., participating in a conversation and initiating a conversation) were inconsistent and did not yield an interpretable pattern. Pre–post staff ratings reflected a substantial increase in social skills and reductions in atypicality, withdrawal, and behavioral symptoms (BASC).
Lopata, Thomeer, Volker, & Nida (2006)	21 (6–13)	6-week treatment program, 5 days per week, four treatment cycles per day. Targets included social skills, face–emotion recognition, interest expansion, and interpretation of nonliteral language. Parent training provided. Additionally, one treatment condition received response–cost/IDN-based feedback while the second received noncategorical feedback.	Randomized pretest-posttest two-treatment design	Significant main effects (improvement) for the overall program on parent- and staff-rated social skills (BASC) and parent-rated adaptability and atypicality (BASC). Staff reported no change in adaptability and an increase in atypicality. No interactions (treatment × time) were significant (based on feedback format). Anecdotal parent reports. Parents reported increased peer interactions, social awareness, and use of skills taught in the program.

(*continued*)

215

TABLE 9.2. (*continued*)

Study	N (ages)	Comprehensive treatment program	Study design	Results
Lopata, Thomeer, Volker, Nida, & Lee (2008)	54 (6–13)	6-week treatment program, 5 days per week, four treatment cycles per day. Targets included social skills, face–emotion recognition, interest expansion, and interpretation of nonliteral language. Parent training provided. Additionally, one treatment condition received response–cost/IDN-based feedback while the second received noncategorical feedback.	Randomized pretest–posttest two-treatment design	Significant main effects (improvement) for the overall program on parent and staff ratings of social skills, adaptive skills (BASC), and targeted social skills (ASC). No significant interactions (treatment × time) were found on these measures. Parent ratings indicated no change in atypicality, however main effects for the overall program were found for both withdrawal and the behavior symptoms index (BASC); no treatment × time interactions for parent ratings on these measures. Significant interactions (treatment × time) favoring the response–cost/IDN group were found for staff ratings of atypicality, withdrawal, and the behavior symptoms index (BASC). These suggested positive effects associated with the response–cost/IDN condition. No significant effect on the child measure of face–emotion recognition (DANVA2).

| Lopata, Thomeer, Volker, Toomey, Nida, Lee, Smerbeck, & Rodgers (2010) | 36 (7–12) | 5-week treatment program, 5 days per week, five treatment cycles per day. Targets included social skills, face–emotion recognition, interest expansion, and interpretation of nonliteral language. Response–cost and IDN administered and parent training provided.

Wait-list controls monitored for other therapeutic programming while awaiting treatment. | RCT pretest–posttest control group design (wait-list control) | Primary measures (direct child measures and parent ratings). Following Bonferroni correction (for the seven primary measures/analyses), five significant posttest differences (ANCOVA controlling for pretest) were found favoring the treatment group on the direct child measures of knowledge of target social skills (SKA) and interpretation of nonliteral language (idiomatic language; CASL), and parent ratings of ASD symptoms (SRS), target social skills (ASC), and withdrawal (BASC2).

Secondary measures (staff ratings). Following Bonferroni correction (for the four secondary measures/analyses), all four pre–posttest comparisons were significant (repeated-measures ANOVA) and indicated decreases in ASD symptoms (SRS) and withdrawal (BASC2) and increases in target social skills (ASC) and broader social skills (BASC2). |

Note. Studies in the table are presented according to their corresponding NIMH-phase trial (instead of chronologically). BASC, Behavior Assessment System for Children (Reynolds & Kamphaus, 1992, 1998); ASC, Adapted Skillstreaming Checklist (formerly Skillstreaming Survey); IDN, individual daily note; DANVA2, Diagnostic Analysis of Nonverbal Accuracy 2 (Nowicki, 1997); SKA, Skillstreaming Knowledge Assessment; CASL, Comprehensive Assessment of Spoken Language (Carrow-Woolfolk, 1999); SRS, Social Responsiveness Scale (Constantino & Gruber, 2005); BASC2, Behavior Assessment System for Children—Second Edition (Reynolds & Kamphaus, 2004).

The initial treatment trials (Lopata et al., 2006, 2008, 2009) were based on a 6-week program schedule that comprised four treatment cycles each day. In the RCT that included the wait-list control condition (Lopata et al., 2010), the same protocol was administered during a 5-week schedule, with five treatment cycles each day. This modification was made to ensure that wait-list-control children were able to complete treatment during the summer (prior to the beginning of the school year). The program described in this chapter (see "Overview of Manualized Summer Program for Children with HFASD" section) is based on the 5-week format evaluated and validated in the 2010 RCT.

program with other children with HFASD. Five operationally defined behaviors were tracked during 20-minute structured game sessions four times per week. Interobserver agreement was evaluated for 12.5% of all observation periods, with average agreement ranging from 91 to 97% for all five behavioral categories. Results indicated clear patterns of improvement over the course of treatment for three of the five behaviors (on-task participation in social activities, whining, and verbal aggression and verbal defiance). Data on two conversational behaviors were variable and did not allow for clear interpretation. Secondary staff ratings reflected substantial improvement in social skills, and decreases in ASD-related behaviors (i.e., atypicality) and problem behaviors. Data suggested that participation in the program was associated with gains and potential therapeutic benefits.

Phase 2: Manual Development and Pilot Testing

Two group-based studies that were completed largely reflect the goals of Phase 2 studies, including establishment of fidelity measures, identification of sensitive and valid outcome measures (primary and secondary), assessment of feasibility (acceptability/satisfaction and fidelity), and finalization of the treatment manual (for use in subsequent RCTs; Smith et al., 2007). Beyond these Phase 2 elements, the two studies were used to gather preliminary outcome data. Smith et al. noted that preliminary outcome studies/data, while not part of the overall model, can be useful prior to RCTs (e.g., securing grant support). Such data assist in demonstrating positive outcomes associated with exposure to the treatment and with power analyses to inform RCTs. In both studies, all children received the same manualized, 6-week program. However, whereas half of the children were randomly assigned to receive performance feedback using the response–cost and IDN procedures, the other half received noncategorical feedback (i.e., specific feedback without point allocations or tracking using the point system and IDN). Given the limited sample size in the first group-based study (n = 21; Lopata, Thomeer, Volker, & Nida, 2006) comparisons were limited to three scales. Pre- and poststudy comparisons reflected significant improvements (main effects) for the overall program for four of the six rating scale comparisons. The most consistent finding was the significant improvement in social skills reported by both parents and staff. While no differences were found based on the feedback format, the small sample size suggested that feedback type should be further examined with a larger sample. Overall treatment fidelity was 87% across the 6-week treatment.

Based on limitations in the original group-based study, a second study (Lopata, Thomeer, Volker, Nida, & Lee, 2008) was conducted with a larger sample (n = 54) and an expanded number of outcome measures, including a satisfaction survey. Significant findings (main effects and/or interactions) were found for 11 of the 12 rating scale comparisons (parent and staff ratings using six scales). While parent ratings reflected significant improvements for all but one scale (i.e., atypicality) and no differences between the feedback formats, staff ratings suggested that the response–cost and IDN procedures may have therapeutic benefits. These benefits were on the negatively oriented scales (problem behavior symptoms, withdrawal, and odd behaviors), and suggested that the contingent and categorically based feedback system may assist in reducing undesired behaviors. Feasibility was supported in high levels of treatment fidelity ($\geq$ 95% across the program) and parent-rated satisfaction with the program. Despite the positive findings, the studies lacked a no-treatment comparison group, relied predominantly on rating scales to assess outcomes, and made no statistical adjustments for multiple comparisons. Additionally, the Atypicality subscale (used as a proxy for ASD symptoms) was yielding inconsistent findings and appeared to lack adequate sensitivity, suggesting the need for a different ASD measure.

Phase 3: RCT

To overcome the weaknesses in the prior trials, Lopata, Thomeer, et al. (2010) conducted an RCT that included a control group. Given the therapeutic benefit associated with the response–cost and IDN feedback formats in the prior study, they were retained in the treatment protocol for the RCT. Direct child measures were added, along with a scale specifically measuring ASD symptoms (i.e., Social Responsiveness Scale [SRS]). Children were randomly assigned to treatment or wait-list control conditions. The protocol was administered in a 5-week format (five treatment cycles per day) in this RCT to ensure that the wait-list children received their treatment following the treatment trial. The seven primary outcome measures comprised three direct child measures and four parent rating scales. These measures assessed skills taught in the program, broader adaptive skills, and ASD symptoms. The secondary outcome measures (i.e., four staff-completed rating scales) were used to corroborate parent ratings. While all seven primary measures yielded significant posttest differences favoring the treatment group, five remained significant following the correction for multiple comparisons, including two of the three direct child measures (i.e., knowledge of target skills and interpretation of nonliteral language skills) and three of the four parent rating scales (i.e., target social skills, ASD symptoms, and withdrawal). Secondary staff ratings were all significant following the correction for multiple comparisons and corroborated parent ratings. Feasibility was supported in high levels of fidelity (≥ 94%) and parent, child, and staff satisfaction. Data were also collected on interobserver agreement for the fidelity measures. Results indicated an average per session agreement (across individual intervention elements) of 97.2%. Effect size estimates were primarily medium to large and uniformly favored the treatment group.

FUTURE DIRECTIONS

Results of these studies have supported the efficacy of the comprehensive summer protocol in reducing ASD symptoms and increasing adaptive performance across a range of areas. While the Phase 3—RCT (Lopata, Thomeer, et al., 2010) provides the strongest evidence of efficacy, results from a single RCT should be viewed not as decisive but rather as a contribution to the larger evidence base (Lord et al., 2005). Our team has since conducted a replication RCT, and preliminary results largely parallel the original RCT. Additional replication RCTs by other research teams would provide important information on exportability and the efficacy of the program. A large-scale, multisite RCT would also be beneficial.

The studies of the summer program described in the previous section were conducted under highly controlled research conditions. According to Lord et al. (2005), nearly all such programs have been university- or research-center-based, with few programs evaluated in community or school settings. Given the support for the summer program in the Phase 3—RCT, a Phase 4—Community Effectiveness Trial was recently completed. According to the NIMH working-group guidelines (Smith et al., 2007), Phase 4 studies involve assessment of "whether similar outcomes can be achieved when the intervention is applied outside specialized research centers, in real world settings by community practitioners" (p. 362). In the Phase 4 trial, the program was conducted by a local ASD service agency that was independent of the study. Preliminary results indicated significant improvements on four of six primary measures (i.e., direct child measure and three parent ratings) and all four secondary staff-rating measures (Lopata, Toomey, Thomeer, et al., 2012). These findings, and the accompanying effect sizes, were remarkably similar to the Phase 3—RCT; however, they should be considered preliminary, because there was no comparison (control) group. A large-scale Phase 4 trial is a logical next step in the evaluation process.

There is also a significant need for comprehensive school-based interventions (CSBIs) for children with HFASD, yet few exist. This is especially challenging in that most educational professionals lack knowledge of or have expertise in HFASD/ASD treatment research (Lord et al., 2005). To address the need for a CSBI for children with HFASD, our team recently completed a 3-year pilot study involving adaptation of the summer program protocol into a CSBI, assessment of feasibility, and initial evaluation of child outcomes. The process and outcomes of the adaptation and component trials are detailed in Thomeer (2012). Results of the 10-month CSBI open-trial (Lopata et al., 2012) indicated significant pre- to poststudy improvements on eight of nine outcome measures (i.e., direct child measures assessing knowledge of target social skills, recognition of emotional expressions taught in treatment, and broader emotion recognition skills; teacher ratings of skills taught in the program and ASD symptoms; and parent ratings of skills taught in the program, ASD symptoms, and broader social skills; effect sizes medium and large). Fidelity ratings for implementation by school staff were consistently high (approximately 90%), and parent and staff ratings of acceptability and satisfaction were also high. Assessment of the CSBI protocol in a randomized trial is the next step in this line of research.

Ongoing work based on the comprehensive psychosocial summer program includes evaluation of new modules within the standard program protocol. Dismantling studies would also provide valuable information on the relative contribution of the different components of the program. This is a challenge for all researchers evaluating comprehensive treatment protocols, because the comprehensive nature of the intervention makes it difficult to pinpoint a specific component(s) or mechanism(s) responsible for gains (Lord et al., 2005). Finally, future studies should attempt to identify features of children with HFASD who show greater responsiveness to the program. While this has been investigated in other autism treatment studies by examining children who exhibited *best outcomes* (e.g., Smith, Groen, & Wynn, 2000), it may also be beneficial to examine predictors of responsiveness across a number of continuous-scale outcome measures (i.e., amount of change) instead of categorically (i.e., best outcomes).

REFERENCES

American Psychiatric Association. (2000). *Diagnostic and statistical manual of mental disorders* (4th ed., text rev.). Washington, DC: Author.

American Psychiatric Association. (2013). *Diagnostic and statistical manual of mental disorders* (5th ed.). Arlington, VA: Author.

Baron-Cohen, S., Jolliffe, T., Mortimore, C., & Robertson, M. (1997). Another advanced test of theory of mind: Evidence from very high functioning adults with autism or Asperger syndrome. *Journal of Child Psychology and Psychiatry, 38*, 813–822.

Bellini, S., Peters, J. K., Benner, L., & Hopf, A. (2007). A meta-analysis of school-based social skills interventions for children with autism spectrum disorders. *Remedial and Special Education, 28*(3), 153–162.

Carothers, D. E., & Taylor, R. L. (2004). Social cognitive processing in elementary school children with Asperger syndrome. *Education and Training in Developmental Disabilities, 39*(2), 177–187.

Carrington, S., Templeton, E., & Papinczak, T. (2003). Adolescents with Asperger syndrome and perceptions of friendships. *Focus on Autism and Other Developmental Disabilities, 18*, 211–218.

Carrow-Woolfolk, E. (1999). *Comprehensive Assessment of Spoken Language.* Circle Pines, MN: American Guidance Service.

Church, C., Alisanski, S., & Amanullah, S. (2000). The social, behavioral, and academic experiences of children with Asperger syndrome. *Focus on Autism and Other Developmental Disabilities, 15*(1), 12–20.

Cohn, J. F., & Ekman, P. (2005). Measuring facial action. In J. A. Harrigan, R. Rosenthal, & K. R. Scherer (Eds.), *The new handbook of methods in nonverbal behavior research* (pp. 9–64). New York: Oxford University Press.

Constantino, J. H., & Gruber, C. P. (2005). *Social Responsiveness Scale.* Los Angeles: Western Psychological Services.

Downs, A., & Smith, T. (2004). Emotional understanding, cooperation, and social behavior in high-functioning children with autism. *Journal of Autism and Developmental Disorders, 34*, 625–635.

Goldstein, A. P., McGinnis, E., Sprafkin, R. P., Gershaw, N. J., & Klein, P. (1997). *Skillstreaming the adolescent: New strategies and perspectives for teaching prosocial skills* (Rev. ed.). Champaign, IL: Research Press.

Howlin, P., Baron-Cohen, S., & Hadwin, J. (1999). *Teaching children with autism to mind-read: A practical guide for teachers and parents.* West Sussex, UK: Wiley.

Klin, A., McPartland, J., & Volkmar, F. R. (2005). Asperger syndrome. In F. R. Volkmar, R. Paul, A. Klin, & D. Cohen (Eds.), *Handbook of autism and pervasive developmental disorders: Vol 1. Diagnosis, development, neurobiology, and behavior* (3rd ed., pp. 88–125). Hoboken, NJ: Wiley.

Klin, A., Sparrow, S. S., Marans, W. D., Carter, A., & Volkmar, F. R. (2000). Assessment issues in children and adolescents with Asperger syndrome. In A. Klin, F. R. Volkmar, & S. S. Sparrow (Eds.), *Asperger syndrome* (309–339). New York: Guilford Press.

Klin, A., & Volkmar, F. R. (2000). Treatment and intervention guidelines for individuals with Aspergers syndrome. In A. Klin, F. R. Volkmar, & S. S. Sparrow (Eds.), *Asperger syndrome* (pp. 340–366). New York: Guilford Press.

Koenig, K., White, S. W., Pachler, M., Lau, M., Lewis, M., Klin, A., et al. (2010). Promoting social skill development in children with pervasive developmental disorders: A feasibility and efficacy study. *Journal of Autism and Developmental Disorders, 40*, 1209–1218.

Laurent, A. C., & Rubin, E. (2004). Challenges in emotion regulation in Asperger syndrome and high-functioning autism. *Topics in Language Disorders, 24*(4), 286–297.

Lindner, J. L., & Rosén, L. A. (2006). Decoding of emotion through facial expression, prosody and verbal content in children and adolescents with Asperger's syndrome. *Journal of Autism and Developmental Disorders, 36,* 769–777.

Lopata, C., Thomeer, M. L., Volker, M. A., Lee, G. K., Smith, T. H., Rodgers, J. D., et al. (2012). Open-trial pilot study of a comprehensive school-based intervention for high-functioning autism spectrum disorders. *Remedial and Special Education.* Available at *http://intl-rse.sagepub.com.*

Lopata, C., Thomeer, M. L., Volker, M. A., & Nida, R. E. (2006). Effectiveness of a cognitive-behavioral treatment on the social behaviors of children with Asperger disorder. *Focus on Autism and Other Developmental Disabilities, 21,* 237–244.

Lopata, C., Thomeer, M. L., Volker, M. A., Nida, R. E., & Lee, G. K. (2008). Effectiveness of a manualized summer social treatment program for high-functioning children with autism spectrum disorders. *Journal of Autism and Developmental Disorders, 38*(5), 890–904.

Lopata, C., Thomeer, M. L., Volker, M. A., Toomey, J. A., Nida, R. E., Lee, G. K., et al. (2010). RCT of a manualized social treatment for high-functioning autism spectrum disorders. *Journal of Autism and Developmental Disorders, 40*(11), 1297–1310.

Lopata, C., Toomey, J. A., Fox, J. D., Volker, M. A., Chow, S. Y., Thomeer, M. L., et al. (2010). Anxiety and depression in children with HFASDs: Symptom levels and source differences. *Journal of Abnormal Child Psychology, 38*(6), 765–776.

Lopata, C., Toomey, J. A., Thomeer, M. L., Fox, J. D., Meichenbaum, D., Volker, M. A., et al. (2012, May). *Phase IV—Community Effectiveness Trial of a Psychosocial Treatment for Children with HFASDs.* Poster presented at the International Meeting for Autism Research (IMFAR) Conference, Toronto, Canada.

Lopata, C., Volker, M. A., Toomey, J. A., Chow, S. Y., & Thomeer, M. L. (2008). Asperger's and other high functioning autism spectrum disorders: A review of group-based social enhancement research and a model for school-based social intervention. In D. H. Molina (Ed.), *School psychology: 21st century issues and challenges* (pp. 299–325). Hauppauge, NY: Nova Science.

Lord, C., Wagner, A., Rogers, S., Szatmari, P., Aman, M., Charman, T., et al. (2005). Challenges in evaluating psychosocial interventions for autistic spectrum disorders. *Journal of Autism and Developmental Disorders, 35*(6), 695–708.

Macintosh, K., & Dissanayake, C. (2006). Social skills and problem behaviors in school aged children with high-functioning autism and Asperger's disorder. *Journal of Autism and Developmental Disorders, 36,* 1065–1076.

Marans, W. D., Rubin, E., & Laurent, A. (2005). Addressing social communication skills in individuals with high-functioning autism and Asperger syndrome: Critical priorities in educational programming. In F. R. Volkmar, R. Paul, A. Klin, & D. Cohen (Eds.), *Handbook of autism and pervasive developmental disorders: Vol. 2. Assessment, interventions and policy* (3rd ed., pp. 977–1102). Hoboken, NJ: Wiley.

McConnell, S. (2002). Interventions to facilitate social interaction for young children with autism: Review of available research and recommendations for educational intervention and future research. *Journal of Autism and Developmental Disorders, 32*(5), 351–372.

McGinnis, E., & Goldstein, A. P. (1997). *Skillstreaming the elementary school child: New strategies and perspectives for teaching prosocial skills* (rev. ed.). Champaign, IL: Research Press.

Nowicki, S. (1997). *Instructional manual for the Receptive Tests of the Diagnostic Analysis of Nonverbal Accuracy 2.* Atlanta: Peachtree.

Odom, S. L., Boyd, B. A., Hall, L. J., & Hume, K. (2010). Evaluation of comprehensive treatment models for individuals with autism spectrum disorders. *Journal of Autism and Developmental Disorders, 40,* 425–436.

Portway, S. M., & Johnson, B. (2005). Do you know I have Asperger's syndrome?: Risks of a non-obvious disability. *Health, Risk and Society, 7*(1), 73–83.

Rao, P. A., Beidel, D. C., & Murray, M. J. (2008). Social skills interventions for children with Asperger's syndrome or high-functioning autism: A review and recommendations. *Journal of Autism and Developmental Disorders, 38*(2), 353–361.

Reichow, B., & Volkmar, F. R. (2010). Social skills interventions for individuals with autism: Evaluation for evidence-based practices within a best evidence synthesis framework. *Journal of Autism and Developmental Disorders, 40*(2), 149–166.

Reynolds, C. R., & Kamphaus, R. W. (1992, 1998). *Behavior Assessment System for Children, manual.* Circle Pines, MN: American Guidance Service.

Reynolds, C. R., & Kamphaus, R. W. (2004). *Behavior Assessment System for Children—Second Edition.* Circle Pines, MN: American Guidance Service.

Safran, S. P., Safran, J. S., & Ellis, K. (2003). Intervention ABCs for children with Asperger syndrome. *Topics in Language Disorders, 23,* 154–165.

Shattuck, P. T., Wagner, M., Narendorf, S., Sterzing, P., & Hensley, M. (2011). Post–high school service use among young adults with an autism spectrum disorder. *Archives of Pediatrics and Adolescent Medicine, 165*(2), 141–146.

Smith, T., Groen, A. D., & Wynn, J. W. (2000). Randomized trial of intensive early intervention for children with pervasive developmental disorder. *American Journal on Mental Retardation, 105*(4), 269–285.

Smith, T., Scahill, L., Dawson, G., Guthrie, D., Lord, C., Odom, S., et al. (2007). Designing research studies on psychosocial interventions in autism. *Journal of Autism and Developmental Disorders, 37*(2), 354–366.

Thomeer, M. L. (2012). Collaborative development and component trials of a comprehensive school-based intervention for children with HFASDs. *Psychology in the Schools, 49*(10), 955–962.

Toomey, J. A., Lopata, C., Volker, M. A., & Thomeer, M. L. (2009). Comprehensive intervention for high-functioning autism spectrum disorders: An in-depth case study. In M. T. Burton (Eds.), *Special education in the 21st century* (pp. 95–118). Hauppauge, NY: Nova Science.

Volker, M. A., & Lopata, C. (2008). Autism: A review of biological bases, assessment, and intervention. *School Psychology Quarterly, 23*(2), 258–270.

Volker, M. A., Lopata, C., Smerbeck, A. M., Knoll, V., Thomeer, M. L., Toomey, J. A., et al. (2010). BASC-2 PRS profiles for students with high-functioning autism spectrum disorders. *Journal of Autism and Developmental Disorders, 40*, 188–199.

White, S. W., Koenig, K., & Scahill, L. (2007). Social skills development in children with autism spectrum disorders: A review of the intervention research. *Journal of Autism and Developmental Disorders, 37*(10), 1858–1868.

10

Cognitive–Behavioral–Ecological Intervention to Facilitate Social–Emotional Understanding and Social Interaction in Youth with High-Functioning ASD

Nirit Bauminger-Zviely

HISTORICAL BACKGROUND AND SIGNIFICANCE OF THE TREATMENT

Social functioning—more specifically, interacting with peers and understanding social situations—is a lifelong struggle for individuals with autism spectrum disorders (ASD) at different levels of functioning. Billstedt, Gillberg, and Gillberg (2007) recently demonstrated the persistence of the social-communicative reciprocity deficit in ASD from early childhood into adulthood. In their study, 15 of 22 symptoms of deficient social interaction skills were still present in adulthood for half or more of their sample. Major difficulties appeared in adults' reciprocal peer interactions, which were infrequent as well as inappropriate, including inappropriate emotional responses to peers; a one-sided, self-centered social approach; infrequent physical expressions of affection; inappropriate conventions; and poor or unfocused eye contact. Predictors of better adult outcomes were speech before 5 years and higher IQ; higher-functioning individuals scored better.

Indeed, ASD research on children has also linked IQ with peer interaction outcomes. For example, children with an IQ over 85 had more friends than those with an IQ under 85 (Mazurek & Kanne, 2010), and higher Verbal IQ correlated with better dyadic friendship qualities such as responsiveness and coordinated play (e.g., Bauminger et al., 2008). Scholars have speculated that this group of children with higher cognitive capabilities may rely on cognitive efforts to deal more effectively with their social and emotional world—termed the *cognitive compensation hypothesis* (e.g., Kasari, Chamberlain, & Bauminger, 2001). Yet in the dynamic, multifaceted world of social-emotional stimuli and behavior, even the stronger cognitive abilities of these children with HFASD cannot fully compensate for their social deficit.

Better social functioning in children with HFASD than in their cognitively lower functioning counterparts presents only part of the complex social deficit in HFASD, because individuals with HFASD continue to lag way behind their typically developing agemates. These gaps in peer interaction, friendship, and social cognition in these individuals with HFASD compared with typical peers seem to correlate with high levels of depression, anxiety, and loneliness, especially in adolescence (e.g., Locke, Ishijima, Kasari, & London, 2010; White & Roberson-Nay, 2009). Recent reports from the Centers for Disease Control and Prevention (2009) indicate that about 60% of U.S. school-age children (age 8+) with ASD function above the retardation level; therefore, children with HFASD comprise a substantial group along the autism spectrum that requires special consideration when designing social interventions.

To set the stage for the proposed intervention guidelines, I first review the multidimensional social deficit in HFASD, as well as recent multimodal social intervention studies designed specifically for HFASD that adopt cognitive-behavioral therapy (CBT) principles. Next, I present a multidimensional social intervention for HFASD that combines CBT with ecological treatment (Bauminger, 2002, 2007a, 2007b), emphasizing its practical aspects and research supporting its efficacy. Finally, I end with suggestions for future research in the area of social intervention for school-age children with HFASD.

THE MULTIDIMENSIONAL SOCIAL DEFICIT IN HFASD: SOCIAL COGNITION AND SOCIAL INTERACTION

The social deficit in HFASD is multifaceted and includes difficulties in understanding social stimuli and cues, as well as difficulties with social-pragmatic behaviors within dyadic and peer-group interactions. Another way to conceptualize the deficit is that it affects input (i.e., cognitive processing of information) and output (i.e., socially directed behaviors) of the individual.

Social Cognition Deficits

Social cognition encompasses the processes undertaken to make sense of social-emotional situations and stimuli. Research has highlighted impairments in HFASD in various social-cognitive capabilities. Specifically, researchers identified social perception deficits, including the very basic prerequisites of social interaction, such as (1) deficits in attending to dynamic social stimuli (e.g., children with HFASD looked less at others' eyes and more at the mouth or body region; Klin, Jones, Schultz, Volkmar, & Cohen, 2002), and (2) deficits in encoding social stimuli (e.g., children with HFASD needed more prompts to recall vignette details and added erroneous information that was not in the vignette; Channon, Charman, Heap, Crawford, & Rios, 2001). Researchers also identified social understanding deficits in children with HFASD, such as (1) limited understanding of social norms, rules, and constructs (e.g., Nah & Poon, 2011); (2) impaired social problem-solving skills, mainly difficulties in understanding the social appropriateness and effectiveness of solutions to social problems (e.g., Channon et al., 2001); and (3) deficient understanding of nonliteral language, such as irony (e.g., Pexman et al., 2011).

Emotional understanding and recognition is another aspect of social cognition that is hampered in HFASD. Whereas the ability to recognize prototypical basic emotions in others (e.g., happiness, sadness, fear, anger) seems relatively intact in HFASD, awareness of one's own negative basic emotions and ability to understand basic emotions' causes are less consistently reported (e.g., Begeer, Koot, Rieffe, Terwoqt, & Stegge, 2008). A more compelling deficit in emotional understanding in HFASD regards understanding socially complex emotions such as pride, embarrassment, or guilt. One cannot identify these emotions by simply focusing on another person's facial expression like one can for basic emotions. The understanding of this class of emotions requires consideration of the social situation, recognition of body gestures and intonations, as well as comprehension of the mental states experienced by the situation's participants (Lewis, 1993). Compared with typically developing agemates, children with HFASD showed a narrower knowledge of complex emotions when asked to provide personal examples; they provided general, scripted examples of such emotions rather than specific, personal ones. They also tended to omit important references to an audience when providing examples of complex emotions such as embarrassment. Thus, the examples they provided of complex emotions (e.g., pride in receiving a video game) were indistinguishable from basic emotions (see reviews in Begeer et al., 2008; Kasari et al., 2001).

Social Interaction Deficits

Another important aspect of the social deficit in HFASD involves children's actual social and emotional behaviors, as manifested during social interaction processes with peers. Ongoing peer and group interactions comprise a unique area of difficulty for HFASD across ages and diagnostic criteria (American Psychiatric Association, 2013). Peer ratings of children with HFASD revealed their socially peripheral status in their classroom and fewer reciprocal friendships than typically developing children (e.g., Kasari, Locke, Gulsrud, & Rotheram-Fuller, 2011; Locke et al., 2010). Recent findings attest to a much greater risk in children with HFASD compared to children without ASD, for being bullied and victimized by peers (e.g., Cappadocia, Weiss, & Pepler, 2012). Low social participation rates in children with HFASD correlate with a poorer quality of peer interaction than that in their typical counterparts, as measured by lower social initiation rates; higher rates of passive social behaviors (e.g., looking or maintaining close proximity); higher frequencies of solitary play and of functional communication (exchange of information) rather than social-interactive-cooperative behaviors (e.g., sharing or helping); and a specific difficulty in co-regulating their own behavior with peers' social behavior to maintain and develop continuous interactions and conversations (e.g., Landa, 2000; Machintosh & Dissnanyake, 2006; van Ommeren, Begeer, Scheeren, & Koot, 2012).

Furthermore, these children's difficulties in understanding other minds, as well as difficulties with executive functioning skills, mainly attention shifting and flexibility (e.g., Volkmar, Lord, Bailey, Schultz, & Klin, 2004), compound the challenges posed by heightened social demands. Thus, the most typical social situations in the school setting, namely, nonstructured social situations (e.g., school recess) and interactions that involve a group rather than a dyad (i.e., one-on-one peer interactions), pose the highest social challenges for children with HFASD. As a result, enhancement of cooperative skills and social conversation skills in dyadic and group peer interactions, located in nonstructured naturalistic social situations (e.g., at school), should comprise basic ingredients of every social intervention for HFASD.

Summary of Multidimensional Deficit

In summary, the deficit in social-cognitive processes in children and adolescents with HFASD is broad and extensive, encompassing social perception processes and social and emotional understanding, as well as social interactive behaviors. Social interventions targeting the domain of social cognition, then, should focus on facilitating children's social-emotional understanding capabilities, with an emphasis on comprehending social constructs, norms, and rules, as well as understanding various emotions at different levels of complexity. Such interventions should teach children with HFASD to attend to and read social cues in diverse social situations; help them learn to provide accurate and socially relevant interpretations of social stimuli and situations; and enhance their ability to judge the social appropriateness of behavioral alternatives for different social tasks.

If children with HFASD indeed compensate for their multidimensional social deficit as suggested (e.g., Kasari et al., 2001), by relying on their relatively higher cognitive capabilities, researchers still have a long way to go in developing effective treatment techniques to help these children use this compensatory mechanism more efficiently. Designing treatments to target children's better understanding of social interactions and more adaptive reciprocal behaviors during social interaction is a great challenge for interventionists, especially because it is hard to devise a consistent, clear set of rules for teaching youngsters about the dynamic social world and the ever-changing social stimuli they might encounter. Treatment, therefore, should be multifaceted, addressing both social-cognitive and social-behavioral deficits. Furthermore, interventions should help children integrate their learned social-emotional knowledge, with its implications for day-to-day spontaneous interactions with peers, and vice versa. All told, social intervention planners need to shift their focus from a skills orientation to a more thorough integration of the various aspects of social functioning, tapping social behavioral skills and social-cognitive understanding. And finally, due to the fact that most school-age children with HFASD are integrated into regular education, where they experience social difficulties on a daily basis, treatment should move from the controlled laboratory setting to more naturalistic, "real life" social settings in the school or community. As I explain in the following section, to design multifaceted social interventions specifically for HFASD, researchers have adopted CBT principles.

MULTIFACETED SOCIAL INTERVENTIONS FOR HFASD

This section reviews prior empirical research on the implementation and evaluation of multifaceted cognitive and behavioral procedures in combination with social skills training to enhance integral social functioning in

HFASD. *Multimodal* studies (see Table 10.1) combined training in both social-cognitive skills and social-interactive skills (rather than focusing on only social-cognitive skills, such as theory of mind [ToM] skills, or behavioral interactive skills, such as collaboration) and were CBT-oriented, using cognitive mediation as a channel for changing social behavior (for expansion on CBT conceptual bases and modifications applied to ASD, see Scarpa & Lorenzi, Chapter 1, and Attwood & Scarpa, Chapter 2, this volume). In the next section, I detail reviewed CBT-based studies' aims and social targets, identified populations, intervention agents and settings, cognitive and behavioral techniques, and outcomes.

Aims and Social Targets of the Reviewed Studies

All of the reviewed studies included training in social-interactive skills to enhance peer interaction, cooperation, and interactive play and/or social conversation. Regarding social-cognitive aims, the most prevalent intervention target in the reviewed research was teaching ToM and perspective taking (77%; $n = 7$); followed by teaching emotion recognition (66%; $n = 6$), with or without emotion regulation and management of anxiety and anger. Only a few studies named the specific target emotions for recognition, hindering estimations of the range of emotions taught. Specified emotions included basic ones (happy, sad, angry, and afraid; e.g., Solomon, Goodlin-Jones, & Anders, 2004) and more complex ones (guilt, embarrassment, suspicion, and teasing: Beaumont & Sofronoff, 2008; pride, guilt, and embarrassment: Solomon et al., 2004). Interventions taught emotion recognition in oneself and others, and in various social situations, including teaching both physiological and situational cues to identify each of the emotions. Two other social-cognitive aims appeared at a lower prevalence: executive functions, such as, problem solving (33%, $n = 3$) and nonliteral language, such as idioms and double meanings (11%, $n = 1$).

HFASD Populations

Six studies (66%) included preadolescents (8–12 years); two (22%) included adolescents (11–14 years); and one included a large age range (6–16 years). Four studies randomly assigned participants into experimental and wait-list control groups, and one control group underwent traditional social skills training unspecific to HFASD. Three other studies implemented pre- and postassessment procedures, and one study had a single-case design. Most interventions ($n = 7$, 66%) used a small-group format comprising only individuals with HFASD; two studies used learning process in a one-on-one

TABLE 10.1. Multidimensional CBT-Oriented Social Intervention in HFASD

Study	Aims	Participants	Agents	Setting	Techniques	Outcomes
Beaumont & Sofronoff (2008)	• Emotion recognition and management (anxiety and anger) • Social conversation • Interactive play • Coping with bullying	Children ages 7.5–11 years • EX: $n = 26$; CA = 9.64 • WL: $n = 23$; CA = 9.81	• Parent–child interaction via computer game • Group social skills for HFASD led by therapists	University	• Affective education (through computer game) • Social problem solving • Modeling • Role play • Homework • Parent training • Group discussion	• EX > WL on parents' social skills questionnaires • EX > WL on emotion management (coping with anxiety and bullying at school) • EX = WL on pre–post facial and body gesture recognition • Due to high attrition rates on teacher questionnaire effect was not clear
DeRosier, Swick, Ornstein-Davis, Sturtz-McMillen, & Matthews (2011)	• Modify the S.S.GRIN (Social Skills Group Intervention) to HFASD • Enhance social skills in: • Communication (verbal–nonverbal social/emotional cues) • Working with others (ToM & cooperation) • Peer interaction	Children ages 8–12 years • EX: $n = 27$; training adapted to HFASD • CO: $n = 28$; traditional social skills training, non-HFASD-specific	• Group intervention for HFASD by trained staff • Parent coached community social missions	• Main treatment: private, community-based practice • Generalization: Community social tasks coached by parents	• Group intervention • Didactic instruction (concept clarification and social learning) • Active practice through • Role playing • Modeling • Homework • Community-based activities • Parent training	• EX > CO on all parents' measures: • Social Responsivenes Scale (SRS): awareness; communication; reduced autistic mannerisms • Social Skills Scale—the Achieved Learning Questionnaire (ALQ) • Social self-efficacy • EX = CO on child's reported loneliness scale and on self-reported social efficacy

232

| Feng, Lo, Tsai, & Cartledge (2008) | • ToM
• Social interaction | Single case (age, 11 years, 6th grade) | • One-on-one training by teachers
• Teacher-led group (with peers having learning disabilities, mild mental retardation) | School, in and out of resource room | • Systematic teaching of ToM
• Active practice through
 ○ Modeling
 ○ Role play
• Performance feedback in one-on-one and group settings | • Pre < post on qualitative ToM measure including eight real-life vignettes on different ToM levels (first- and second-order false belief)
• Pre < post on social interaction and its generalization, based on observations (in class during teaching and outside class at lunchtime and recess); showing higher frequency and better quality of socially appropriate behaviors at lunchtime and recess after treatment |
| Lopata, Thomeer, Volker, Toomey, Nida, Lee, Smerbeck, & Rodgers (2010) | Social skills development:
• Interest expansion
• Face–emotion recognition
• Interpretation of nonliteral language | Children ages 7–12 years
• EX: $n = 18$; CA = 9.39
• WL: $n = 18$; CA = 9.56 | Groups led by professionals (students in education and psychology) | Summer program on college campus using group rooms | • Learning; direct instruction, modeling, role-playing, performance feedback, and learning transfer
• Affective education
• Problem solving
• Concept clarification of nonliteral language
• Practicing;
Cooperative dyadic and group activities, modeling, role play, performance feedback, and homework | • EX > WL on parent rating scales:
• SRS
• Adapted Skillstreaming Checklist (ASC) assessing skills taught in the social program
• Behavior Assessment System for Children (BASC-2) assessing withdrawal
• EX > WL on children's scales:
• Skillstreaming knowledge assessment (SKA) of skills taught in the social program
• Idiomatic Language (CASL) |

(continued)

233

TABLE 10.1. (*continued*)

Study	Aims	Participants	Agents	Setting	Techniques	Outcomes
					• Response–cost behavioral system to increase prosocial behavior and decrease problematic behaviors • Small-group treatment of only HFASD • Parent training	• Staff reports (only for EX): • Pre > post on SRS, BASC-2 Withdrawal • Pre < post on ASC, BASC-2 Social Skills
Mackay, Knott, & Dunlop (2007)	• Social understanding (social and emotional perspective taking) • Social interaction (conversation skills, friendship skills)	Children ages 6–16 years $n = 46$	Groups led by diverse professionals (e.g., educators, psychologists)	In school during afterschool hours	• Teaching ToM • Concept clarification of social terms, skills, and norms (e.g., social conversation, friendship) • Group discussion • Role play • Small- and large-group activities and group games • Generalization through community outings (e.g., restaurant), homework • Feedback meeting with parents	• Pre < post on social skills questionnaires for parents and children (only for $n = 20$ pupils and $n = 38$ parents) • Pre < post on 65% of the identified skill deficits rated by parents; areas of major change included reduction in inappropriate social behavior and increase in awareness of, listening to, and acknowledgment of others' views

| Ozonoff & Miller (1995) | • ToM
• Social interaction
• Conversation skills | Children age 13 years
• EX: $n = 5$; CA = 13.8
• CO (no treatment): $n = 4$; CA = 13.6 | University staff

University | • Teaching ToM and perspective taking
• SST: Structured learning, modeling, role play, reinforcement, and feedback on performance of learned social skills; group discussions and activities | • EX > CO on composite score of false belief tasks; at posttest 65.4% of EX passed tasks that they did not pass at pretest, versus 23.5% in CO
• Pre = post for EX and for CO on parent and teacher reports of social competence |
| Solomon, Goodlin-Jones, & Anders (2004) | • ToM
• Executive function/problem solving
• Emotion recognition and regulation
• Conversation skills | Children ages 8–12 years
• EX: $n = 9$; including younger (CA = 8; FSIQ = 115) and older (CA = 10; FSIQ = 86) groups
• WL–CO: $n = 9$; Two groups matched on age and FSIQ | • Groups led by university staff (psychologists, psychiatrist, and a speech and language pathologist)
• Male university students who videotaped activities were instructed to serve as role models for participants

University | Group intervention (only EX):
• Affective education
• Problem solving
• Modeling
• Role play
• Group activities
• Psychoeducational training for parents | • EX > WL on:
• Emotional awareness as measured by facial expression recognition for simple emotions
• Executive functions as measured by problem-solving skills
• For EX only:
• Pre > post on self-reported depression for older group and for less cognitively able
• Tendency toward pre > post on mother-reported child depression
• Pre < post on parent-reported child problematic behaviors |

(continued)

TABLE 10.1. (*continued*)

Study	Aims	Participants	Agents	Setting	Techniques	Outcomes
Stichter, Herzog, Visovsky, Schmidt, Randolph, & Schultz, & Gage (2010)	SCI-A: Social Competence Intervention for Adolescents • ToM • Executive functions/problem solving • Emotion recognition and regulation • Conversation skills	Adolescents ages 11–14 years *n* = 27; CA = 12.57	Groups led by trained staff in special education	University	Group SCI-A adapted to HFASD: • Affective education • Structured, scaffolded learning that taught each skill based on former skills, and reinforced skills via the learning process • Skills modeling • Practice in structured and naturalistic activities • Parent education program (*n* = 17)	• Pre < post on: • SRS: awareness, cognition, motivation, communication, reduced autistic mannerisms • Behavior Rating Inventory of Executive Function (BRIEF; Parent Report): behavior regulation and metacognition • Emotion recognition through facial and eye express on • Test of Problem Solving (TOPS): making inferences on causes of problems, identifying potential solutions; however, participants were still below normative sample means
Stichter, O'Connor, Herzog, Lierheimer, & McGhee (2012)	SCI-E = SCI-A for elementary students	Children ages 6–10 years *n* = 20; CA = 8.77	Trained staff	University	SCI-E adapted to elementary-age children	• Pre < post on: • SRS-Parent—all subscales • SRS-Teacher—total; communication; motivation; reduced autistic mannerisms • TOPS-3: sequencing the problem scenarios • ToM: recognizing social mistakes (*faux pas* test)

Note. EX, experimental group; WL, wait-list group; CO, control group; CA, chronological age; CASL, Comprehensive Assessment of Spoken Language; FSIQ, Full Scale IQ.

(parent–child or teacher–student) format followed by social skills group treatment.

Agents and Settings

In all studies (except Feng, Lo, Tsai, & Cartledge, 2008) (88%), trained staff provided the treatment (psychology students, special education teachers), and the interventions took place at a university or private clinical diagnostic center. In Feng et al.'s single-case study, the agent was the child's teacher, in the school setting. To increase generalization, seven of the studies (66%) involved parents in psychoeducational training that scaffolded their interactions with their child and supported ongoing homework and activities in the home and community. One study (Beaumont & Sofronoff, 2008) involved teachers through handouts about treatment contents.

CBT Techniques

The reviewed studies implemented a mixture of cognitive and behavioral techniques. Cognitive techniques were mostly implemented during the didactic phase for social-cognitive skills rather than social-interactive skills. These included affective education (i.e., expanding the child's emotional repertoire and helping the child to recognize emotions in self and others, Attwood, 2004); problem solving (e.g., providing the child with schemas to perceive and analyze social situations by defining problems presented in short social vignettes, finding alternative solutions, and considering their social consequences; Bauminger, 2002); direct teaching of skills such as ToM and concept clarification, and expansion of social constructs (e.g., What is friendship?); and structured social learning (building social-cognitive capabilities in hierarchical order from basic to more complex skills, such as teaching first-order before second or higher order ToM; see Stichter et al., 2010).

CBT behavioral techniques appeared frequently for practicing and experiencing interactive cooperative skills and social conversation (across the different described studies in Table 10.1). Usually the teaching process in the different studies, included modeling of the targeted social behavior, followed by practice and rehearsal in a safe environment (e.g., within the small group through role play), followed by homework to apply the learned social behavior outside the treatment milieu (e.g., at home or in the community). Children received feedback and positive reinforcement for demonstrating newly acquired social behaviors. Groups were the most frequent treatment setting; indeed, almost all studies incorporated group discussions, cooperative activities, and games to increase social motivation and social engagement (for expansion on CBT technique, see Attwood & Scarpa, Chapter 2, this volume).

Outcomes

Per treatment objectives, research outcomes focus on (1) improvement in social-cognitive skills; (2) improvement in social-interactive cooperative skills and social conversation; and (3) generalization of treatment effects to children's natural social environments.

Social-Cognitive Outcomes

Interestingly, although ToM was a major stated aim in seven of the nine studies, treatment effects remained unclear. Not all of these studies directly evaluated ToM progress (e.g., DeRosier, Swick, Ornstein-Davis, Sturtz-McMillen, & Matthews, 2011; Mackay, Knott, & Dunlop, 2007), and those that did include ToM measures showed mixed results. In Ozonoff and Miller (1995), whereas 65.4% of children in the experimental group passed false-belief tasks at posttest that they had failed at pretest, only 23.5% in a wait-listed control group did so. Similarly, the single child studied in Feng et al. (2008) qualitatively improved on a test of real-life vignettes tapping different levels of ToM (i.e., first- and second-order false beliefs). However, in Solomon et al. (2004), both the experimental and wait-list groups showed better ToM performance at the posttest; thus, improvement in ToM could not be attributed to treatment. Furthermore, the adolescents with HFASD in Stichter et al. (2010) marginally improved their ability to attribute a mental state to another person by viewing only that person's eyes, whereas preadolescents with HFASD in Stichter, O'Connor, Herzog, Lierheimer, and McGhee (2012) did not replicate this improvement.

Importantly, children's ability to generalize their posttraining improvement in ToM to their actual social-interactive skills has yet to be determined. In Ozonoff and Miller (1995), parents and teachers reported no improvement in children's overall social skills, despite improvement in paper-and-pencil false-belief measures. However, in Stichter et al. (2012) parents reported improvement on the Social Responsiveness Scale (SRS; Constantino & Gruber, 2005), including improvement in social communication, which may indicate gains in children's actual social behaviors at home. Thus, effects of ToM training should be further examined, specifically children's ability to transfer theoretical understanding of others' mental states into a more pragmatic understanding of how to use this knowledge to develop more reciprocal peer interactions. Also, future research should compare the usefulness of teaching ToM directly through didactic methods to teaching ToM indirectly by emphasizing reciprocity during interactions experienced in the treatment process.

Recognition of simple emotions using the Diagnostic Analysis of Non-Verbal Accuracy 2—Child Facial Expressions (DANVA 2-CF; Nowicki & Carton, 1993) improved after treatment in both the experimental and the wait-list control groups in Solomon et al. (2004) and in the HFASD sample in Stichter et al. (2010). Yet Lopata et al. (2010) and Stichter et al. (2012) failed to replicate this improvement using a similar measure. Also, in Beaumont and Sofronoff (2008), both the experimental and wait-list control groups improved their emotion recognition capabilities from pretest to posttest, based on children's perceptions of facial expressions (e.g., happy, sad, angry, afraid, disgusted, and nicely surprised) and on posture cues, but the experimental group surpassed the wait-list group on emotional management and regulation. Altogether, although several studies did demonstrate progress in emotion recognition, treatment effects must be clarified, especially regarding the previously unexplored ability to recognize complex emotions or understand emotions in social situations.

Several interventions revealed participants' gains in different areas of social understanding, such as (1) problem solving (i.e., making inferences about problems' causes and finding potential solutions: Stichter et al., 2010; sequencing a problem scenario: Stichter et al., 2012, but participants remained below normative sample means; (2) global executive functions such as metacognition and behavior regulation (Stichter et al., 2010); and (3) understanding of idiomatic language and of social concepts (e.g., DeRosier et al., 2011; Lopata et al., 2010; Makay et al., 2007). Differences in research methodologies (e.g., controlled vs. uncontrolled, pre- and post-methodology; only HFASD participants; case study) preclude conclusions about general treatment effects for social-cognitive skills. Likewise, the interventions targeted different social-cognitive skills to represent broader capabilities in emotional and social understanding. Thus, although social-cognitive skills comprise the core of social interaction and may be improved through treatment, such interventions' effects on children's actual social-interactive skills require further inquiry.

Social-Interactive Outcomes

Inasmuch as almost no researchers observed children's peer interactions in their natural social environments, such as schools (other than Feng et al. [2008] for their single participant), or children's social conversation skills (the major behavioral goal of almost all the reviewed Interventions), it is difficult to establish a clear-cut picture about children's actual improvement in interactive skills such as conversational and cooperative capabilities. Studies mostly used adults' reports (typically, parents), including general social skills questionnaires and ratings of problematic behaviors, and self-reports (of loneliness, depression, and general social skills). These showed improvement, to some extent, in children's overall social skills and problematic behaviors. However, in some studies, parent informants were also part of the intervention or were well aware of treatment goals and procedures through psychoeducational training or homework assignments (e.g., Beaumont & Sofronoff, 2008; DeRosier et al., 2011; Lopata et al., 2010; Mackay et al., 2007; Solomon et al., 2004; Stichter et al., 2010, 2012). Indeed, in Ozonoff and Miller (1995) teachers and parents who were not actively involved in the treatment reported no improvement of the experimental group versus the wait-list group. Thus, parents are an important source of information on children's social skill gains, but their reports should be verified by objective measures such as direct observation of actual child behavior. Interestingly, Feng et al.'s (2008) observations revealed clear improvement in social interaction and its generalization, showing a higher frequency and quality of socially appropriate behaviors during lunchtime and recess interactions with peers. Importantly, parents in DeRosier et al. (2011) reported gains in their children's social efficacy after treatment, whereas children's self-reports showed no such improvement in social efficacy or in loneliness ratings. Thus, the insertion of objective observations into future research could close the gap between the various informants. To sum up, reports pinpointed improvement on general measures of social skills, but more objective evaluations of children's peer interaction skills and social conversations should provide a more robust picture of treatment effects.

Generalization and School-Based Outcomes

Each of the reviewed social interventions aimed to help children implement the learned skills in diverse social situations (e.g., group and dyadic interactions with a broad range of peers), in various social environments (e.g., home, community, school), and in coping with different social stimuli and tasks (e.g., developing a conversation, maintaining an interaction, reading and correctly using verbal and nonverbal social cues). However, it is still unresolved whether these multifaceted CBT-based social intervention procedures effectively led to the desired transfer and generalization. Parents' reports indicated some generalization of skills that were not directly taught in the treatment, perhaps implying some transfer of treatment gains into the home environment; however, information is lacking on generalization of treatment gains to the school environment. These shortcomings call for implementation of interventions in children's natural social environments, such as schools, to assess improvement during authentic, naturally occurring peer interactions. Indeed, a review demonstrated that single-case studies implemented in a child's typical classroom setting produced significantly higher intervention, maintenance, and generalization effects than interventions that involved removing the child from the classroom (Bellini, Peters, Benner, & Hopf, 2007).

The benefits of conducting treatments in the school setting are numerous. Schools offer spontaneous natural social settings for peer interaction, thereby enabling integration of learned social skills within children's actual social behaviors to increase generalization. School settings also integrate children's different social partners—teachers, parents, typical peers—and may incorporate trained professionals such as teachers, therapists, and psychologists as agents of social intervention. Most importantly, locating interventions in schools squarely addresses the social deficit of children with HFASD, which interferes with their social relationships, their adaptive functioning, and even their academic performance (e.g., Bellini et al., 2007). However, school-based social interventions for HFASD pose weighty challenges for school personnel due to limited time, resources, training, and supervision in the implementation of such treatments. They also pose methodological difficulties related to the need for randomized controlled trials or no-treatment control groups and to achieving treatment fidelity because of the multiple change agents involved (Mesibov & Shea, 2011). Thus, intervention effectiveness in school-age children's natural environments requires further study.

COGNITIVE-BEHAVIORAL-ECOLOGICAL INTERVENTION: PRACTICAL CONSIDERATIONS AND OVERVIEW OF SESSIONS

Conceptual Basis for the Intervention

The cognitive-behavioral-ecological intervention (CBE), a multifaceted social treatment that strives to enhance both social-cognitive capabilities and social-interactive skills, is based on the conceptual principles of CBT, which highlight the interplay between how children think, feel, and behave in social situations (e.g., Hart & Morgan, 1993). Also, CBE presumes (based on CBT) that cognitive processes mediate between social events and the person's typical enacted behavioral or emotional responses during those events. For example, a child who experienced social rejection may incorrectly interpret a peer's actions and emotions (e.g., misinterpreting the peer's smile and eye contact, intended as an invitation to play, as a hostile or mocking smile). Such misperceptions most likely lead to a set of incorrect social responses (e.g., fight-or-flight reactions). Within the CBE framework, treatment focuses on changing the child's cognitive-meditational processes, such as distorted thoughts or misperceptions of the social world and of social stimuli, including verbal and nonverbal social and emotional behaviors (Bauminger, 2002, 2007a, 2007b). Another theoretical assumption of CBE based on CBT is that social perception processes can influence behavior (Hart & Morgan, 1993). Thus, better cognitive understanding of the social world and modifications of thinking processes lead to more adaptive interpersonal functioning by modifying how children respond to social events, and by increasing children's understanding of their own emotional and behavioral reactions through the systematic implementation of cognitive strategies. CBE's adaptation of the CBT notion of the child as an active "cognitive constructor" of his or her social world corresponds to the "compensation hypothesis" for children with HFASD, which suggests that such children make cognitive efforts to learn about their social-emotional life through their relatively higher-functioning cognitive channel (Kasari, Chamberlain, & Bauminger, 2001). Therefore, in CBE, efforts are made to help children use their relatively advanced cognitive capabilities (versus low functioning ASD) in a more efficient ways. In the ecological theoretical framework (Bronfenbrenner, 1979), also the basis of CBE, treatment is taking place in the child's natural environment (school) and includes the child's main social-interactive agents (teachers, peers, and parents).

Main Components of the Intervention

Over the last decade, I developed a multidimensional, school-based CBE social intervention (CBE treatment; Bauminger 2002, 2007a, 2007b) that teachers implement in regular education school settings across Israel (for expansion on the CBE curriculum and procedures, see Bauminger-Zviely, 2013) . The integral CBE social intervention blends two intervention models: the CBE-dyadic social intervention (Bauminger, 2002, 2007b), and (2) the CBE-group social intervention (Bauminger, 2007a). Both CBE models are multidimensional and strive to facilitate children's social-cognitive capabilities (social and emotional understanding) and peer interaction capabilities (as in cooperation and social conversation). The CBE-dyadic model aims to facilitate one-on-one dyadic peer interaction, with an emphasis on both social initiation and the more basic emotional and social understanding capabilities (e.g., understanding basic emotions such as happiness, sadness, anger, and fear; understanding basic social concepts, such as what a friend is). The CBE-group intervention aims to facilitate peer group social interaction, with an emphasis on developing and maintaining such interactions and on the more advanced social-emotional understanding capabilities (e.g., understanding complex emotions such as embarrassment, pride, and loneliness, as well as irony, cynicism, and hidden emotions) and coping abilities (e.g., coping with group pressure and rejection). Both CBE social intervention models were implemented by children's special education teachers in schools for a full academic year, as part of the curriculum.

The CBE-Dyadic Intervention

This intervention model included three teacher–child lessons per week (totaling 3 hours) for 7 months, beginning with two preliminary stages: (1) concept clarification of important social constructs (e.g., What is social listening? Why are friends important?) and (2) emotional understanding and recognition (taught through affective education focusing mainly on basic emotions). The lessons then focused on teaching 10 social initiations essential for peer interaction, such as initiating a conversation with a friend; sharing experiences, thoughts, and feelings with a friend; and asking for help from a friend. The teacher introduced each type of social initiation as a problem to solve through several short social vignettes. For example, the following vignette illustrates how to initiate a conversation: "John went out at recess time and saw his friend Steve sitting alone. John would like to start a conversation with Steve, but he doesn't know how." Then the teacher and the child worked through the social problem-solving stages as follows: (1) recognizing the problem (the targeted social goal or task); (2) identifying the related emotion (e.g., anxiety when starting a conversation); (3) generation of social solutions to the problem (i.e., planning possible actions); (4) considering the social appropriateness of solutions based on their consequences ("What will happen if . . . ?"); and (5) choosing the social solution that best fits the defined social problem. Practice of the selected, desired solution (e.g., calling a friend and starting a conversation with him or her) included several stages: (1) with the teacher, through role play during the training sessions; (2) with a typical peer aide who met with the target child twice weekly, once at home and once during a school recess, while the teacher supervised, guided, and supported the peer aide along the different social tasks; and (3) with parents and siblings in the home environment, as homework. Involvement of typical peers who were "enforced collaborators" reduced the anxiety related to experiencing social tasks with an unfamiliar child. The teacher maintained ongoing contact with the parents, notifying them about the targeted social tasks, and obtaining feedback from them on the child's performance of the requested homework.

Thus, the teacher in the CBE-dyadic intervention had three main roles: (1) teaching the social problem model, affective education, and social understanding in the allotted 3 hours per week; (2) selecting, supporting, and guiding an assigned typical peer aide for each child participating in the training; and (3) informing the child's parents and the assigned peer aide about each targeted social skill that should be practiced with the child, and eliciting feedback on the child's performance. Teachers received training prior to the intervention that provided theoretical background on the unique social-emotional characteristics of children with HFASD, as well as practical training in CBT techniques. In addition, once or twice per month teachers were observed and supervised in the schools to provide support and ensure fidelity.

The CBE-Group Intervention

This intervention model included small, teacher-led social groups that met twice per week for 7 months at school. Each group comprised one to three children with HFASD and two typical agemates. Each child with HFASD had a third individual meeting with the teacher to work on intervention social tasks (e.g., preparing the child in advance, strengthening the learned skills, clarifying issues raised in the group session). The group social curriculum included 50 lessons on five main intervention topics: (1) understanding of social constructs (e.g., What is a group? Why is it important to participate in a group?) and of nonliteral language (e.g., humor); (2) emotional understanding (e.g., the recognition of complex emotions); (3) developing social conversation skills within a group and making group entry; (4) developing cooperative and joint engagement skills with peers, as well as prosocial behaviors (e.g., sharing, negotiating); and (5) developing strategies for managing stressful social situations. The group intervention, like the dyadic intervention, employed a mixture of cognitive CBT techniques (e.g., problem solving, concept clarification, affective education) and behavioral CBT techniques (e.g., modeling of the learned skill by the teacher or by group members; practice and rehearsal through group role play and cooperative social activities and games). As in the CBE-dyadic training, teachers received prior training on social-emotional characteristics of children with HFASD, on CBT treatment techniques, and on group interventions. Teachers' group work was observed and supervised throughout the school year, once or twice per month, to provide support and ensure fidelity.

RESEARCH TO DATE ON THE TREATMENT

Three empirical studies thus far have examined CBE's effectiveness in enhancing integral social competence in children with HFASD.

Research on the CBE-Dyadic Intervention

The main goals of the school-based CBE-dyadic interventions were to examine improvement from pretest to posttest on social-emotional understanding and on spontaneous dyadic social interactions among children with HFASD. A pilot study (n = 15; Bauminger, 2002) and a replication of the dyadic model with minor modifications, mainly to the methodology (n = 19; Bauminger, 2007b), both included children with an average or above Verbal IQ, but Verbal IQ in the pilot study (M = 84.87; range: 69–106) were somewhat lower than those in the replication study (M = 101.74; range: 75–128). The replication study also included a more limited age range (pilot: 8.05–17.33 years; replication: 7.7–11.6). Intervention procedure, structure, and content were similar in the two studies, but some evaluation measures and procedures differed.

The following four measures appeared in both studies. Two scales measured overt social behavior:

1. Observations of social interaction during school recesses with peers unrelated to the treatment assessed three social interaction domains (Bauminger, 2002).
   a. Positive social interaction (e.g., eye contact with smile, sharing experiences, talk that reflects an interest in another child).
   b. Negative social interaction (e.g., physical or verbal aggression, avoidance, looking away).
   c. Low-level social interaction (e.g., looking, standing in close proximity, functional communication of needs).
2. The Social Skills Rating System—Teacher version (SSRS-T; Gresham & Elliot, 1990) assessed three social skills dimensions: cooperation, assertion, and self-control.

Two scales were used to measure social cognition:

1. The Problem Solving Measure (PSM; Lochman & Lampron, 1986),
   assessing social problem solving and social understanding through
   nine hypothetical social problems (e.g., coping with teasing), each
   containing a beginning and an end, to which the child is asked
   to compose possible solutions. Solutions underwent coding for
   social and non-social content, relevancy, and passivity (the problem
   resolved itself) or activity (the child solved the problem).
2. The Emotion Inventory Measure (EIM; Seidner, Stipek, & Feshbach, 1988) assessed emotional knowledge by asking children to
   provide examples of a time they experienced basic (e.g., happy,
   sad) and complex emotions (e.g., proud, embarrassed). Responses
   underwent coding for knowledge of the emotions, inclusion of an
   audience, and specificity of the example (general stereotypical vs.
   specific personally experienced).

Several measures were unique to the replication study. The Affective Matching Measure (AMM; Bauminger, Shorr-Edelsztein, & Morash,
2005), assessing children's ability to recognize emotions from their social
context, exposed children to 12 different pictures depicting social scenarios
of different basic and complex emotions (sad, angry, proud, lonely). In each
picture, one figure (a child) lacked facial expression; thus, children needed
to identify the emotion based on the social context. Coding focused on
accuracy of identification and relevancy of the child's explanation for the
identified emotion. Two self-reports assessed children's loneliness feelings:
the Loneliness Rating Scale (Asher, Hymel, & Renshaw, 1984) and the Self-
Perception Profile of Children (Harter, 1985), which includes six domains:
Scholastic and Athletic Competence, Social Acceptance, Physical Appearance, Behavioral Conduct, and General Self-Worth. Other additions to the
replication study included (1) using observers and data collectors who were
blind to the intervention's specific aims; (2) collecting reports of children's
progress in social skills by regular teachers who were unrelated to the social
skills training implementation; and (3) observing social interactions not
only immediately at posttest but also 4 months later.

Findings from both studies indicated that children with HFASD pro-
gressed from pretest to posttest in both social-cognitive and social-interactive capabilities. Social-cognitive improvement emerged for the problem-
solving measure, in which children in both studies provided more relevant
solutions to the hypothetical social problems and suggested fewer nonsocial
solutions after treatment. Problem solving in the replication study was even
better, with children showing less passivity in their solution profile (i.e.,
they understood that social events occurred for a reason) and furnishing

a higher number of appropriate social solutions. Emotional understanding also improved in both studies, with interesting results demonstrating significant improvement in the quality of children's examples of emotional experiences. Change was more robust with regard to the understanding of complex emotions: After intervention, children provided examples for more complex emotions than they could before, included more attributions to an audience (which may imply gains in their sensitivity to others), and gave more specific examples related to personal experience rather than general dictionary one (perhaps implying better awareness of their inner emotional experiences). The addition of the emotion recognition measure in the replication study strengthened this line of results by showing better recognition of complex emotions in the pictured social scenarios after treatment. Thus, altogether, the CBE-dyadic treatment proved very effective in fostering children's knowledge of complex emotions and ability to solve social problems, both of which comprise specific deficits among children with HFASD.

Results of the two studies with regard to pre- and posttreatment change in social-interactive skills were also promising. Overall, observed spontaneous peer interactions during school recesses identified progress after treatment in positive social behaviors, specifically, increases in eye contact and sharing behaviors. In the pilot study only, pre- and posttreatment improvement also emerged for talk that reflected interest in another child. In addition, reductions in children's ritualistic behaviors and increases in children's functional communication emerged in the pilot study. Results of the replication supported this tendency but did not reach significance.

Long-term progress (4 months after treatment) measured in the replication study revealed a tendency for improvement in positive social interaction compared to pretest and immediate posttest. Also, low-level behaviors (e.g., social behaviors that are passive or not efficient) significantly decreased between the pretest and the 4-month interval. This continued improvement in children's interactive behaviors, even months after treatment terminated, may suggest a cumulative or "late bloomer" effect deserving further inquiry.

Last, reports by both regular and special education teachers in the replication study indicated pre- to posttreatment gains in these children's cooperation, assertion, and self-control. Social skill progress reported by regular teachers may reflect generalization of the child's newly learned social behaviors to other peers in regular classrooms. The regular education teachers were not part of the treatment, usually led by a special education teacher. Reports by the special education teachers in the pilot study resembled those of the replication study regarding children's improved cooperation and assertion.

Research on the CBE-Group Intervention

The main goals of the school-based CBE-group interventions were to examine improvement from pretest to posttest on advanced social-emotional understanding and on spontaneous peer-group social interactions among children with HFASD (Bauminger 2007a). In order to increase the number of participants for the group intervention, two groups (n = 26) of children with HFASD participated in this intervention: 11 children who had participated in the CBE-dyadic training in the previous year (chronological age [CA]) = 8.75 years; Verbal IQ = 104.09), and 15 new recruits (CA = 9.00 years; Verbal IQ = 110.62). Groups were matched according to CA; all IQ dimensions (Full Scale, Verbal, and Performance); and all Autism Diagnostic Interview—Revised dimensions—Social, Communication, and Repetitive Behaviors (Lord, Rutter, & LeCouteur, 1994).

The multidimensional study measures for the CBE-group intervention included social-cognitive and social-interactive assessments to examine children's pretest versus posttest change:

1. Direct treatment effects on children's social cognition were measured by three scales employed in the CBE-dyadic research: problem-solving using the PSM (Lochman & Lampron, 1986), emotional understanding using the AMM (Bauminger et al., 2005) and the EIM (Seidner et al., 1988).
2. Two indirect measures assessed generalization of treatment effects to crucial socio-cognitive areas that were not directly taught:
   a. ToM, assessed using five of Happé's (1994) Strange Stories (Lie, White Lie, Persuade, Double Bluff, and Hiding Emotions).
   b. Executive function, assessed using the Delis–Kaplan Executive Function System (D-KEFS; Delis, Kaplan, & Kramer, 2001), a nonsocial sorting subtest that asked children flexibly to reconstruct concepts by shape, size, and verbal content. The D-KEFS examined changes in children's general ability for concept formation and cognitive flexibility as a result of treatment.
3. Assessment of overt interactive-cooperative capabilities with peers within and outside of the group included two measures:
   a. The instrument for observations of spontaneous dyadic and group peer interaction during school recesses (Bauminger, 2002) used in the CBE-dyadic research.
   b. A companionship measure that evaluated children's cooperative behaviors within the group (e.g., mutual planning, cooperative behavior, negotiating, eye contact, and sharing) while drawing a shared picture with their groupmates.

Main findings revealed robust changes in both direct and indirect measures of social-cognitive capabilities for the two groups of participants, and mixed results with regard to their social-interactive capabilities. On the problem-solving measure, children in both groups suggested significantly more social solutions with the child as an initiator after treatment than before treatment. Children also demonstrated better recognition of both basic and complex emotions, and provided more accurate and relevant explanations for these correctly recognized emotions after treatment. As for the CBE-dyadic treatment, findings for the CBE-group treatment indicated that progress in emotional knowledge and understanding emerged mainly for complex emotions. Children provided more examples of complex emotions, with more attributions to an audience. Yet unlike the CBE-dyadic findings, no change emerged in the specificity of the emotional examples provided. Surprisingly, the indirect social-cognitive measures revealed pre- to posttreatment gains, in which children were better able to justify others' mental states on the Strange Stories measure (to assess ToM) and showed improved executive function by supplying richer conceptualizations of their sorting strategies and recognizing more sorting strategies generated by the examiner. Moreover, their own flexible cognitive conceptualizations (reflected in their sorting ability) tended to increase after treatment. Thus, treatment appeared to be effective in promoting the social perception and problem-solving capabilities that are essential components of social cognition.

With regard to social-interactive skills, results were mixed. Children showed increased cooperative behaviors within the group, specifically, their global cooperative capabilities and specific behaviors such as eye contact, mutual planning, and sharing experiences within the group. However, unfortunately, their overall spontaneous social interactive skills outside the group (e.g., during school recess) did not change. The improvement on sharing within the group is particularly interesting, perhaps implying that because friendships evolved between the children within the group, they felt more secure to share. This lack of generalization from the small-group setting to outside social activities (e.g., spontaneous dyadic or group interactions with peers who were not associated with the treatment, during recesses in school) is especially interesting in light of generalizations demonstrated by former research (e.g., Bauminger, 2002, 2007b). Perhaps the fact that children's social agents outside the intervention group (e.g., parents and peers) were not actively involved in the CBE-group study (but were involved in the CBE-dyadic interventions) reduced the children's ability to generalize what they learned in the small group to their day-to-day interactions with peers during recesses. It appears that in the case of children with

HFASD, social interventions may need to include direct mediation to different natural social settings within schools and maybe even outside school, to increase the likelihood of generalization to children's spontaneous social interaction capabilities.

Summary of CBE

Taken together, multimodal CBE, whether individual and/or group oriented, seems to present promising direct effects (e.g., progress in emotional and social understanding) and indirect effects (e.g., executive function and ToM) on social cognition. However, the enhancement of authentic, spontaneous peer interaction appears to require careful consideration of setting and social agents' generalization within CBE for this population. Use of an ecological model—involving children's different social agents (parents, peers, and teachers) in the treatment (e.g., Bronfenbrenner, 1979)—seems to hold potential for increasing such spontaneous peer interactions. Specifically, the insulated, semistructured, small-group intervention may serve to enhance children's cooperative capabilities and friendships.

CBE also poses several limitations, such as relatively small sample size and the lack of comparison condition. It is also important to include in future studies direct comparison of CBE (dyadic or group) with other CBT-based (but not ecological) interventions to delineate the relative importance of the ecological models.

SUMMARY, CONCLUSIONS, AND FUTURE DIRECTIONS FOR SCHOOL-BASED SOCIAL CBT FOR HFASD

This chapter has reviewed multidimensional, CBT-based social interventions and presented a school-based CBE intervention model with promising efficacy. Overall, encouraging results have emerged from prior research on treatments targeting the social-cognitive and social-interactive capabilities of children with HFASD, but children's spontaneous transfer of the learned social-interactive skills to their natural environments such as school remains uncertain. Also, selection of the optimal social skills targets and techniques to be incorporated into such interventions requires further inquiry. For example, which of the core social deficits should be taught directly and which should be taught indirectly? This question stems, for instance, from the inconsistent findings that emerged from most of the reviewed studies that taught ToM directly, in contrast to the progress obtained by the CBE intervention that taught ToM indirectly by emphasizing reciprocity. Another example is the possible progress in executive function that seemed to stem from teaching problem-solving skills (Bauminger, 2007a; Solomon et al., 2004; Stichter et al., 2010). Yet it was not clear whether teaching emotional recognition resulted in progress in other social-cognitive skills such as ToM or social understanding. Learning about the differential usefulness of the various CBT techniques for various social capabilities, and generalization within the different social-cognitive skills, and between them and the social-interactive skills, is an important future task.

Despite the significant need for school-based interventions in HFASD, multimodal social interventions within the school environment remain rare. Assimilation of a social curriculum into children's general school curriculum is a major challenge, requiring the design of both effective and feasible procedural and methodological mechanisms, while considering also financial resources and a commitment from teachers. Some issues/questions that need to be addressed, for example, are as follows:

Who is the most appropriate or efficient professional to provide the treatment?

Who should supervise these teachers as they implement the intervention?

Who will mentor parents' collaboration and peer involvement?

How can comparative research into a yearlong school intervention succeed logistically in the face of ethical considerations and parents and staff who resist wait-listing of eligible children?

What steps can increase treatment fidelity across different classes or schools?

Finally, effective implementation of an ecological model seems to emphasize the need to include diverse intervention settings (i.e., school, home) and social agents (i.e., teachers, parents, typical peers). Future research should explore collaborations between such settings and agents (e.g., parents–teachers/home–school; treatment provider and other teachers or staff in the school; small-group and large-class social activities) that may lead to more efficient social interventions for HFASD. In summary, in line with extensiveness of the multidimensional social deficit in individuals with HFASD, although rapidly evolving CBT-based multimodal social interventions present promising results, future empirical efforts are still needed to strengthen their effectiveness.

REFERENCES

American Psychiatric Association. (2013). *Diagnostic and statistical manual of mental disorders* (5th ed.). Arlington, VA: Author.

Asher, S. R., Hymel, S., & Renshaw, P. D. (1984). Loneliness in children. *Child Development, 55*, 1456–1464.

Attwood, T. (2004). Cognitive behaviour therapy for children and adults with Asperger's syndrome. *Behavior Change, 21*, 147–161.

Bauminger, N. (2002). The facilitation of social-emotional understanding and social interaction in high functioning children with autism: Intervention outcomes. *Journal of Autism and Developmental Disorders, 32*, 283–298.

Bauminger, N. (2007a). Group social-multimodal intervention for HFASD. *Journal of Autism and Developmental Disorders, 37*, 1605–1615.

Bauminger, N. (2007b). Individual social-multi-modal intervention for HFASD. *Journal of Autism and Developmental Disorders, 37*, 1593–1604.

Bauminger, N., Schorr-Edelsztein, H., & Morash, J. (2005). Social information processing and emotional understanding in children with learning disabilities. *Journal of Learning Disabilities, 38*, 45–61.

Bauminger, N., Solomon, N., Aviezer, A., Heung, K., Gazit, L., Brown, J., et al. (2008). Children with autism and their friends: A multidimensional study of friendship in high-functioning autism spectrum disorder. *Journal of Abnormal Child Psychology, 36*, 135–150.

Bauminger-Zviely, N. (2013). *Social and academic abilities of children with high-functioning autism spectrum disorders.* New York: Guilford Press.

Beaumont, R., & Sofronoff, K. (2008). A multi-component social skills intervention for children with Asperger syndrome: The Junior Detective Training Program. *Journal of Child Psychology and Psychiatry, 49*, 743–753.

Begeer, S., Koot, H. M., Rieffe, C., Terwogt, M., & Stegge, H. (2008). Emotional competence in children with autism: Diagnostic criteria and empirical evidence. *Developmental Review, 28*, 342–369.

Bellini, S., Peters, J. K., Benner, L., & Hopf, A. (2007). A meta-analysis of school-based social skills interventions for children with autism spectrum disorders. *Remedial and Special Education, 28*, 153–162.

Billstedt, E., Gillberg, C., & Gillberg, C. (2007). Autism in adults: Symptom patterns and early childhood predictors: Use of the DISCO in a community sample followed from childhood. *Journal of Child Psychology and Psychiatry, 48*, 1102–1110.

Bronfenbrenner, U. (1979). *The ecology of human development: Experiment in nature and design.* Cambridge, MA: Harvard University Press.

Cappadocia, C. M., Weiss, J. A., & Pepler, D. (2012). Bullying experiences among children and youth with autism spectrum disorders. *Journal of Autism and Developmental Disorders, 42*(2), 266–267.

Centers for Disease Control and Prevention. (2009, December 18). Surveillance summaries. *Morbidity and Mortality Weekly Report, 58*(SS-10), 1–20.

Channon, S., Charman, T., Heap, J., Crawford, S., & Rios, P. (2001). Real-life problem-solving in Asperger's syndrome. *Journal of Autism and Developmental Disorders, 31*, 461–469.

Constantino, J. N., & Gruber, C. P. (2005). *Social Responsiveness Scale (SRS)*. Los Angeles: Western Psychological Services.

Delis, D. C., Kaplan, E., & Kramer, J. H. (2001). *Delis–Kaplan Executive Function System (D-KEF)*. San Antonio, TX: Psychological. Corporation.

DeRosier, M. E., Swick, D. C., Ornstein-Davis, N., Sturtz-McMillen, J., & Matthews, R. (2011). The efficacy of a social skills group intervention for improving social behaviors in children with high functioning autism spectrum disorders. *Journal of Autism and Developmental Disorders, 41*, 1033–1043.

Feng, H., Lo, Y., Tsai, S., & Cartledge, G. (2008). The effects of theory of mind and social skill training on the social competence of a sixth grade student with autism. *Journal of Positive Behavior Interventions, 10*, 228–242.

Gresham, F. M., & Elliott, S. N. (1990). *Social skills rating system (SSRS)*. Circle Pines, MN: American Guidance Service.

Happé, F. G. E. (1994). An advanced test of theory of mind: Understanding of story characters' thoughts and feelings by able autistic, mentally handicapped, and normal children and adults. *Journal of Autism and Developmental Disorders, 24*, 129–154.

Harter, S. (1985). *Self-perception profile for children*. Unpublished manual, University of Denver, Denver, CO.

Hart, K. J., & Morgan, J. R. (1993). Cognitive behavioral therapy with children: Historical context and current status. In A. J. Finch, W. M. Nelson, & E. S. Ott (Eds.), *Cognitive behavior procedures with children and adolescents: A practical guide* (pp. 1–24). Boston: Allyn & Bacon.

Kasari, C., Chamberlain, B., & Bauminger, N. (2001). Social emotions and social relationships in autism: Can children with autism compensate? In J. Burack, T. Charman, N. Yirmiya, & P. Zelazo (Eds.), *Perspectives on development in autism* (pp. 309–323). Hillsdale, NJ: Erlbaum.

Kasari, C., Locke, J., Gulsrud, A., & Rotheram-Fuller, E. (2011). Social networks and friendships at school: Comparing children with and without ASD. *Journal of Autism and Developmental Disorders, 41*, 533–544.

Klin, A., Jones, W., Schultz, R., Volkmar, F., & Cohen, D. (2002). Visual fixation patterns during viewing of naturalistic social situations as predictors of social competence in individuals with autism. *Archives of General Psychiatry, 59*, 809–816.

Landa, R. (2000). Social language use in Asperger syndrome and in high-functioning autism. In A. Klin, F. R. Volkmar, & S. S. Sparrow (Eds.), *Asperger syndrome* (pp. 121–155). New York: Guilford Press.

Lewis, M. (1993). The emergence of human emotions. In M. Lewis & J. M. Haviland (Eds.), *Handbook of emotions* (pp. 223–235). New York: Guilford Press.

Lochman, J. E., & Lampron, L. B. (1986). Situational social problem solving skills and self-esteem of aggressive and nonaggressive boys. *Journal of Abnormal Psychology, 14*, 605–661.

Locke, J., Ishijima, E. H., Kasari, C., & London, N. (2010). Loneliness, friendship quality and the social networks of adolescents with high-functioning autism in an inclusive school setting. *Journal of Research in Special Educational Needs, 10*, 74–81.

Lopata, C., Thomeer, M. L., Volker, M. A., Toomey, J. A., Nida, R. E., Lee, G.

K., et al. (2010). RCT of a manualized social treatment for high-functioning autism spectrum disorders. *Journal of Autism and Developmental Disorders, 40,* 1297–1310.

Lord, C., Rutter, M., & LeCouteur, A. (1994). Autism Diagnostic Interview—Revised: A revised version of a diagnostic interview for caregivers of individuals with possible pervasive developmental disorders. *Journal of Autism and Developmental Disorders, 19,* 185–212.

Machintosh, K., & Dissnanyake, C. (2006). A comparative study of the spontaneous social interactions of children with high-functioning autism and children with Asperger's disorder. *Autism, 10,* 199–220.

Mackay, T., Knott, F., & Dunlop, A. (2007). Developing social interaction and understanding in individuals with autism spectrum disorder: A groupwork intervention. *Journal of Intellectual and Developmental Disability, 32,* 279–290.

Mazurek, M. O., & Kanne, S. M. (2010). Friendship and internalizing symptoms among children and adolescents with ASD. *Journal of Autism and Developmental Disorders, 40,* 1512–1520.

Mesibov, G., & Shea, V. (2011). Evidence-based practices and autism. *Autism, 15,* 114–133.

Nah, Y., & Poon, K. (2011). The perception of social situations by children with autism spectrum disorders. *Autism, 15,* 185–203.

Nowicki, S., & Carton, J. (1993). The measurement of emotional intensity from facial expressions. *Journal of Social Psychology, 133,* 749–750.

Ozonoff, S., & Miller, J. N. (1995). Teaching theory of mind: A new approach to social skills training for individuals with autism. *Journal of Autism and Developmental Disorders, 25,* 415–433.

Pexman, P. M., Rostad, K. R., McMorris, C. A., Climie, E. A., Stowkowy, J., & Glenwright, M. (2011). Processing of ironic language in children with high-functioning autism spectrum disorder. *Journal of Autism and Developmental Disorders, 41,* 1097–1112.

Seidner, L. B., Stipek, D. J., & Feshbach, N. D. (1988). A developmental analysis of elementary school-aged children's concepts of pride and embarrassment. *Child Development, 59,* 367–377.

Solomon, M., Goodlin-Jones, B. L., & Anders, T. F. (2004). A social adjustment enhancement intervention for high functioning autism, Asperger's syndrome, and pervasive developmental disorder NOS. *Journal of Autism and Developmental Disorders, 34,* 649–668.

Stichter, J. P., Herzog, M. J., Visovsky, K., Schmidt, C., Randolph, J., Schultz, T., et al. (2010). Social competence intervention for youth with Asperger syndrome and high functioning autism: An initial investigation. *Journal of Autism and Developmental Disorders, 40,* 1067–1079.

Stichter, J. P., O'Connor, K. V., Herzog, M. J., Lierheimer, K., & McGhee, S. D. (2012). Social competence intervention for elementary students with aspergers syndrome and high functioning autism. *Journal of Autism and Developmental Disorders, 42*(3), 354–366.

van Ommeren, T. B., Begeer, S., Scheeren, A. M., & Koot, H. M. (2012). Measuring reciprocity in high functioning children and adolescents with autism spectrum disorders. *Journal of Autism and Developmental Disorders, 42*(6), 1001–1010.

Volkmar, F. R., Lord, C., Bailey, A., Schultz, R. T., & Klin, A. (2004). Autism and pervasive developmental disorders. *Journal of Child Psychology and Psychiatry, 45*, 135–170.

White, S. W., & Roberson-Nay, R. (2009). Anxiety, social deficits, and loneliness in youth with autism spectrum disorders. *Journal of Autism and Developmental Disorders, 39*, 1006–1013.

PART IV

SEXUALITY AND AFFECTION

11

Expressing and Enjoying Love and Affection

A Cognitive-Behavioral Program for Children and Adolescents with High-Functioning ASD

TONY ATTWOOD

The referral of a person with an autism spectrum disorder (ASD), especially Asperger syndrome or mild autism, for the treatment of a mood disorder is usually due to concerns regarding the intensity of anxiety, sadness, and anger. However, extensive clinical experience with children and adolescents with ASD suggests a fourth domain of socioemotional difficulty that is of parental, personal, and sometimes clinical concern, namely, the ability to understand and express feelings of love and affection. Children and adolescents with ASD are often not instinctive or intuitive in expressing their liking or love for someone, or their understanding that family members and friends need affection (Attwood, 2007). Despite recognition by clinicians, families, and those with ASD of the need for progams for this domain of social-emotional difficulties, there is to date very little empirical research on the communication of affection by children and adolescents with ASD or resource material designed to improve the ability of those with ASD to express love and affection.

HISTORICAL BACKGROUND
AND SIGNIFICANCE OF THE TREATMENT

Affection in Childhood

The communication of affection is a core human need (Rotter, Chance, & Phares, 1972), essential for the development of interpersonal relationships (Guerro & Floyd, 2006) and the encouragement of friendships (Furman & Masters, 1980; Newcomb, Bukowski, & Pattee, 1993). Within families and among friends, there is an expectation of mutually enjoyable, reciprocal, and beneficial exchanges of words and gestures that express affection. From very early in life, typical infants seek and enjoy affection from their parents, and toddlers are able to read the signals when someone expects affection (e.g., crying) and to recognize when to give affection. Indeed, one of the early signs that clinicians use to diagnose ASD is a lack of gestures or words of comfort when a parent is distressed (LeCouteur, Lord, & Rutter, 2003).

As the typical child matures, there is an intuitive understanding of the type, duration, and degree of affection that is appropriate for the situation and the person involved. Children under age 2 know that words and gestures of affection are perhaps the most effective emotional restorative for themselves and for someone who is sad (Banham, 1950). However, the child with ASD may be confused as to why a parent or friend responds to his or her distress with an expression of affection, such as a hug; and unfortunately, some children with ASD experience a hug as an uncomfortable and restricting physical sensation, such that they may soon learn not to express their distress (e.g., cry) for fear of eliciting a "squeeze" from someone. Conversely, some children with ASD perceive a hug as enjoyable and relaxing due to the deep pressure—but not as a gesture to share or alleviate feelings (see section below on sensory experiences and affection).

We have social conventions regarding the expression of affection, and many children with ASD do not follow the social "rules" for expressing and responding to love and affection within themselves and others. Young boys and girls with ASD, for example, may prefer to play with hard toys, such as plastic models of dinosaurs and metal vehicles, rather than soft toys that represent human characteristics and tend to elicit strong feelings and gestures of love and affection in typical children and even adults (Attwood, 2007). Children with ASD are notorious for not sharing when playing with peers, and difficulties in sharing imaginative play is one of the DSM-5 diagnostic criteria for ASD (American Psychiatric Association, 2013). Sharing an activity or toy is perceived by typical children as an indication of their liking for someone, while an aversion to sharing can lead to the perception that they are not being friendly and do not like someone. Children with ASD may also not recognize the social conventions regarding affection; for example, they might express and expect in return the same degree of affection from a teacher as they would get from their mothers. There are also gender differences in the expression of affection between friends, with typical girls anticipating that affection will be integrated within their mutual activity. The absence of affection in the play of a girl with ASD can be a barrier to friendship. Regardless of gender, however, appearing to be indifferent or aloof to the affection of peers can inhibit social inclusion and contribute to the loss of potential friendships for both boys and girls.

Based on clinical experience, it appears that some children with ASD may enjoy and express very brief and low-intensity expressions of affection but become confused or overwhelmed when greater levels of expression are experienced or expected. The reverse may occur in some children with ASD, however, where they need almost excessive amounts of affection, sometimes for reassurance or sensory experience. These children might express affection that is too intense or immature. In addition, the person with ASD may not perceive the nonverbal signals and contextual cues that indicate when to stop showing affection, leading to potential feelings of discomfort, embarrassment, or even fear in the other person.

As a result, parents may perceive their child as either inadequate or excessive in expressing affection. When parents express their love for their child with ASD, perhaps with an affectionate hug, the child's body may stiffen rather than relax to match and mold into the body shape of the parent. The child may also not be soothed by words and gestures of affection when distressed. When an expression of love and affection is rejected or is not comforting, parents may wonder what they can do to repair the distress, or whether their son or daughter actually loves or even likes them. The child's rare use of gestures and words of affection may be lamented by parents and friends, who may feel affection-deprived and not obviously liked or loved by their child (Charlop & Walsh, 1986). For example, a mother of a girl with HFASD said that her daughter's lack of affection to family members was "basically breaking her father's heart; he's devastated." Another parent said, "It really hurts that you can't have the relationship you wanted." If affection is not reciprocated, a parent may try to elicit a greater degree of affection by increasing the intensity and frequency of his or her expressions of affection. This can lead to even greater withdrawal by the child and mutual despair. Another characteristic is that a child with ASD may have a strong attachment to one parent and only accept and express affection with that parent. This can lead to feelings of rejection and jealousy in the other parent.

When it comes to expressing affection, children with ASD have a limited repertoire of actions and gestures. Moreover, the emotional expressions they possess often tend to lack subtlety, and (in the case of adolescents) may be inappropriate for their age or developmentally immature. Their expression of affection and of liking or loving someone may be perceived by family members or friends as too little or too much—feast or famine. To illustrate this problem, an adolescent with HFASD said, "We feel and show affection, but not often enough, and at the wrong intensity." Each person has a capacity for expressing and enjoying affection. For a typical person, this capacity can be metaphorically conceptualized as a bucket, but for someone with an ASD, the capacity is a cup that is quickly filled and slow to empty. If the parent fills the affection cup to capacity, the child or adolescent with ASD may feel saturated with affection and be unable to return the same degree of (or sometimes any) affection.

The current theoretical models of ASD may explain some of the reasons for difficulties expressing love and affection. Impaired theory of mind abilities (Baron-Cohen, 1995, 2001) may explain the difficulty in reading subtle body language that a loving and affectionate response is anticipated. It may also explain the difficulty in perceiving whether not enough or too much affection has been expressed. The weak central coherence theory (Frith & Happé, 1994) may explain the greater attention to detail when processing social-emotional information conveyed in facial expressions and body language, and not knowing the relevant and redundant cues for affection. This can lead to misinterpreting someone's feelings by overlooking crucial cues or not combining the cues to achieve a higher-order interpretation: for example, focusing attention on someone's nose, which conveys little information, or not combining tone of voice with facial expressions, body language, and context to recognize that someone feels embarrassed rather than hot. Problems with executive function (Prior & Hoffmann, 1990; Ozonoff, South, & Provencal, 2005; Russell, 1997) can explain the tendency to impulsively respond to social-emotional cues that indicate a specific, anticipated level of affection, and a lack of self-reflection and monitoring can affect how affection is being communicated and perceived. If social-emotional cues are processed intellectually rather than intuitively, there might be a delay in processing information until there are a sufficient number of clear cues. A recent study on recognition of facial expressions by adolescents with ASD indicated that they required more intense facial expressions to identify accurately that someone is expressing sadness (Wallace et al., 2011). Because affection is an anticipated response to someone feeling sad, this may partially explain the reports of parents that the child with HFASD appears indifferent to their distress (Attwood, 2007).

Affection in Adolescence

The teenager with ASD may not understand the value in an adolescent friendship of mutual and reciprocal exchanges of appreciation and affection that range from liking to loving. Such teenagers may have learned a vocabulary of words and gestures to express affection in very early childhood with their parents, but may not have modified the actions in recognition of maturity and social conventions. For example, they may invade personal space and not know which parts of someone's body are now inappropriate to touch. The teenager with ASD may also not know how to progress beyond a reciprocal but platonic friendship, or how to express deeper feelings of affection.

In addition, although adolescents with ASD likely achieve the physical changes associated with puberty within the same age range as their peers, their social and emotional maturity and adaptive functioning may be delayed by several years (Klin et al., 2007). Thus, there may be a strong drive for romantic/sensual experiences but a lack of appreciation and understanding of age-appropriate peer codes of conduct.

Because the adolescent with ASD is often rejected and ridiculed by peers and has fewer social encounters (Attwood, 2007), a rare act of friendship from someone who expresses liking a quality or ability of the adolescent with ASD may be misperceived as meaning more than was intended. The adolescent with ASD can then pursue that person for more similar experiences. The degree of companionship may not be reciprocal, and often the typical peer can be very polite and subtle in expressing nonverbal signals of wanting only a platonic relationship. These signals may go unnoticed by the adolescent with ASD, who is perceived as having developed a "crush" and may be accused of incessantly annoying or stalking the person. Parents and teachers may notice that the adolescent with ASD seems excessively focused on that person, wanting to accompany them, learn all about them and frequently talk about them. The depth of attentiveness suggests the evolution to a new level of expression of a special interest, namely, a fascination with a person (Attwood, 2007).

The associated pleasure of thinking about, talking about, or being with the person can become intoxicating for the adolescent with ASD (not unlike other self-stimulatory behaviors), who can become extremely agitated when denied access to that person. It is then difficult to determine whether the adolescent is expressing liking in a friendly or in a romantic way, is desperate to end feelings of loneliness, or has "matured" to a new expression of special interest. In some cases, these sorts of special interests can become irresistible (i.e., they seem uncontrollable to the person) and have some characteristics associated with an obsessive–compulsive disorder (OCD). Because of the difficulties associated with these strong urges toward other people, the adolescent may be referred for treatment for any of a number of reasons; for example, the clinician may receive a referral for anger management when the adolescent is thwarted in achieving access to the person, for treatment of OCD, or for advice in managing a conduct disorder. Whatever the reason for the infatuation with the person, in all these cases, the adolescent with ASD needs guidance for the underlying difficulty with expressing interest and affection. Without this understanding, his or her actions could lead to further alienation from peers and sanctions from school or the legal system.

Typical adolescents have many friends to provide guidance about expected and appreciated levels of affection in a romantic relationship. Clinical experience has indicated that adolescents with ASD can become increasingly aware of the expressions of affection that occur between their peers, and the apparent enjoyment of physical/sensory experiences between romantic partners. Such relationships can be elusive for a teenager with ASD, but he or she may have an intellectual and emotional curiosity, and a longing to have similar experiences. The adolescent may seek information and guidance about expressing affection to peers from television programs, which tend to emphasize dramatic expressions of affection; or from pornography on the Internet, which portrays age-inappropriate or illegal actions. When such behavior is imitated with peers, the adolescent with ASD can be in serious trouble. Immature and naive expressions of affection from a girl who has ASD, for example, can be misinterpreted by boys as indicating a desire for greater intimacy, which was not her intention. This can lead to accusations of "leading someone on," and to serious and traumatic experiences. Another concern for some adolescent males with ASD is knowing when to stop expressing affection in a romantic relationship. Typical teenagers recognize the verbal and nonverbal signals, the "amber" or "red light" signals that indicate there is no consent to continue. If these signals are not recognized, then there can be accusations of assault and subsequent legal implications (see also Hénault, Chapter 12, this volume). We now have for adolescents with HFASD (and what was formerly known as Asperger's syndrome) literature that provides a guide to dating and adolescent romantic relationships (Attwood, 2008; Uhlenkamp, 2009).

In their desire to be popular, adolescents with ASD are vulnerable to being "set up" by malicious peers. Because of difficulties with theory of mind and understanding the intentions of others, as well as difficulties using context to interpret sarcasm or humor, individuals with ASD can be easily misled. In this way, persons with ASD may be deliberately misinformed of someone's romantic interest but believe it as fact. When this false assumption leads to unwelcome advances or suggestions, the adolescent may be confused and even accused. In contrast, some adolescents with ASD are confused by aspects of affection and may develop fears or avoidance of experiencing, or even seeing, expressions of affection. The person is then perceived as prudish or puritanical.

Affection to Repair Feelings

Although I am not aware of research on this topic, it is likely that most typical children and adolescents probably rate affection as their primary emotion repair strategy. However, clinical experience suggests that for someone with ASD the most effective emotional repair strategies are being alone, being with animals, or engaging in a special interest. It is interesting that, as reported in several autobiographical accounts, youth with ASD seem able to relate to and express affection and love more easily to animals than to people (Grandin, 1995; Holliday Willey, 2012; Lipsky, 2012). Thus, parents may observe that the child or adolescent with ASD can and often does express affection for a pet to a level far greater than that expressed for a parent. This can lead to envy of the pet and resentment that the person can indeed express love, but not for the parent. From the perspective of the person with ASD, people have complex needs, they can deceive or tease you, or interrupt and prevent you from engaging in your preferred activities. In contrast, animals are loyal, respectful, predictable, and so pleased to see you that it is easy to make them feel happy. The alternative emotional repair mechanisms to affection often used by children and adolescents with HFASD also may include seeking solitude or engaging in a special interest (Attwood, 2007). Both of these strategies can be viewed as attempts to escape or avoid social interactions, or they may simply be easier for the child/adolescent. Parents, on the other hand, often prefer to repair emotions using affection, which may not fit with the strategy preferred by their child with ASD.

Frequency of Affection Expression

In general, we learn to anticipate compliments and frequent words or gestures of affection to confirm and consolidate a relationship or friendship. For the child or adolescent with ASD, however, this frequency of affection can be perceived as repetitive, and the reiteration of the obvious as illogical and a waste of time. In other words, the child may question why, once a statement has been made, should it have to be repeated? A mother complained to her adolescent son, for example, that he never said he loved her. In defense, he became very annoyed and replied that he had said he loved her when he was 6 years old. Why would he need to say it again? Was she developing signs of Alzheimer's? This may reflect impaired theory of mind abilities and a lack of appreciation of how someone's mood and happiness can be improved by expressing words and gestures of affection. Explanations for this sort of misinterpretation of others' needs deserve further exploration in research.

Sensory Sensitivity and Affection

It is important that family members and friends recognize that a particular aspect of ASD affects the ability to enjoy and express affection, namely hyper- or hyporeactivity to sensory experiences. These characteristics are now included in the new diagnostic criteria for ASD in DSM-5. For example, some individuals with ASD have tactile sensitivity such that light touch on their skin can be perceived as an extremely unpleasant sensory experience (Blakemore, Tavassoli, & Calo, 2006). This will obviously affect enjoyment of and response to gestures of affection, such as the touch of a person's hand or arm during a conversation to emphasize a point or express compassion (Cascio, McGlone, & Folger, 2008). Unanticipated touch, due to not reading the signals that this is about to occur (such as a pat on the back or a hug from behind), can elicit a startle response. A kiss can also be perceived as an unpleasant tactile sensation. There may be olfactory sensitivity, such that when experiencing a hug, the person with ASD can be hyperaware of someone's perfume or body odor, perceiving it as an extremely unpleasant sensation. All this can explain why some demonstrative family members are avoided.

The Neurology of Affection

The amygdala is known to regulate a range of emotions, including anger, anxiety, sadness and affection. Amygdalar pathology has been suggested as one of the neurological explanations for the unusual emotional profile associated with ASD (Baron-Cohen et al., 2000; Damasio & Maurer, 1978). Histological studies (Bauman & Kemper, 1985), stereological studies (Schumann & Amaral, 2006), and structural MRI studies (Nacewicz et al., 2006; Schumann, Barnes, Lord, & Courchesne, 2009) have identified structural and functional abnormalities of the amygdala in children and adults with ASD. Thus, theoretical and neuroanatomical evidence suggests that there will be problems with the perception and regulation of emotions, including love and affection. Temple Grandin (2005) explained:

> My brain scan shows that some emotional circuits between the frontal cortex and the amygdala just aren't hooked up—circuits that affect my emotions and are tied to my ability to feel love. I experience the emotion of love, but it's not the same way that most neurotypical people do. Does this mean my love is less valuable than what other people feel? (Grandin & Barron, 2005, p. 40)

A COGNITIVE-BEHAVIORAL THERAPY PROGRAM FOR AFFECTION

We recognize that affection is essential for physical and mental health (Oliver, Rafferty, Reeb, & Delaney, 1993), and an important means of initiating and maintaining friendships and relationships, and avoiding loneliness (Downs & Javidi, 1990). Although clinicians are rarely asked to help a typical person express affection, clinicians who work often with people who have ASD increasingly are recognizing that these clients need information and guidance to understand and express affection (Attwood, 2007). Research studies have indicated that children with ASD can learn to be more affectionate (Apple, Billingsley, & Schwartz, 2005; Charlop & Walsh, 1986; Twardosz, Nordquist, Simon, & Botkin, 1983), but no study has examined whether a cognitive-behavioral therapy (CBT) program can be used for children whose parents are concerned about their perceived lack of affection.

The program and manual described herein were originally designed by Michelle Garnett and myself (Attwood & Garnett, 2013). We designed a CBT program comprising five, 2-hour sessions, called the Affection Program, which is primarily to enable children 5–13 years old with ASD to express and enjoy affection within friendships and family. However, young adolescents with ASD who are conspicuously immature may also benefit from the activities and strategies used in the program. Adults with ASD may also benefit from aspects of the program that can be modified to be age-appropriate.

Three small group pilot programs facilitated the design and evaluation of strategies to enable participants explore the ability to express and experience affection with parents and friends. The Affection Program emphasizes on affective education, especially explaining the value of affection within a family and between friends, and the benefits of expressing affection from the child's perspective. Children with ASD are more responsive to a factual learning style (Attwood, 2007). Thus, the presentation of information and strategies was designed to be practical and logical rather than intuitive and inferential. Parents of the children participated in parallel sessions in a large group to discuss issues in the family associated with the expression of and response to affection, the content of the program, and the children's responses to components of each session. They were also informed of a homework project to be completed between sessions.

Aims of the CBT Affection Program

The aims of the program were as follows:

- Help each child discover how expressing and experiencing affection can improve friendships and relationships.
- Help each child to identify not only his or her own comfort and enjoyment range for gestures, actions, and words of affection, but also those of friends and family members.
- Improve for each child the range of expressions for liking and loving someone, appropriate to each relationship and situation.
- Explain to parents and friends the challenges faced by a person with ASD in reading signals that indicate when expressions of affection are needed and appreciated.

The program is currently being evaluated using a randomized controlled study with over 70 children with a diagnosis of Asperger syndrome per DSM-IV (American Psychiatric Association, 2000). The results of a smaller pilot trial with 21 subjects who have Asperger syndrome have been published (Sofronoff, Eloff, Sheffield, & Attwood, 2011). The pilot trial produced a significant increase in parent-identified appropriateness of the children's affectionate behavior toward family members and people outside the immediate family, and a significant improvement in the children's understanding of the purpose of affection.

Practical Considerations

When the CBT Affection Program was originally designed, there were no standardized measures of affection that could be applied to children and adolescents with ASD. A team of psychologists at the University of Queensland, Australia, developed and evaluated three measures of affection that explored the ability of typical children and adolescents, and those with an ASD, to communicate affection and measured any changes attributable to a CBT program (Lee, Sofronoff, Sheffield, & Attwood, 2011). The three questionnaires completed by parents were the following.

Affection for You Questionnaire

The Affection for You Questionnaire (AYQ) is a 19-item questionnaire that examines giving and receiving affection, and the communication of empathy, to the parent completing the questionnaire. There are five subscales: Giving Verbal Affection, Giving Physical Affection, Receiving Verbal Affection, Receiving Physical Affection, Communicating Empathy.

There are two parts to each question, the first asks the parent to rate how often the child expressed the gesture of affection on a scale from 1, *Never,* through 7, *Twice a day or more.* The second part asks the parent to provide a description of the amount (ranging from 1, *Not enough,* to 7, *Too much.* A total score is calculated by adding the totals for each subscale.

The Affection for Others Questionnaire

The Affection for Others Questionnaire (AOQ) is a 20-item questionnaire that also examines giving and receiving affection and the communication of affection, but to classmates, friends and family members. There are five subscales: Giving Verbal Affection to Others, Giving Physical Affection to Others, Receiving Verbal Affection from Others, Receiving Physical Affection from Others, Communicating Empathy to Others.

Each subscale includes four questions with two parts. The first asks parents to rate whether their son or daughter was able to complete each of the affectionate gestures appropriately (ranging from 1, *Never appropriate,* to 7, *Always appropriate*). The second part asks parents to provide a description of the degree to which their child displayed this affectionate gesture, with responses ranging from 1, *Not enough,* to 7, *Too much.* Total Appropriateness and Total Amount scores are calculated by adding the totals for each subscale.

General Affection Questionnaire

The General Affection Questionnaire (GAQ) is a 12-item questionnaire that examines aspects of affection communication, such as expressing inadequate or excessive affection, the importance of affection in the person's daily life, and the degree to which teaching and support regarding affection are required.

The GAQ has 12 statements that assess the amount of affection in which the child engages (e.g., *He or she shows a lack of affection*), the appropriateness of the affection experienced by the child, and the impact of problems with affection on various aspects of the child's life. The scale ranges from 1, *Strongly disagree*, to 7, *Strongly agree*. The sum of all 12 items provides a Total Difficulty with Affection score.

Story: A Walk in the Forest

The Walk in the Forest measure, designed to assess the child's understanding of affection, is a hypothetical scenario of the child walking in a forest, coming across a space ship that has crash landed, and meeting an alien who has been observing humans. The alien is curious to know why humans seem to need to communicate that they like or love one another, and the child is asked to explain to the alien why humans are affectionate to each other. This can elicit the child's depth of understanding of the value of affection. The scoring system allocates 1 point to each appropriate response.

Overview of Sessions

Session 1

The activities and experiences that you like.
People whom you like or love.
How do those people express that they like you or love you?
How we feel, think, and behave when someone likes or loves us.
What would life be like without being liked or loved?
List some of the things that are not so nice about being liked or loved.
Project: To collect pictures of people expressing affection.
Family project: To identify those family situations in which affection is expected and you have difficulty expressing your liking or love for someone.

Session 2

Review Session 1.
A Social Story™ about how liking or loving someone can affect your feelings, thoughts, and abilities based on the information provided in Session 1.
The "like and love" thermometer: using the thermometer to measure the degree of expression.
What can you say and do to show that you like someone?

What can you say and do to show that you love someone?

Project: To use these ideas at home to express liking or loving a member of the family.

Session 3

Review the affection project from Session 2.

Why do we give compliments?

Compliments for specific people.

Types of compliment.

How often should you give someone a compliment?

How do you reply to a compliment?

Practice giving and receiving compliments.

When might a compliment be embarrassing?

Project: To create a diary of compliments.

Session 4

Review the compliment diary.

Why do we give affection?

What would happen if nobody showed you that they liked or loved you?

What would happen if you stopped showing your friends that you liked them?

If you did not get enough affection, how could you make yourself feel better?

How do you feel when . . . ?

Project: To complete a diary of receiving and giving affection.

Session 5

Review of Session 4 and the affection diary.

Different types of affection in different situations.

How can you tell if someone needs affection?

How can you tell if you have given too much affection?

How can you tell if you have *not given enough* affection?

What are the three most important things you have learned about affection?

Complete the postprogram assessments.

Express affection to someone in the group with a compliment or gesture, such as a hug.

Awards: Each participant to receive a certificate of knowledge.

The cognitive profile of children with ASD was recognized in the design of the CBT Affection Program. The profile can include remarkable visual reasoning abilities, such that activities are enhanced with the use of pictures and drawing, thereby placing less emphasis on conversation. Due to problems with generalization associated with ASD, role plays and practice in real-life situations need to be included in the program to a greater extent than would occur with a typical child. The theme of the program was to encourage participants to be scientists investigating why we have emotions such as affection, discovering how to identify and measure emotions, and discovering new strategies to communicate and manage emotions. This approach appeals to the logical thinking of children and adolescents with ASD.

The program includes a workbook in which participants record information, although this was deliberately kept to a minimum due to the recognition that children with an ASD often have poor handwriting skills and prefer to listen, watch, and do rather than write. If there is a genuine aversion to writing, the person conducting the program can listen to the participant's spoken comments and answers, and write them in the workbook.

At the end of each session, the project to be completed before the next session is explained, and the information obtained from the project is discussed at the start of the subsequent session. The project was designed to obtain more information or data and to apply strategies in real situations. Children with an ASD often have an aversion to the concept of homework from bitter school experiences, so the person conducting the program needs to emphasize the importance of completing the project, with clear encouragement from the presenter and parents to do so. There also needs to be good collaboration between home and school with regard to expressing affection to friends. It is important for teachers to be aware of the program and how they can contribute to the knowledge base of expressing and responding to affection, and the successful implementation of strategies.

If the program is using a group format there may need to be careful selection of group participants. We recognize that children and adolescents with ASD are at risk of additional diagnoses, especially attention-deficit/hyperactivity disorder (ADHD) and oppositional defiant disorder (Tonge, Brereton, Gray, & Einfeld, 1999). A dual diagnosis may impact the cohesion of the group. It is also important to consider the personality of each participant and his or her emotional and intellectual maturity to encourage group cooperation, mutual support, and the possibility of encouraging the development of friendships within and after the group sessions. If a group format is used, the recommended ratio of one leader or presenter to two participants allows monitoring and facilitation of group interactions and attention.

The program includes time at the end of each session for participants' parents to exchange information regarding their son's or daughter's responses and abilities during the activities, to explain the project, and to seek information on particular issues that could be addressed in a subsequent session. It is also essential to encourage family members to respond positively and appropriately to participants' new abilities and understanding of affection, and to facilitate the successful application of strategies learned in the program to real-life situations. Clinical experience of the program has indicated that some family members of a person with ASD may also have problems communicating affection, and group discussion with parents may encourage solutions to problems experienced by other family members.

Research to Date on the CBT Affection Program

While the open (nonrandomized), pilot study that evaluated the Affection Program with 21 children with Asperger's syndrome has been published (Sofronoff, Eloff, Sheffield, & Attwood, 2011), data of the randomized controlled trial with over 70 subjects are currently being analyzed. There were three children in each group, with two therapists (postgraduate clinical psychology students) to run the group. Assessments were conducted just before the start of the program, immediately after the program, and again at 3-month follow-up.

In the first, open trial, using the GAQ, the mean total scores increased over time (mean score 68.67 at preprogram assessment, 84.91 at postprogram assessment, and 83.43 at 3-month follow-up), but did not reach a statistically significantly difference. However, the sample size was relatively small, and the larger study will provide data based on three times the number of subjects in the pilot study. The AOQ, which measures the expression of affection to others (i.e., people other than immediate family), showed statistically significant improvement from pre- to postintervention ($p < .001$). The parents reported an increase in appropriateness of affectionate interactions between the children and others that was maintained at follow-up. The results of the Giving Affection subscales of the AOQ showed that mean scores were significantly different from pre- to postintervention ($p < .001$), but in contrast, the results from the Receiving Affection subscales of the AOQ showed that mean scores were not significantly different from pre- to postintervention in the pilot study. Results from the "Communicating Empathy to Others" subscale of the AOQ showed that mean scores were significantly different from pre- to postintervention ($p < .005$). The positive result was maintained at follow-up.

Three groups were derived, based on parent-reported scores on the AOQ and AYQ: high affection, adequate affection, and low affection. Participants with baseline scores of 59 and below on the AOQ and of 57 and below on the AYQ were categorized as the low affection group. The subjects with baseline scores between 59 and 100 on the AOQ and between 57 and 95 on the AYQ were designated the adequate affection group. Participants with baseline scores of 101 and over on the AOQ and 96 and over on the AYQ were regarded as the high affection group. There was only one participant with ASD allocated to this group. There was a substantial increase from pre- to postintervention in the number of children reported by parents to be expressing more adequate levels of affection to others, with eight children (38.1%) moving from the low affection to the adequate affection category, and this was maintained at follow-up. Total Amount scores on the AYQ at pre- and postintervention also indicated a marked increase in the number of children perceived by their parents to be expressing adequate levels of affection to them. Nine children (42.86%) moved from the low affection to the adequate affection group.

There are also qualitative findings from the pilot study. With a questionnaire examining parents' experience of the program, researchers found that the majority of parents observed and enjoyed improvements in their children's communication of affection. Children with Asperger syndrome were judged to have greater awareness and appreciation of the need for affection within the family and with friends. Their parents also reported higher levels of their children giving verbal affection, especially compliments, and nonverbal affection such as hugs and kisses. There was also increased tolerance in the children of being the recipient of verbal and nonverbal affection, and an increased repertoire of ways to express affection.

The pilot study also confirmed a significant increase in understanding of the value of affection between pre- and postintervention, using the Walk in the Forest story ($p < .001$) The Walk in the Forest was scored by allocating one point for each appropriate response. Two independent examiners evaluated interrater reliability, which was 98%. After the program, the children were able to provide significantly more reasons why humans benefit from expressing affection.

The program primarily focuses on the child initiating appropriate expressions of affection and was fairly successful in achieving this goal. However, parents reported less improvement in children's responses to affection initiated by others, with most of the children continuing to show apparent tolerance rather than enjoyment. Gestures of affection may be unexpected in children with Asperger's syndrome, due to delayed theory of mind abilities and less attention to social information in the environment. Because of these difficulties, they may not be able to read the subtle body language and contextual cues that an expression of affection is imminent, and they may continue to have a startle response. The tactile sensitivity associated with ASD may also include a startle response to being touched, which can be an aversive experience that is difficult to inhibit. The program would benefit from activities to improve the ability to predict when a gesture of affection is likely and strategies to teach muscle relaxation, in order to enable relaxation and enjoyment of the experience.

FUTURE DIRECTIONS AND CONCLUSIONS

The next stage is to design a program for older adolescents and young adults based on the same principles but using situations and issues for this age group. In the present program love is expressed between a child and his or her parent. A subsequent program for older adolescents and young adults needs to focus on expressing love for a boyfriend or girlfriend and recognizing the signals of mutual love.

Overall, the program effectively increased the affectionate behavior of children who initially had an unusually low level of affect expression; thus, it is consistent with previous studies that found children with Asperger syndrome can learn to be more affectionate (Apple et al., 2005; Charlop & Walsh, 1986; Twardosz et al., 1983). The majority of parents were extremely pleased at the subsequent level and type of affection expressed by their son or daughter with ASD. Thus, a CBT affection program for children with Asperger syndrome has clinical value and could be incorporated into the repertoire of treatment programs for clinicians who specialize in ASD.

REFERENCES

American Psychiatric Association. (2013). *Diagnostic and statistical manual of mental disorders* (5th ed.). Arlington, VA: Author.

Apple, A. L., Billingsley, F., & Schwartz, I. S. (2005). Effects of video modelling alone and with self-management on compliment-giving behaviors of children with high-functioning ASD. *Journal of Positive Behavior Interventions, 7,* 33–46.

Attwood, T. (2007). *The complete guide to Asperger's syndrome.* London: Jessica Kingsley.

Attwood, S. (2008). *Making sense of sex: A forthright guide to puberty, sex and relationships for people with Asperger's syndrome*. London: Jessica Kingsley.

Attwood, T., & Garnett, M. S. (2013). *From like to love within friendships and family: Cognitive behaviour therapy to understand and express affection*. London: Jessica Kingsley.

Banham, K. (1950). The development of affectionate behaviour in infancy. *Pedagogical Seminary and Journal of Genetic Psychology, 76,* 283–289.

Baron-Cohen, S. (1995). *Mind blindness: An essay on autism and theory of mind*. Cambridge, MA: MIT Press.

Baron-Cohen, S. (2001). Theory of mind and autism: A review. In L. M. Glidden (Ed.), *International review of research in mental retardation: Autism*. San Diego: Academic Press.

Baron-Cohen, S., Ring, H. A., Bullmore, E. T., Wheelwright, S., Ashwin, C., & Williams, S. C. (2000). The amygdala theory of autism. *Neuroscience Biobehavioral Review, 24,* 355–364.

Bauman, M., & Kemper, T. L. (1985). Histoanatomic observations of the brain in early infantile autism. *Neurology, 35,* 866–874.

Blakemore, S. J., Tavassoli, T., Calo, S., et al. (2006). Tactile sensitivity in Asperger syndrome. *Brain and Cognition, 61,* 5–13.

Cascio, C., McGlone, F., Folger, S., et al. (2008). Tactile perception in adults with autism: A multidimensional psychophysiological study. *Journal of Autism and Developmental Disorders, 38,* 127–137.

Charlop, M. H., & Walsh, M. E. (1986). Increasing autistic children's spontaneous verbalizations of affection: An assessment of time delay and peer modelling procedures. *Journal of Applied Behavior Analysis, 19,* 307–314.

Damasio, A. R., & Maurer, R. G. (1978). A neurological model for childhood autism. *Archives of Neurology, 35,* 777–786.

Downs, V. C., & Javidi, M. (1990). Linking communication motives to loneliness in the lives of older adults: An empirical test of interpersonal needs and gratifications. *Journal of Applied Communication Research, 18,* 32–48.

Frith, U., & Happé, F. (1994). Autism: Beyond theory of mind. *Cognition, 50,* 115–132.

Furman, W., & Masters, J. C. (1980). Affective consequences of social reinforcement, punishment and neutral behavior. *Developmental Psychology, 16,* 100–104.

Grandin, T. (1995). *Thinking in pictures*. New York: Doubleday.

Grandin, T., & Barron, S. (2005). *Unwritten rules of social relationships*. Arlington, TX: Future Horizons.

Guerro, L. K., & Floyd, K. (2006). *Nonverbal communication in close relationships*. Mahwah, NJ: Erlbaum.

Holliday Willey, L. (2012). *Safety skills for Asperger women*. London: Jessica Kingsley.

Klin, A., Saulnier, C. A., Sparrow, S. S., Ciccheti, D. V., Volkmar, F., & Lord, C. (2007). Social and communication abilities and disabilities in higher functioning individuals with autism spectrum disorders: The Vineland and ADOS. *Journal of Autism and Develeopmental Disorders, 37,* 748–759.

LeCouteur, A., Lord, C., & Rutter, M. (2003). *The Autism Diagnostic Interview—Revised (ADR-R)*. Los Angeles: Western Psychological Services.

Lipsky, D. (2012). Talking to the animals. In J. Santomauro (Ed.), *Autism all-stars*. London: Jessica Kingsley.

Nacewicz, B. M., Dalton, K. M., Johnstone, T., Long, M. T., McAuliff E. M., & Oakes, T. R. (2006). Amygdala volume and nonverbal social impairment in adolescent and adult males with autism. *Archives of General Psychiatry, 63*, 1417–1428.

Newcomb, A. F., Bukowski, W. M., & Pattee, L. (1993). Children's peer relations: A meta-analytic review of popular, rejected, neglected, controversial and average sociometric status. *Psychological Bulletin, 113*, 99–128.

Oliver, J. M., Rafferty, M., Reeb, A., & Delaney, P. (1993). Perceptions of parent–offspring relationships as a function of depression in offspring: Affectionless control, negative bias, and depressive realism. *Journal of Social Behavior and Personality, 8*, 405–424.

Ozonoff, S., South, M., & Provencal, S. (2005). Executive functions. In F. Volkmar, R. Paul, A. Klin, & D. Cohen (Eds.), *Handbook of autism and pervasive developmental disorders: Third edition*. Hoboken, NJ: Wiley.

Prior, M., & Hoffmann, W. (1990). Neuropsychological testing of autistic children through an exploration with frontal lobe tests. *Journal of Autism and Developmental Disorders, 20*, 581–590.

Rotter, J. B., Chance, J. E., & Phares, E. J. (1972). *Applications of a social learning theory of personality*. New York: Holt, Rinehart & Winston.

Russell, J. (1997). *Autism as an executive disorder*. Oxford, UK: Oxford University Press.

Schumann, C. M., & Amaral, D. G. (2006). Stereological analysis of amygdala neuron number in autism. *Journal of Neuroscience, 26*, 7674–7679.

Schumann, C. M., Barnes, C. C., Lord, C., & Courchesne, E. (2009). Amygdala enlargement in toddlers with autism related to severity of social and communication impairments. *Biological Psychiatry, 66*, 942–949.

Sofronoff, K., Eloff, J., Sheffield, J., & Attwood, T. (2011). Increasing the understanding and demonstration of appropriate affection in children with Asperger syndrome: A pilot trial. *Autism Research and Treatment, 2011*, Article 214317.

Tonge, B. J., Brereton, A. V., Gray, K. M., & Einfeld, S. L. (1999). Behavioral and emotional disturbance in high-functioning autism and Asperger syndrome. *Autism, 3*(2), 117–130.

Twardosz, S., Nordquist, V. M., Simon, R., & Botkin, D. (1983). The effect of group affection activities on the interaction of socially isolate children. *Analysis and Intervention in Developmental Disabilities, 3*, 311–338.

Uhlenkamp, J. (2009). *The guide to dating for teenagers with Asperger syndrome*. Shawnee Mission: Kansas Autism Asperger.

Wallace, G. L., Case, L. K., Harms, M. B., Silvers, J. A., Kenworthy, L., & Martin, A. (2011). Diminished sensitivity to sad facial expressions in high functioning autism spectrum disorders is associated with symptomatology and adaptive functioning. *Journal of Autism and Developmental Disorders, 41*, 1475–1486.

12

Understanding Relationships and Sexuality in Individuals with High-Functioning ASD

ISABELLE HÉNAULT

HISTORICAL BACKGROUND
AND SIGNIFICANCE FOR THE TREATMENT

The sexual development of individuals diagnosed with HFASD is a subject that deserves particular attention. Over the last few years, several authors (Hellemans & Deboutte, 2002; Hénault, 2006; Holmes, Isler, Bott, & Markowitz, 2005; Newport & Newport, 2002) have made us increasingly aware of the importance of this topic by proposing various intervention strategies, therapeutic tools, and sociosexual educational programs adapted for individuals with HFASD. Sexuality constitutes an important factor in the healthy development of individuals, and quality of life is partly indicated by how satisfied individuals are with their sexual lifestyles (Holmes et al., 2005).

The issue of whether individuals with HFASD are able to experience sexual desire is no longer debated. In the 1970s and 1980s, the common belief was that such individuals were not capable of experiencing sexual desire. Currently, researchers (Attwood, 2007; Haracopos & Pedersen, 1999, in Hellemans, 2002; Hénault & Attwood, 2002; Hénault, 2006) believe that individuals with HFASD do experience sexual desire, and that many wish to have intimate relationships. The main difficulty lies in the disparity between their needs, their social skills, and their level of maturity. Therefore, individuals with AS must have education programs that are specifically adapted to their level of functioning and to their sociosexual profiles (Hellemans & Deboutte, 2002; Hénault & Attwood, 2002).

The sexual development of individuals with ASD comprises several aspects, including behaviors, intimacy, emotions, communication skills, self-esteem, sexual knowledge, and experiences. Despite the difficulties they encounter in communicating and interacting socially, their interest in sexuality is very similar to that of adolescents and young adults in the general population. However, the cognitive profile (naiveté, egocentrism, etc.) and symptoms associated with the syndrome must be considered in order to fully understand their sexual development.

Several causal factors can affect the sexual development of individuals with ASD and other, coexisting conditions such as developmental disorders or Down syndrome: lack of sociosexual knowledge, lack of experience, prior history of abuse, current and past environments, policies relating to sexuality, medical and behavioral history, selection of partner, frustrations, imagination, modeling and imitation (Griffiths, Quinsey, & Hingsburger, 1989). A detailed analysis of these factors and of existing sexual behaviors is necessary in order to prepare the individual for sexual education, and in certain cases, for an individual or group intervention (Haracopos, 2009).

Lack of sociosexual knowledge is the first of these causal factors. Sociosexual knowlege plateaus around the age of puberty; individuals with ASD rarely attain the maturity of a young adult. They do not have the same experiences as adolescents in the general population, whether at the level of gender identity (sense of belonging to one's gender) or in interactions with other teenagers, especially with those of the opposite sex. These youngsters are prisoners of social asexualization; their sexuality is not recognized. It is as if their condition eliminates the possibility of sexuality. The hypersexualization observed in some adolescents can be viewed as occurring due to a lack of understanding about social rules and the notion of consent. Their environment frequently denies that they have sexual needs. In addition, they have little social support: With whom can they share their experiences and feelings? Peers and parents may be uncomfortable with the subject of sexuality, which further contributes to isolation during social situations. One the one hand, they have sexual needs that they attempt to express; on the other hand, sexual behaviors are punished. This conflict often causes inappropriate behaviors to appear (Griffiths et al., 1989). Adolescents with AS and ASD score lower on a sexual knowledge questionnaire (Durocher & Fortier, 1999) than do those in the general population (Hénault, Forget,

& Giroux, 2003). Some have a very elaborate fund of information on some precise subjects (anatomy, transsexualism, hormones, etc.), but the general concepts surrounding sexuality are often misunderstood.

Sexual segregation is experienced by many individuals with ASD, be it in specialized establishments, support groups, or at school. Given the ratio of four to five men to one woman (which can increase to 10:1 in clinical settings; Attwood, 2003), the possibility of interacting with members of the opposite sex remains quite limited. Adolescents are confronted with this reality and the lack of choice among available female partners. Homosexual and masturbatory behaviors can therefore result from unsatisfying or limited contact with members of the opposite sex. Griffiths, Richards, Fedoroff, & Watson (2002) has stated that if sexual segregation were replaced by integration, these behaviours would change and resemble those observed in the general population. Social activities and contact need to be encouraged. The greater the social network, the better the chance of meeting someone with whom common interests can be shared.

Environmental restrictions are frequently found in the policies of establishments, among staff members, and in the formal and informal rules surrounding the sexuality of individuals with ASD. If no precise rules exist, who determines whether the behavior is acceptable? Individuals are frequently bombarded with inconsistent messages. Frequent punitive interventions decrease the likelihood of acquiring responsible behavior. Teams that work with adolescents should create an open atmosphere around sexuality by preventing sexual abuse, providing sexual education, and recognizing the possibility of sexual contacts (Griffiths, Quinsey, & Hingsburger, 1989). It is of critical importance to educate staff, counselors, youth workers, and parents who may otherwise impart incorrect information about sexuality (Hingsburger, 1993).

Intimacy refers to the possibility of being alone with a romantic or sexual partner. Such occasions are rare for adolescents with ASD and other conditions (Griffiths, Quinsey, & Hingsburger, 1999). Intimate moments are not reserved for sexual contact. They also make it possible for teens to broaden their repertoires of interpersonal experiences. The goal is to provide them with time and opportunities to develop intimate relationships with others. Adolescence can be difficult due to hormonal changes, the desire for independence, and the marked need to explore. For some, intimacy is not deemed necessary or important and is replaced by attempts for physical closeness that are frequently frustrating for the partner. In other cases, sexuality becomes an obsession and a fixed behavioral routine lacking in diversity and intimacy (Edmonds & Worton, 2006).

Certain inappropriate sexual behaviors are part of the sexual repertoire of some individuals with ASD. The majority of these behaviors consist of sexual acts performed in public, touching or fondling, lack of respect for consent, sexual assault, excessive or inadequate masturbation, and sexual obsessions and compulsions (Haracopos & Pedersen, 1999; Ruble & Dalrymple, 1993). These are the most common inappropriate behaviors reported in the literature and clinical observations. The lack of sociosexual knowledge is a major consideration given that due to a lack of understanding or misinterpretations of social and sexual contexts it can contribute to an inappropriate act. In addition, many individuals are confused with regard to issues of privacy, especially those related to behaviors of an intimate nature. Thus, a detailed and concrete description of sexual acts and intimate areas of the body has to be given to most adolescents and young adults with ASD. The majority of these individuals have very limited experience with intimate and interpersonal relationships, and the onset of puberty risks creating much stress and frustration with regards to sexual issues. In addition, social pressure and the desire to be accepted in a group might exacerbate the stress and frustration felt by these individuals.

Finally, ASD affects the notion of consent in relation to theory of mind skills (i.e., one's ability to recognize different mental states and the existence of thoughts, beliefs, and emotions in others; Baron-Cohen, 1995, 2002). The individual with AS may assume without first confirming that others share the same thoughts and desires. Therefore, many inappropriate sexual acts result from poor judgement, lack of information, and limited abilities relating to Theory of Mind. For instance, an adolescent with AS may experience a strong crush on a student in his class. He decides to prove his love for her by offering her a gift and trying to kiss her. He is convinced that she feels the same love for him despite the lack of any evidence that she shares his feelings. She is surprised, and informs him that she already has a boyfriend. He feels sad, angry, and confused by her response. This example is common and, unfortunately, can precipitate inappropriate behaviors or strong emotional reactions. When the topic of sexuality has been addressed in the literature, it has usually been restricted to a discussion of problem behaviors (e.g., compulsive masturbation, inappropriate sexual interactions). Such a perspective is limited, in that it fails to consider the complexity of sexuality in general. As in any other context, sexuality in AS consists of intimacy, friendship, pleasure, communication, love, dating, desire, identity, and sexual behaviors.

The topic of sexuality is often ignored, and parents often wait until it emerges by itself. They often express fears that their adolescent will engage in more sexual experiences if his or her knowledge about sexuality increases. In fact, having a solid sexual knowledge base contributes to better decision-making skills and therefore less confusion and inappropriate behaviors (Griffiths et al., 1989; Haracopos, 2009). Sexual curiosity and interest are an integral part of the normal development of adolescents, and we have recently begun to recognize that individuals with ASD have the right to experience and fulfill this important part of life. Adolescents with ASD have a genuine need to learn about sexuality; they are curious and seek information and opportunities to experiment with sexuality. They are like other adolescents with regard to sexual development, interests, and needs.

For the majority of individuals with AS, sexual behaviors are perceived to be like any other behavior, free of social rules and convention. In contrast, parents and professionals often view sexuality in a much different manner. For them, sexuality may be taboo, value-laden, and a source of malaise. The need to protect the adolescent may be so strong that the subject of sexuality is avoided or banned altogether. There is also a tendency to define everything with respect to AS. This perspective fails to consider that adolescence, as a developmental period, brings about a variety of changes, new behaviors, and a need for discovery. The knowledge of sexuality can be found at the extremes for those with AS. Some have a special interest in sexuality and pornography, and great factual knowledge but almost no personal experience. Others have no knowledge or experience and a very limited social network. Clearly, this is an opportune and appropriate time to provide them with sexual education.

Sexuality on the Internet

The Internet contains millions of sites with sexual content, including pornography, erotica, and information about sex. Supervision by parents and educators is essential given that individuals with AS may lack judgment and experience when it comes to understanding the material they might encounter and the risk of inadvertently discovering illegal pornography. In addition, sexual images on the Internet, when viewed during masturbation, often become habitual and can form part of a ritual that is then difficult to break. Repeated exposure to sexual content also increases the risk of developing specific sexual interests, along with sexual obsessions and compulsions (Carnes, Delmonico, & Griffin, 2007; Hénault, 2006).

An additional risk involves the presence of sexual predators who tend to frequent sites where "chatting" or encounters take place (Carnes et al., 2007; Edmonds & Worton, 2006). Individuals with AS are more vulnerable to such risks; therefore, rules must be clearly explained to ensure their security, and supervision must be constant. In their book, Edmonds and

Worton (2006) list a series of suggestions to ensure the protection of those with autism and AS. They suggest, for example, parental or peer supervision to increase safety and to ensure that limits placed when "chatting" are respected. Due to their tendency to be naive, these individuals risk discovering inappropriate or illegal sites on the Internet when such precautions are not observed. In addition, their naiveté places them at greater risk of being targeted and having their confidence abused by predators. According to guidelines taught in a number of sexual education programs (Basso, 1997; Hénault, 2006; University of Calgary, 2009), conversations on the Internet that include sexual content (i.e., words, intentions, images, and videos) must not be tolerated. This also includes meeting an individual (even one who is considered a friend) one has met on the Internet, unless accompanied by parents or a responsible adult in a public place. Under no circumstances should personal information be shared (name, address, telephone number, bank or credit card information).

Interpersonal Relations and Emotions

With the exception of masturbation, sexual behavior expresses itself in the context of a relationship. Individuals with ASD must therefore show socially acceptable behavior, such as good communication and healthy expressions of emotions and intimacy. Unfortunately, many individuals have difficulty not only interpreting and understanding their feelings (Attwood, 2005), but also interpreting facial expressions and the emotions they are meant to convey (Baron-Cohen, 2002). This has a major impact on the establishment of interpersonal and intimate relationships.

When individuals with ASD become emotionally overwhelmed, their thoughts typically become illogical, and they become fixated on them. They do not think before reacting but react impulsively, which often leads to the expression of inappropriate behaviors. Given that the majority of these individuals have difficulty processing their emotions, interventions aimed at expressing, decoding, and understanding them become necessary (Attwood, 1999, 2005; Hess, 1998).

The initial goal of interventions is to create relationships based on the specific needs and interests of individuals with AS. It is then possible to establish good rapport based on trust. The main objective is to teach individuals how to recognize and identify a variety of emotions to help them express what they are feeling. Their emotional rigidity limits their expression (Attwood, 1999). In cases when verbal expression is difficult, written expression (use of a keyboard by individuals with fine motor difficulties) can be helpful. Essential is the use of whatever means possible to enable the expression of affect (e.g., music therapy or art therapy) (Attwood, 1999). These interventions help them discover the range of emotions that can be experienced between joy and anger.

The concept of *emotional intelligence* includes recognizing one's emotions, understanding them within their context, and identifying feelings expressed by others and interacting with them (Hess, 1998). Because some individuals with AS have only a technical understanding of emotional reactions, they tend to experience difficulties when attempting to integrate and assimilate them. They tend to focus on others' facial details (especially the mouth) when trying to identify emotions, which renders the task more difficult. Consistent effort must therefore focus on the essentials to enable individuals to decode and identify emotions adequately in others, simplifying the wealth of information that goes into such a task and thereby making it easier to accomplish. Neuroanatomical and imaging research (Channon, Charman, Heap, Crawford, & Rios, 2001; Klin, Jones, Schultz, Volkmar, & Cohen, 2006; Young, 2001) on those with autism and AS show dysfunction in the amygdala. This has led researchers to question whether technical knowledge alone is sufficient for the facial recognition of emotions to take place. To address these difficulties, several teaching activities are very useful. Computer software programs such as Mind Reading (Baron-Cohen, 2002), The Transporters (*www.thetransporters.com*) by Simon Baron-Cohen, along with Exploring Feelings (Attwood, 2005) and Cat-Kit (Callisen, Moller Nielsen, & Attwood, 2006) are all helpful in teaching expression of emotions in individuals with AS (Sofronoff et al., 2005, 2007; Eloff, 2009). These tools address specific needs, such as identifying and recognizing emotions conveyed by facial expressions, as well as exploring and understanding feelings, not to mention recognizing the signs associated with changes from one emotion to another.

Identifying and expressing emotions help individuals with ASD learn about intimacy and sexuality. With the help of images, photos and role playing, participants are asked to identify emotions, imitate facial expressions, and identify situations that produce a range of emotional responses. In addition, participants explore the fluctuations in their own feelings during a given day, and learn to understand the intensity of their feelings using the metaphor of a thermometer. Once these steps are completed, emotions that are more difficult to tolerate (e.g., anger, sadness, frustration, anxiety) are "repaired" using a *toolbox* metaphor (Atwood, 2005). A series of physical activities, relaxation exercises, social scenarios, and positive thoughts (i.e., antecdotes) are written in a workbook. During role play, participants learn the sequence of "repairs" by first identifying the emotion (or the combination of emotions) that needs to be "repaired," making use of content from their toolboxes, and reevaluating the intensity of their feelings once they have gained better control over them. The objective is therefore to reflect on their feelings, identify them, and proceed to "repair" them. Otherwise, they risk expressing their more intense feelings with potentially impulsive and inadequate behaviors. Once this objective is reached, individuals can then proceed to the next step, which involves acquiring more advanced social skills.

An important component of sociosexual education also involves helping individuals with ASD develop better social skills. The objective is to help these individuals become comfortable in social contexts, express appropriate behaviors in a variety of settings (schools, community centers, family gatherings, etc.), and enlarge their circle of friends. An exercise called Social Circles (Walker-Hirsh & Champagne, 1986) allows a visual and concrete exploration of the different spheres of intimacy, family, and social relations. In addition, the concept of a stranger is broached with regards to specific individuals, appropriate behaviours to expect, and adequate physical distances to maintain within each sphere. Colors are used (green, yellow, red and black) to make learning more concrete. Each color relates to a circle representing a group of desired behaviors depending on specific social contexts (Hénault, 2006). Social skills training also aims to refine and increase the repertoire of possible behaviors while favoring adapted and positive behaviors. Needless to say, certain basic skills are indispensable for individuals with HFASD. Such skills include initiating contact with another person, maintaining a discussion, expressing emotions, and decoding nonverbal language, among others. This training is best when offered in the context of a group setting. In fact, "group therapy" is preferred by some professionals (Barrett, 2003).

The educational program Making Waves, available at *www.ucalgary. ca/resolve/violenceprevention/english/reviewprog/youthdprogs.htm*, is a useful resource for adolescents and adults with HFASD. In a simple and effective way, the individual is asked to reflect on different sorts of relations that can exist between two people. An initial questionnaire evaluates basic knowledge of participants, such as appropriate times for affection, sexuality, and friendship. Depending on the results obtained, interpersonal relationships are explored to evaluate various limits of knowledge, as well as abuse scenarios in the section "About Relationships." This tool includes many examples, suggestions, and resources (i.e., links with several organizations, helpful tips regarding prevention of abuse, websites). Throughout the interventions, individuals with HFASD are called upon to participate in a concrete way, through role-playing scenarios. Special capacities and strengths are encouraged, in order to maintain interest and motivation.

PRACTICAL CONSIDERATIONS

In order to inform the sexual education of adolescents with ASD, it is important to identify the critical elements of general sexual education programs. Several subjects have been recommended as being essential to address in sexual education programs for typically developing adolescents. Here are some examples (Sex Information and Education Council of the United States, 1992) at *www.siecus.org/index.cfm?fuseaction=page.viewpage&pageid=472*):

- Sexual organs of both sexes: names, functions, and concrete descriptions
- Bodily changes that accompany puberty
- Self-esteem
- Information on nocturnal emissions
- Values and steps to decision making
- Intimacy: private and public settings
- Sexual health: behaviors and initial examination of sexual organs/gynecological examination
- Communication about dating, love, intimacy, and friendship
- How alcohol and drug use influence decision making
- Sexual intercourse and other sexual behaviors
- Masturbation
- Sexual orientation and identity
- Birth control, menstruation, and the responsibilities of childbearing
- Condoms, contraception, and disease prevention
- Emotions related to sexuality, since they motivate many behaviors.

The first step in intervention and sexual education programs involves general knowledge, tailored to the individual's chronological and developmental age. This information allows the individual to make informed choices. It also enables the person to understand better the limits within his or her learned behaviors that can be explored and experienced, while respecting his or her own values and those of others. The goal of the intervention is to provide both a structure for appropriate sexual behaviors and many opportunities to learn and obtain enriching experiences. The main goal is to adapt and teach sex education, while taking into account the ASD profile.

The objectives of the intervention are primarily the following:

- Acquire better knowledge about social and sexual expectations in the adolescent years
- Cope with changes in body, thinking, and friendship
- Develop one's own limits and judgment
- Decode situations: interpersonal and intimate contexts
- Improve social and sexual skills
- Decrease problem behaviors and inappropriate sexual conduct
- Empower the adolescent and increase self-esteem

Basic sex education is called for prior to adolescence. Young children of 7 or 8 can be taught about body parts, privacy, positive and inappropriate behaviors, and so forth. Once they reach the teenage years, these topics should be explored in more detail. The books *The Underground Guide to Teenage Sexuality* (Basso, 1997) and *Making Sense of Sex: A Forthright Guide to Puberty, Sex and Relationships for People with Asperger's Syndrome* (Attwood, 2008), written for adolescents, provide clear and respectful information on topics such as affectionate and sexual relationships, anatomical differences between men and women, personal transformations during adolescence, conception, pregnancy, and delivery, and myths related to sexuality. The books also provide information for parents. *Life Horizons I, II* programs (Kempton, 1999) for adults and adolescents include a series of slides on physiology and the sexual organs. Such photos should accompany all explanations to make the information more concrete and to avoid misunderstanding. Information presented in a visual way is recommended for individuals with ASD; it captures their attention, it is practical and concrete, and easier to understand. Spoken information has more chance to be confusing and intangible. Details on the program can be found at *www.stanfield.com*.

It is important to use the exact terms of the technical jargon (anatomical, medical) and their popular counterparts when discussing these various topics. The individual with ASD likely knows several of the scientific terms to describe sexuality (especially if he or she is fond of encyclopedic information), but it is preferable to use the more popular terms to allow association of more than one word with a given concept. The popular jargon of other, same-age youth must be accessible, so that he or she can also interact with his or her peer group. This certainly does not mean that vulgar language should be used to talk about sexuality. The idea is to be open regarding popular culture to avoid stigmatization or rejection by peers.

According to Family Planning Queensland (2001) and the National Information Center for Children and Youth with Disabilities (1992), sex education programs should provide information, develop values, encourage and develop interpersonal skills, and help individuals learn to be responsible. Sexuality should also be considered in its entirety and include notions of intimacy, desire, communication, love, deviance, and satisfaction (Griffiths, Richards, Fedoroff, & Watson, 2002; Haracopos & Pedersen, 1999). Intervention programs should also discuss sexual and gender identity, sexual needs, and sexual development. As suggested in the literature (Cornelius, Chipouras, Makas, & Daniels, 1982; Griffiths et al., 1989; Hellemans, 1996), a structured and adapted education program designed to meet the needs of the ASD population must be part of the services offered and extended. The National Information Center for Children and Youth with Disabilities (1992), Kempton (1993), and Hingsburger (1993) all state that the more individuals are informed about sexuality, the better they are able to make informed and autonomous choices. This not only decreases the risk of sexual abuse but also allows individuals with autism and HFASD access to a rewarding social and sexual life.

Several authors have recognized the need for sexual education for individuals with ASD (e.g., Attwood, personal communication, June, 1998; Gray, Ruble, & Dalrymple, 1996; Haracopos & Pedersen, 1999; Hellemans, 1996; Hingsburger, 1993). Unfortunately, most sex education programs are limited and the educational material is insufficiently concrete. Other social skills programs (e.g., Ouellet & L'Abbé, 1986; Soyner & Desnoyers Hurley, 1990) are explicit about socialization but only briefly address the notions of sexuality and intimacy. La SexoTrousse (Lemay, 1996), Programme d'éducation à la vie affective, amoureuse et sexuelle (Desaulniers, 2001) and the Life Horizons I, II (Kempton, 1999) programs, developed for people with intellectual disability and ASD, have the advantage of including concrete material and pertinent activities but are not adapted to the needs of individuals with ASD without intellectual disability.

The Programme d'Éducation Sexuelle (Durocher & Fortier, 1999) appears to be most promising given the sexual and cognitive profile of individuals with ASD. Activities are concrete, full of imagery, and require high levels of participation. The program, designed to be administered in a group format, focuses on interpersonal exchanges and social contacts. It has been used to help individuals with a variety of behavioral problems, such as aggression, oppositionality, and hyperactivity (Bouchard, Keller, & Saint-Jean, 1988).

This program therefore constitutes the foundation for the sociosexual education program for individuals with ASD presented here. The program can be offered on an individual basis, but the section on social skills needs to be modified, since the activities were designed to be administered in a group format. All the instructions about the program are provided in the book (Hénault, 2006): age for the participants, number of participants in each groups, and information for the group leader. A detailed description of the 12 workshops (goals, timing of the activities, material required, worksheets, and tips for the leader) is provided in the manual. Although each workshop takes place over a 90-minute period, a group leader might easily divide it into two 45-minute workshops. Activities and exercises may also be repeated and extended over 20 workshops or more. Other modifications of the 12-session pedagogical formula may also be made according to the discretion of the group leader.

Materials can be adapted, both visually and practically, to help with the learning process. Films, computer programs, photos, diagrams, games and Social Stories™ are referred to throughout the intervention. Sexual education can be offered in mixed groups (usually six to 10 participants, males and females). Individual sessions are also possible in due course of therapeutic interventions with individuals with ASD. For example, fact sheets, questionnaires, and games can be used to address different topics and explore the knowledge and experience of an individual with ASD. Many clinicians have reported the use of the program in clinical settings.

OVERVIEW OF SESSIONS FROM THE SOCIOSEXUAL SKILLS EDUCATIONAL PROGRAM

The following themes, which are adapted to the reality of adolescents and adults with ASD, cover characteristics linked to their social and sexual development (Hénault, 2006):

- Information on nocturnal emissions
- The value of and stages involved in making decisions
- Intimacy: both private and nonprivate parts of the body; different environments
- Sexual health and initial examination of genital organs—or gynecological exam
- Communication: interpersonal, intimate, love, and friendly relationships
- The effect of alcohol and drugs on the ability to make decisions
- Sexual relations and other sexual behaviors
- Self-stimulation (masturbation)
- Sexual orientation and identity
- Planning for pregnancy, menstruation, and parental responsibilities

- Condoms, contraception, and the prevention of sexually transmitted diseases and infections
- Hygiene
- Friendship: recognition of abusive/unfriendly relationships
- Dangerous relationships: age difference, intention, bullying, aggression
- Qualities of a healthy relationship: sharing, communication, pleasure, interest, respect
- Intensity of relationships: finding a balance and learning the limits
- Social skills: presentation, interactions, reciprocity, sharing, and so forth
- Boundaries and the notion of informed consent

The sociosexual education program presented here draws on the activities of Durocher and Fortier's (1999) program and is divided into 12 topics related to sexuality. The program was developed specifically to meet the needs of the HFASD population. Numerous additions were made and include more concrete activities, increased visual support, and the repetition of exercises to allow participants to integrate the material better. Various tools are also used, such as the Mind Reading software (Baron-Cohen, 2002), pictures from the *La SexoTrousse* (Lemay, 1996), Social Stories (Gray, 1995), and so forth. The sociosexual educational program (Hénault et al., 2003; Hénault, 2006) has been validated in more than 20 groups of adolescents and young adults with HFASD. Specifically, this program was evaluated through independent observations, charts, and questionnaires used throughout the sessions with defined groups. Since the publication of the book, many organizations and schools have used the program and replicated the results. The proposed themes are divided into 12 workshops that last 90 minutes each. The activities in each workshop are varied and incite active participation from the participants. The themes not only reflect the experiences of participants but also respect the criteria outlined in the sexual education of the National Information Center for Children and Youth with Disabilities (1992) and those defined by Haracopos and Pedersen (1999), and Kempton (1993):

1. Assessment and introduction to the program
2. Introduction to sexuality and communication
3. Love and friendship
4. Physiological aspects and the sexual response cycle
5. Sexual intercourse and other behaviors
6. Emotions
7. Sexually transmitted diseases and infections, HIV, and prevention

8. Sexual orientation
9. Alcohol, drugs, and sexuality
10. Sexual abuse and inappropriate behaviors
11. Sexism and violence
12. Managing emotions and theory of mind related to romance, love, and intimacy

Each workshop includes a support sheet for the group leader, the required materials, and all instructions. Activities can be adapted depending on the group (as a function of age, special needs, receptivity, etc.). In general, groups are based on participants' ages (16 to 20 years, 20 to 30 years, 30 to 40 years, etc.), and include both males and females. Males are always curious to hear what females think, and vice versa.

By nature, individuals with ASD need to be taught social skills explicitly. Given that social skills training represents one of their greatest challenges, parents and professionals cannot take for granted that individuals with AS are able to learn these simply by being in a group or reading a book. It is also recommended that those in charge remain flexible and adapt the intervention to the reality and needs of these adolescents' and participants' personal experiences. Role playing and modeling are essential techniques, because they provide a "safe learning experience" for participants, and the professional can provide them with immediate feedback regarding their performance. In this way, the intervention in terms of sexual education responds to their needs.

Positive reinforcement is important throughout the sexual education and intervention program. It can be verbal or nonverbal (signs of appreciation from the leader, cumulative points on a chart, etc.), with feedback given both during and at the end of each session, and should respect the content and the structure of each session. It is important to follow instructions about the topics and activities of each workshop, especially in a group format, and to take into account the possibility of many interactions (social, verbal) between the participants. Social reinforcement is also important when activities are done in a group format. For example, at the end of the program, a special activity can be organized (picnic at the park, movie, museum, etc.) with the group as a way to encourage social skills and the development of friendship.

RESEARCH TO DATE ON THE TREATMENT

The program has been evaluated using a variety of measures. The Australian Scale for Asperger's Syndrome (Garnett & Attwood, 1995, as cited in Attwood, 1998) was used for diagnostic purposes (Hénault et al., 2003). The Aberrant Behaviour Checklist (Aman & Singh, 1986) identified participants' inappropriate behaviors. The Friendship Skills Observation Checklist (Attwood & Gray, 1999a) was used to observe participants' appropriate and inappropriate behaviors related to social and personal skills. The Sociosexual Information Questionnaire (Durocher & Fortier, 1999) assessed general knowledge about pre- and post-program sexual activities. Finally, the Derogatis Sexual Functioning Inventory (Derogatis & Melisaratos, 1982) assessed generalization of gains 3-months postintervention. Given the intrusive nature of the questionnaire (many questions about sexual experience, behaviors, preferences, etc.), it was only administered to participants who were older than 18 years of age. The questionnaire was not appropriate for younger participants, as recommended by the ethical committee of the University of Quebec at Montreal.

The application of the sociosexual educational program (Hénault et al., 2003) has allowed the development of different skills and has altered inappropriate sexual behaviors. The aim of the study was to observe the effects of the treatment program on individual subjects in four different experimental groups with distinct baseline levels. The four groups were built by shifting the onset of the treatment program. The whole experiment took place over a period of 1 year. The second group started the program 1 month after the first group. The third group started 4 months after the second group. The fourth group started 3 months after the third group. This multi-level design has the advantage of avoiding withdrawal followed by reintroduction of the treatment program in the *same group*.

The study tested three main hypotheses related to the effect of the treatment program: enhancement of adaptive interpersonal skills, decrease of inappropriate sociosexual behaviors, and generalization of acquired behaviors in the everyday living environment. Analysis of results included (1) mean frequencies of friendship and privacy skills, and of inappropriate behaviors; (2) analyses of variance (ANOVA); and (3) post hoc analyses (Scheffé's test) to evaluate the effect of the Friendship Skills Observation Checklist and the Aberrant Behavior Checklist. A polynomial regression analysis was then performed to study a potential correlation between selective variables, such as "compromise," "intimate relationship," and "accepting criticisms." The third hypothesis on generalization of acquired behaviors was tested using the Derogatis Sexual Function Inventory.

The principal results can be grouped into three categories:

1a. Improvement of social skills in terms of:
  • Presentation
  • Conversation/reciprocity
  • Eye contact
  • Helping/empathy
  • Nonverbal skills
1b. Increased general knowledge and better judgement about sexuality in general
2. Reduction in problem behaviors:
  • Isolation (more contact with participants, involvement in activities, more conversation)
  • Impulsivity
  • Inappropriate sexual behaviors (masturbation in public, touching others, sexual obsessions and/or compulsions, etc.)
3. Generalization (3-month follow-up measures)
  • Better sociosexual knowledge
  • Development of interpersonal relationships, interest in forming friendships
  • Positive attitude about sexuality
  • Increase in self-confidence

By virtue of the training program, friendship and intimacy skills significantly increased, whereas the frequency of inappropriate behaviors decreased (Hénault et al., 2003). An improvement in skills including introducing oneself, maintaining conversation, communicating nonverbally, was seen over the course of the intervention. Helping and empathy behaviors were observed more frequently at the end of the program. The development of friendships among the participants and openness to others was also observed during the workshops. The sociosexual education program also helped to decrease the frequency of inappropriate behaviors, such as inappropriate masturbation, sexual obsessions, voyeurism, fetishism, and exhibitionism), as reported by the parents, teachers, and professionals in the different environments of the participants with ASD. Parent sessions (before and after the program) and phone contacts were conducted to gather external information about sexual behaviors. In addition withdrawal and isolation behaviors were replaced by greater reciprocity among group members. Impulsive behaviors such as self-mutilation and tantrums were not significantly represented during and after the treatment. These results confirmed the hypothesis that aggressive behaviors are rarely present in the behavioral repertoires of individuals with AS and high-functioning autism. Generalization of treatment gains was shown at 3-month follow-up. An increase in general sexual knowledge and a positive attitude toward sexuality was observed in the participants.

Few programs offer social skills training in combination with sexual education. The collaboration, respect, and interest shown are an indication of participants' motivation to take part in such a program. Most participants were self-referred in response to advertisements mailed to parent associations and community services. A small number of participants were referred due to their inappropriate sexual behaviors. The subject of sexuality itself evoked much curiosity, in that such a program was new to most of them. The intervention program responded to and met a specific need. In light of the nature of the intervention and the topics addressed, personal questions and disclosure on the part of the participants were to be expected. Each workshop was followed by a 30-minute period in which participants were invited to discuss any concerns. On one occasion, an adolescent expressed his fetishistic tendencies. Similarly, following the workshop on sexual abuse, another adolescent revealed the inappropriate behaviors of one of his family members. In order to facilitate these interventions, each workshop is accompanied by "notes for the group leader." These offer suggestions on how to address a variety of difficult issues that may come up subsequent to a meeting. As such, the overarching goal of fostering the expression of a healthy sexuality is maintained parallel to the group activities.

The program's format is also a significant strength. The fact that the intervention takes place over 12 consecutive weeks enables participants to socialize with one another while developing friendships. This is especially obvious during the last two sessions. Qualitative observations reveal that friendships develop among participants. For example, two participants discovered that they shared a common passion for wrestling. They exchanged magazines and began meeting one another outside of the group context. In another group, three adults engaged in activities together on a weekly basis. One participant introduced her favorite activity, bowling, to the group. Two adults in one group discovered their common passion for computers, and an adolescent in another group introduced someone to drawing. Many participants reported less social anxiety at school or at the workplace. Some adolescent males also mentioned more success in initiating and maintaining conversation with females. Such experiences, observed in all four groups, indicate the advantage of group activities in helping group members to become close. The need to socialize makes it possible for friendships to develop and for the quality of interpersonal relationships to improve within the group.

Group participation also helps people develop less self-centered, narcissistic attitudes. Social skills enable them to become more open to the experiences of others, which decrease attitudes, such as "I know everything" or "Everyone is ignorant," observed in certain individuals. Peer reactions are very useful during the workshops. For example, following a video on sexual abuse, the comments of some participants influenced those who tended more toward sexual aggression. Similarly, a discussion and a short video on masturbation allowed an adolescent with high-functioning autism to change his inappropriate behavior, which his mother later confirmed. The change was maintained until the last follow-up, 3 months posttreatment.

The use of stimulating visual materials (videos, photos, computer programs) and the group activities maintained participants' interest and increased appropriate gazing behaviors such as the Mind Reading software (Baron-Cohen, 2002), Emotions Pictures (Lemay, 1996), and many role-playing activities from our program (Hénault, 2006). In general, staring behaviors need to be addressed in these populations, because they are among one of the most frequently observed difficulties (Soyner & Desnoyers Hurley, 1990).

Evaluation of the sociosexual skills education program (Hénault et al., 2003) revealed that participants had acquired technical skills necessary for the expression of emotion (i.e., read, decode, and manage emotions), but that applying the skills was more difficult. Individuals with AS tended to get distracted by facial details, which made it more difficult for them to recognize and label a specific emotion. Continued education would be required to help them reduce and organize information when attempting to decode faces.

FUTURE DIRECTIONS

Individuals with AS must be guided with respect to sexual issues. An extended definition of sexuality takes into account factors linked to sexual development, puberty, and symptoms associated with the autism condition. A positive approach that respects the personal and cultural values is favored over an attitude of condemnation, which risks increasing social stigmas and taboos faced by these individuals. Parents and professionals play a key role in terms of the education and support that they can offer, but they also need the necessary tools to intervene effectively.

An open and receptive attitude of parents and professionals favors open communication and a possibility for individuals with AS to share their experiences and questions, and express their preoccupations toward sexuality. The sexual education and intervention program aims not only to teach adolescents and young adults to become responsible but also offers them the necessary tools to develop interpersonal relationships. This process therefore helps them develop a healthy and enriching sexual lifestyle.

One limitation faced by all education and intervention programs involves the generalization of gains over the long term. As mentioned by Griffiths et al. (1989), generalization involves therapist implications, support networks, and community intervention. The therapist works on interventions in the natural setting. As such, in addition to offering activities in the workshop context, *in vivo* training that takes place helps the individual confront real situations. The second phase comprises creating a support network (family member, friend, counselor, youth worker, etc.) that helps to extend learning, provides social support, and maintains the link with the principal therapist. Finally, community interventions, such as hobbies, support groups, and other services, are offered. Future studies should include these three phases of follow-up to ensure that gains are maintained over the long term.

Support systems need to be established within the existing community services. On several occasions, my services were requested for therapy and follow-up purposes. The intervention program therefore opens avenues to creating psychological and sexological services adapted to the specific needs of individuals living with AS.

In conclusion, specialized education professionals and therapists need to understand the issues involved in the sexuality of individuals with AS. These individuals' sexual development and interest in sexuality are comparable to those of individuals in the general population. However, their social and sexual profiles differ on several levels. Considerable difficulties related to social skills, communication, interpersonal relationships and developmental immaturity can be found. They present with several needs that may be addressed by sociosexual education. Intervention programs specific to their needs must therefore be made available to them, using the premise that sexuality is an important contribution to their quality of life.

REFERENCES

Aman, M. G., & Singh, N. N. (1986). *Aberrant behavior checklist: Manual.* East Aurora, NY: Slosson Educational.

Attwood, S. (2008). *Making sense of sex: A forthright guide to puberty, sex and relationships for people with Asperger's syndrome.* London: Jessica Kingsley.

Attwood, T. (1998). *Asperger's syndrome: A guide for parents and professionals.* London: Jessica Kingsley.

Attwood, T. (1999). *Cognitive behaviour therapy to accommodate the cognitive profile of people with Asperger's syndrome.* Retrieved March 15, 1999, from *www.tonyattwood.com.au.*

Attwood, T. (2003). Cognitive behavior therapy. In L. Holliday Willey (Eds.), *Asperger syndrome in adolescence* (pp. 38–68). London: Jessica Kingsley.

Attwood, T. (2005). *Exploring feelings on anger and anxiety.* Arlington, TX: Future Horizons.

Attwood, T. (2007). *The complete guide to Asperger's syndrome.* London: Jessica Kingsley.

Attwood, T., & Gray, C. (1999a). *Understanding and teaching friendship skills.* Retrieved January 20, 1999, from *www.tonyattwood.com.au.*

Baron-Cohen, S. (1995). *Mind blindness: An essay on autism and theory of mind.* Cambridge, MA: MIT Press.

Baron-Cohen, S. (2002). *Mind reading: The interactive guide to emotions.* Cambridge, MA: Human Emotions.

Barrett, L. (2003, January). Lessons from the little professor: Asperger's syndrome: Wired differently—not defectively. *The Washington Post.* Available at *www.washingtonpost.com.*

Basso, M. J. (1997). *The underground guide to teenage sexuality.* Minneapolis: Fairview Press.

Bouchard, P., Keller, Y., & Saint-Jean, N. (1988). *Dans les coulisses et l'intimité sexuelle [Behind the scene of intimacy].* Montréal: Fondation Jeunesse 2000.

Carnes, P., Delmonico, D. L., & Griffin, E. (2007). *In the shadows of the net.* Center City, MN: Hazelden.

Channon, S., Charman, T., Heap, J., Crawford, S., & Rios, P. (2001). Real-life problem-solving in Asperger's syndrome. *Journal of Autism and Development ment Disorders, 31,* 461–469.

Cornelius, D. A., Chiparas, S., Makas, E., & Daniels, S. M. (1982). *Who cares?: A handbook on sex education and counseling services for disabled people.* Baltimore: University Park Press.

Derogatis, L. R., & Melisaratos, N. (1982). *Derogatis Sexual Functioning Inventory.* Retrieved March 12, 2000, from *www.derogatis-tests.com.*

Desaulniers, M. P. (2001). *Programme d'éducation à la vie affective, amoureuse et sexuelle.* Trois-Rivières: Centre de Services en Déficience Intellectuelle de la Mauricie et du Centre-du-Québec.

Durocher, L., & Fortier, M. (1999). *Programme d'éducation sexuelle [Sex education program].* Montréal: Les Centres Jeunesses de Montréal et la Régie Régionale de la Santé et des Services Sociaux, Direction de la santé publique. Centre Universitaire à Montréal.

Edmonds, G., & Worton, D. (2006). *The Asperger love guide.* London: Paul Chapman.

Eloff, J. (2009). *A trial of a cognitive behavioural intervention for problems with the affectionate communication in children with Asperger syndrome.* University of Queensland, Australia.

Family Planning Queensland. (2001). Retrieved from *www.fpq.asn.au.*

Gray, C. (1995). *Social stories.* Grandville, MI: Jenison Public Schools.

Gray, S., Ruble, L., & Dalrymple, N. (1996). *Autism and sexuality: A guide for instruction*. Carmel: Autism Society of Indiana.

Griffiths, D., Quinsey, V. L., & Hingsburger, D. (1989). *Changing inappropriate sexual behaviour*. Baltimore: Brookes.

Griffiths, D., Richards, D., Fedoroff, P., & Watson, S. L. (2002). *Ethical dilemmas: Sexuality and developmental disability*. New York: NADD Press.

Haracopos, D. (2009, May). *Sex education for individuals with autism spectrum disorders*. Paper presented at the conference for the Greek Society for Autism, Athens.

Haracopos, D., & Pedersen, L. (1999). *The Danish Report*. Copenhagen: Society for the Autistically Handicapped.

Hellemans, H. (1996). *L'éducation sexuelle des adolescents autistes [Sex education for adolescents with autism]*. Paper presented at the Belgium Conference on Autism, Brussels.

Hellemans, H., & Deboutte, D. (2002, November). *Autism spectrum disorders and sexuality*. Paper presented at the World First Autism Congress, Melbourne, Australia.

Hénault, I. (2006). *Asperger's syndrome and sexuality*. London: Jessica Kingsley.

Hénault, I., & Attwood, T. (2002). *The sexual profile of adults with Asperger's syndrome*. Paper presented at the World First Autism Congress, Melbourne, Australia.

Hénault, I., Forget, J., & Giroux, N. (2003). *Le développement d'habiletés sexuelles adaptatives chez des individus atteints d'autisme de haut niveau ou du syndrome d'Asperger*. Doctoral thesis, University of Québec at Montréal.

Hess, U. (1998). *L'intelligence émotionnelle [emotional intelligence*. Notes de cours dans le cadre du baccalauréat en psychologie, Département de psychologie, Université du Québec a Montréal.

Hingsburger, D. (1993). *Parents ask questions about sexuality and children with developmental disabilities*. Vancouver: Family Support Institute Press.

Hingsburger, D. (1995). *Hand made love: A guide for teaching about male masturbation through understanding and video*. Newmarket, BC: Diverse City Press. Retrieved June 6, 2000, from *www.diverse-city.com*.

Holmes, D. L., Isler, V., Bott, C., & Markowitz, C. (2005, Winter–Fall). Sexuality and individuals with autism and developmental disabilities. *Autism Spectrum Quarterly*, pp. 30–33.

Kempton, W. (1993). *Socialization and sexuality: A comprehensive training guide*. Santa Barbara, California: Author.

Kempton, W. (1999) *Life Horizons I, II*. Santa Barbara, CA: James Stanfield.

Klin, A., Jones, W., Schultz, R., Volkmar, F., & Cohen, D. (2006). Visual fixation patterns during viewing of naturalistic social situations as predictors of social competence in individuals with autism. *Archives of General Psychiatry, 59*(9), 809–816.

Konstantareas, M. M., & Lunsky, Y. J. (1997). Sociosexual knowledge, experience, attitudes, and interests of individuals with autistic disorder and developmental delay. *Journal of Autism and Developmental Disorders, 27*, 113–125.

Lemay, M. (1996) *La SexoTrousse*. Maniwaki, Canada: Pavillon du Parc.

National Information Center for Children and Youth with Disabilities. (1992).

Sexuality education for children and youth with disabilities. *NICHCY News Digest, 17,* 1–37.

Newport, J., & Newport, M. (2002). *Autism–Asperger's and sexuality: Puberty and beyond.* Arlington, TX: Future Horizons.

Ouellet, R., & L'Abbé, Y. (1986). *Programme d'Entraînement aux Habiletés Sociales.* Eastman: Éditions Behaviora.

Ruble, L. A., & Dalrymple, J. (1993). Social and sexual awareness of persons with autism: A parental perspective. *Archives of Sexual Behavior, 22,* 229–240.

Sex Information and Education Council of the United States. (1992). *Developing guidelines for comprehensive sexuality education.* Retrieved from *www.siecus.org/_data/global/images/guide.intl.pdf.*

Sofronoff, K., Attwood, T., & Hinton, S. (2005). A randomized controlled trial of a CBT intervention for anxiety in children with Asperger syndrome. *Journal of Child Psychology and Psychiatry, 46,* 1152–1160.

Sofronoff, K., Attwood, T., Hinton, S., & Levin, I. (2007). A randomized controlled trial of a CBT intervention for anger management in children diagnosed with Asperger syndrome. *Journal of Autism and Developmental Disorders, 37,* 1203–1214.

Soyner, R., & Desnoyers Hurley, A. (1990) L'apprentissage des habiletés sociales [Developing social skills]. *Habilitative Mental Healthcare Newsletter, 9*(1), 1–5.

University of Calgary. (2009). *Making Waves.* Retrieved January 17, 2009, from *www.ucalgary.ca/resolve/violenceprevention/English/reviewprog/youthdprogs.htm.*

Walker-Hirsch, L., & Champagne, M. P. (1986). *Circles I, II & III.* Santa Barbara, CA: James Stanfield.

Young, E. (2001, March). A look at theory of mind. *The New Scientist,* pp. 21–26.

PART V

CONCLUDING REMARKS

What Do We Know about Psychosocial Interventions for Youth with High-Functioning ASD, and Where Do We Go from Here?

SUSAN WILLIAMS WHITE, ANGELA SCARPA,
AND TONY ATTWOOD

Autism spectrum disorders (ASD) are pervasive, chronically impairing, and—most importantly—treatable. Although a cure, or symptom abatement to levels at which the individual no longer meets diagnostic criteria, is typically not a feasible goal, quality of life and daily functioning can be significantly improved. Research in this area over the last 20 years has been dominated by a focus on early detection, accurate diagnosis, and a search for biological and other causal factors (Mazefsky & White, in press). We now have well-validated diagnostic tools at our disposal and a wealth of knowledge on myriad genetic, biological, and environmental pathways involved. More recently, we have seen mounting interest in treatment development and evaluation. It is critical that research on ASD intervention be supported as it evolves and matures given the inevitable, growing demand for effective therapeutic services due to rising identification and diagnosis rates. Throughout this book, we have brought together experts from around the world on cognitive-behavioral treatment of ASD-related difficulties to share clinically relevant suggestions based on sound empirical research. The preceding chapters demonstrate both the appeal of cognitive-behavioral approaches for people with ASD, and the rising evidence base for their use.

After initially describing our theoretical understanding of cognitive-behavioral therapy (CBT) and its adaptation for assessing and treating youth with ASD (particularly high-functioning), we divided this book into sections that explore new CBT programs for commonly noted difficulties of children and adolescents with ASD, including anxiety and behavior, social competence, and sexuality/affection problems. In this closing chapter, we synthesize the previously presented material to draw conclusions on the current status of CBT for treating youth with ASD. In so doing, we also provide specific suggestions for further scientific and clinical investigation based on the state of the current research.

THEORETICAL GROUNDING AND CONCEPTUALIZATION

Scarpa and Lorenzi (Chapter 1) summarized the considerable body of research indicating that psychosocial intervention, most notably CBT, can be effective in treating adults and children across a wide number of diagnostic categories. They have provided a primer on CBT, including its history (e.g., roots in constructivist thought) and the approach's guiding principles (e.g., collaborative client–therapist relationship, goal-oriented structure). Applications of CBT to child problems other than ASD, such as childhood anxiety, were provided to highlight some of the specific adaptations necessary when working with children and teens (e.g., creatively building self-motivation for treatment, to improve outcomes).

Specific adaptations to CBT for working with young people with ASD were provided by Attwood and Scarpa (Chapter 2), including *when* and *how* to address some of the most common deficits seen in ASD, which often adversely impact therapeutic progress. Issues such as poor self-awareness and variable self-control are critical considerations. Sensitivity to the unique qualities of the client's learning profile, such as attentional and executive difficulties (e.g., problems with set shifting) and inadequate sense of self (i.e., lack of perceived self-efficacy), is necessary to consider in treatment planning. Failure to do so might exacerbate the client's frustration or contribute to hostility (toward self or others). Likewise, proceeding with thought challenging when the client is overly aroused, anxious, or "stuck" in a repetitive thought pattern can prove quite unproductive. It is akin to trying to derail a train at full-speed on a single track. Yet another challenge often faced by therapists working with this population is the client's poor connection to his or her own emotions and the emotional world in general. This is a challenge given the weighty role that emotion recognition and monitoring play in CBT. Necessary, though likely not sufficient, qualities that therapists must possess in order to work successfully with clients on the spectrum include patience (for the client's perspective and pace) and the ability to think sequentially and logically, to mirror and model a rational approach to problem solving and living.

Mazefsky and White (Chapter 3) have distilled the vast literature on diagnostic assessment into usable suggestions for empirically based assessment. First, it is clear that we lack a solid, or multifaceted, cadre of valid measures with which to assess change with treatment. This is perhaps the greatest hindrance to our field as we endeavor to advance treatment efficacy and begin to explore moderators and mediators of treatment response. For use in clinical trials and clinical practice, we must develop valid measures that are sensitive to change (Lord et al., 2005). Second, although we are more cognizant of the presence of co-occurring problems (depression, eating disorders), we have little guidance on how to assess secondary symptoms in people with ASD. Finally, the chapter offers specific suggestions for therapists to consider in conceptualization of a given behavior or problem, such as carefully attending to the temporality of the presenting problems to determine whether the behavior is a true departure from baseline functioning or a modified expression of something that has been there all along (i.e., heterotypic continuity; Rutter & Sroufe, 2000).

Although the importance of modifications to CBT for ASD is commonly stressed in the literature, the empirical necessity or incremental value of such modification has not been adequately studied. There are well over 500 documented treatments available for children and adolescents from which therapists may choose (Kazdin, 2000). For clients with ASD, we need also to determine empirically *which* modifications, as well as *when* and *for whom* these modifications are critical or helpful. There are surely multiple paths we might take to address such sensitive and important questions. For example, we might explore the impact of treatments established for other clinical populations (e.g., mood disorders in adolescents) on young people with ASD or, via a bottom-up or additive approach, determine the incremental benefit of specific enhancements or modifications. This is a critically important scientific endeavor given the resources, time, and money spent on treatment development and modification, therapist training, and the mind-boggling plethora of stand-alone treatment manuals from which therapists must select (Chorpita, Becker, & Daleiden, 2007), as well as the lack of guidance on how to translate evidence into practice in practical terms, answering questions such as "Will this treatment work in my clinic?" and "Will the clients I tend to serve find this approach accept-able?" (Chorpita, Bernstein, & Daleiden, 2011).

Further work is also needed to determine which clients are likely to benefit from CBT, using appropriate screening and assessment instruments developed and normed for the ASD population. Although emergent research indicates that those with average cognitive abilities can benefit from CBT (Lickel, MacLean, Blakeley-Smith, & Hepburn, 2012), whether it is possible to adapt CBT for individuals with impaired cognitive functioning remains an open question. Ultimately, we hope to be able to develop an empirically based rubric for making decisions to guide treatment planning based on client preferences, problems, developmental level, and functioning, and to be able to assess change in treatment outcome research adequately.

CBT FOR ANXIETY
AND BEHAVIORAL PROBLEMS IN ASD

Several of the chapters address the treatment of anxiety in young people with ASD. This is important because anxiety is such a common co-occurring problem (van Steensel, Bogels, & Perrin, 2011; White, Oswald, Ollendick, & Scahill, 2009) and one that appears to exacerbate core ASD impairments (Chang, Quan, & Wood, 2012). Green and Wood (Chapter 4) observe that although anxiety is quite common in ASD, we do not fully understand its etiology, but there is evidence that mechanisms underlying the anxiety are similar to those seen in children without ASD (e.g., elevated cortisol). They describe their treatment program, Behavioral Interventions for Anxiety in Children with Autism (BIACA; Wood et al., 2009), including the adaptations they made from an evidence-based program for children without ASD (Wood & McLeod, 2008), and adding modules to target social deficits, adaptive skills growth, and stereotyped interests. Green and Wood also indicate the utility of future trials to compare CBT to medication, or to compare adapted CBT to other treatments that do not directly target anxiety to determine differential impact.

In Chapter 5, Reaven and Blakeley-Smith describe the value of parental involvement in treating anxiety in higher-functioning children with ASD. They describe the developmental course of anxiety, based on research with typically developing children, as well as potential, complex pathways to anxiety that may exist in ASD, which as yet are largely unexplored (e.g., parental transmission, social learning). Parental pathology (and heightened expressed emotion) is far from a universal phenomenon in ASD, but it provides evidence of greater stress and psychiatric difficulties among parents of children with ASD compared to parents of children without ASD. The value of a strength-based model (developing resilience, highlighting the generally low levels of criticism and high maternal warmth these families possess) may provide a fruitful undertaking in clinical settings. Reaven and Blakeley-Smith also describe research on parental involvement in their Facing Your Fears (FYF; Reaven, Blakeley-Smith, Nichols, & Hepburn, 2011) program, in which parents are heavily involved in treatment delivery (e.g., taught how to facilitate exposure and not allow children to avoid fearful situations). From this chapter, it is clear that we need to explore empirically parental involvement and family-based intervention for young people with ASD. There is mixed evidence for the importance, or necessity, of parental involvement in treatment for childhood anxiety (Silverman, Pina, & Viswesvaran, 2008). However, parental involvement in treatment may be of utmost importance for young people who have ASD given their strong reliance on their parents, typically beyond the age at which most adolescents start to pull away and develop greater independence. We also need to examine the potential bidirectional influences between parent mental health and child outcome with treatment.

Chapter 6 (White, Scahill, & Ollendick) provides an integrative discussion on the relationship between anxiety and social disability, the core deficit domain on ASD. There is considerable between- and within-individual heterogeneity, as well as temporal change, in social functioning in young people with ASD, all of which can complicate clinical decision making with respect to effective intervention for social disability. Anxiety may be viewed as a within-person moderator, because it can influence the effect of treatment to improve social ability, via social avoidance and inability. White and colleagues assert that anxiety and social disability exert bidirectional impact and highlight the paucity of research on adolescents with ASD. In the chapter, they describe the Multimodal Anxiety and Social Skills Intervention (MASSI; White et al., 2010), which integrates group and individual treatment, and adopts a flexible, modular implementation model. Summarized results from one open pilot trial and one randomized controlled trial on MASSI indicate support for the program. It is suggested that MASSI may be adapted for school-based implementation, and that anxiety reduction, even in cases when anxiety is not manifested as a psychiatric comorbidity, may facilitate treatment to improve social function (e.g., social skills training).

The Stress and Anger Management Program (STAMP; Scarpa, Wells, & Attwood, 2013) is described by Scarpa, Reyes, and Attwood in Chapter 7, was developed for young children (ages 5–7) to promote emotion regulation skills and to decrease emotional outbursts. In the chapter, Scarpa et al. provide a frame of reference with the typical process of emotional development in which children develop competence in their ability to modulate their own emotions. Scarpa et al. then summarize empirical evidence indicating heightened emotionality, negative affect, and dysregulation or lability in children with ASD. STAMP is a downward adaptation of the Exploring Feelings program (for 9- to 12-year-olds; Attwood, 2004), with heavy parent involvement, administered in groups of two to six children. There is preliminary support from a small randomized controlled trial (RCT) indicating that the program has promise, though replication is needed.

Together these studies demonstrate the benefits of CBT for improving anxiety and behavioral agitation in children and adolescents with high-functioning ASD, and also potentially improving social function—directly and as a result of anxiety reduction. Several key questions remain to develop this line of work further. Parents tend to be involved in all of the described approaches, but level of involvement is variable. How much parental involvement is needed for anxiety and behavioral improvements to be seen? Does the utility of parental involvement change as the person with ASD matures from early childhood to adolescence? This also leads to additional questions related to how cognitive, emotional, and physical development impact the effect of CBT for these problems. The age range noted for the treatments reviewed herein is from 5 to 18. It would be fruitful to identify the developmental mechanisms that support change in these programs, and eventually to determine common elements of change at different levels of developmental functioning. Finally, depression, an additional disorder often seen in adolescents with ASD, has been identified as perhaps the most common co-occurring problem in this population (Ghaziuddin, Ghazziuddin, & Greden, 2002), affecting approximately 40% of adolescents with diagnosed ASD (Lopata, Toomey, et al., 2010). Yet we know of no studies that have examined the use of CBT for treating depression in youth with ASD. Since CBT has promise for the reduction of emotional and behavioral difficulties related to anxiety and anger in ASD, it seems likely that it can also help with depressive symptomatology.

SOCIAL COMPETENCE

In Chapter 8, Beaumont and Sofronoff summarize development and research on a multimodal intervention for social skills training in students with ASD, the Secret Agent Society (SAS; Beaumont, 2009, 2010), developed for 8- to 12-year-old higher-functioning children with ASD. It employs an innovative interactive computer game that utilizes a virtual social environment to teach emotion recognition and regulation skills. SAS also includes weekly small-group meetings and parent sessions. A rigorous RCT (Beaumont & Sofronoff, 2008) reported improvement in social skills and emotion regulation, both at endpoint and at 5-month follow-up (compared to a treatment-as-usual group). This highly individualized treatment uses the child's interests and strengths to make the activities interesting to him or her. Users "become a detective," with the task of developing mind-reading skills, progressing through more difficult levels of the game as they learn. The SAS program clearly has great potential: It can be modified to fit other contexts (e.g., school), and it is highly flexible and intuitively appealing for children with ASD. The chapter also offers excellent practical suggestions for clinical implementation (e.g., strategies to decrease boredom in the group) and provides suggestions for subsequent expansion and testing of SAS, such as enhancing the technology and conducting cross-cultural trials.

Lopata, Thomeer, Volker, and Lee (Chapter 9) describe their comprehensive treatment program, which targets the core features of ASD (e.g., social deficits) and development of adaptive skills. This intensive program, delivered 5 days a week in structured, 70-minute cycles over either 5 or 6 weeks', integrates didactic skills instruction with interactive therapeutic activities. It teaches skills drawn from the Skillstreaming (McGinnis & Goldstein, 1997) curriculum and is delivered in a highly sequenced fashion by trained staff. This manualized intervention has been tested in four different studies, including a recently completed RCT (Lopata, Thomeer, et al., 2010). Results, collectively, are quite promising. Directions for future evaluation of this comprehensive summer program are suggested by the authors, including larger-scale RCTs and evaluation in community settings.

In Chapter 10, Bauminger-Zviely describes the cognitive-behavioral-ecological intervention (CBE; Bauminger, 2002, 2007), a school-based treatment implemented by teachers that integrates CBT with ecological treatment. The CBE program, which conceptualizes social disability in ASD as multidimensional, addresses both impaired social cognition (e.g., perceiving and encoding others' gestures and verbal communication) and impaired social behavior (e.g., engaging with peers in groups). CBE is implemented via two modalities—a dyadic component and a group component. In the dyadic component, student participation in multiple, weekly teacher–student lessons during the school year progresses from psychoeducation and explanation of basic social phenomena to emotion understanding and recognition, to teaching specific behavioral skills for social interaction. Alongside these dyadic lessons, children participate in teacher-led groups (the group component) to practice social skills. Results from three trials of CBE demonstrate improvement in social skills use, as well as social-cognitive skills with some evidence of maintained improvement 4 months after treatment. Children's spontaneous use of learned skills in natural environments, however, remains to be demonstrated. This ecological program's use of naturally occurring social agents (e.g., teachers) and contexts (e.g., preestablished peer groups, schools) clearly has merit. The work summarized here by Bauminger-Zviely provides a model for how to develop, implement, and evaluate school-based treatment programs for students with ASD. More of this type of work is needed as we strive to promote skills generalization outside the therapy context (e.g., Gresham, Sugai, & Horner, 2001) and bridge the science–translation gap (e.g., Garland, Hawley, Brookman-Frazee, & Hurlburt, 2012).

While these programs impressively document improvement in social functioning, they raise some additional questions regarding this core feature of ASD. First, none of these programs effectively reduces social deficits to nonclinical ranges. Is it simply not reasonable to expect that degree of social change in ASD, or are there additional elements that can be added to improve upon these findings? Second, all of these studies focus on school-age children. Since ASD begins in infancy and early childhood, how can these programs be modified, or new program developed, to treat social competence at earlier ages? Third, some programs focus specifically on social behaviors, while others also include cognitive processes, such as social understanding or theory of mind. To what degree are these separate, but related, skills of social competence? Are they both needed for the full benefits of CBT to occur? Fourth, it is evident from the interventions presented that programs to promote social competence can involve vastly different levels of intensity as well as occur in a variety of settings. The SAS (Beaumont & Sofronoff, Chapter 8) computer-based program is based on weekly "missions," the Summer Treatment Program described by Lopata et al. (Chapter 9) involves 5–6 weeks of daily intervention in a day camp setting, and the CBE intervention (Bauminger-Zviely, Chapter 10) works with students (both in dyads and in groups) in a school setting over the entire academic year. All show benefits in social functioning, but do different intensities and different settings show differential improvement? As our field continues to explore such questions, it is exciting to launch into a new era of understanding the ways CBT can improve social competence in youth with ASD.

SEXUALITY/AFFECTION

In Chapter 11, Attwood describes a CBT program for young people with ASD that facilitates understanding and acceptable expression of positive feelings toward others. There has been very little scientific exploration on this topic, as Attwood attests. People with ASD do not intuitively perceive others people's expressions of caring or affection, and it is often difficult for them to know how to express it appropriately, even if they have the desire to do so. Some children are excessively affectionate—inappropriately so, whereas others rarely or never show love or affection toward loved ones. The Affection Program (Attwood & Garnett, 2013), is a CBT-based, time-limited program for children with ASD, targets the age-appropriate expression and enjoyment of positive emotions, such as affection toward family members. In the program, children participate in five group sessions to explore feelings of affection, while their parents participate in concurrently run group sessions to discuss issues related to the expression of affection in their families. Preliminary findings from an open trial indicate support for the Affection Program, based on pre- to posttreatment change in parent-reported questionnaires about children's expressions of affection.

Finally, the chapter by Hénault (Chapter 12) is dedicated to one of the most clinically relevant yet understudied areas in our field—sexuality. Sexuality has largely been overlooked, perhaps sometimes ignored, by clinicians and families of people with ASD until very recently. This is unfortunate, because of its important role in healthy adult functioning and intimate interpersonal relationships. It is especially problematic in ASD given the pervasiveness of social deficits, immaturity, and the high male-to-female ratio, which contributes to limited opportunities for men with ASD to meet or interact with women with ASD. This issue is currently especially pertinent, given the magnitude of information, and misinformation, available online to people with ASD, and without parents' knowledge. In this chapter, Hénault provides practical suggestions that are developmentally sensitive, ranging from basic education on sexuality to skills training to develop intimate relationships. She describes a sociosexual education program for people with ASD that can be delivered individually or in groups— the Sociosexual Educational Program (Hénault, Forget, & Giroux, 2003; Hénault, 2006). The program teaches social skills that are age-appropriate, as well as sex education (e.g., the sexual response cycle) and the value of intimate relationships.

These two programs on affection and sexuality in youth with ASD are pioneering efforts in the field. No other interventions have been developed to address intimacy in young people with ASD. The Affection Program and the Sociosexual Education Program are promising first efforts, but it is clear that this work is still in its very early stages of research. Continued scientific investigation to replicate and extend these preliminary findings is critically needed.

WHERE ARE WE
AND WHERE DO WE GO FROM HERE?

In summary, it was our intent to assemble a body of empirically based, promising CBT-based treatment programs developed for young people with ASD. As is apparent in the preceding synthesis, CBT has been applied to diverse treatment targets and areas of functioning, and the evidence base is growing. We are hopeful about the direction this research is taking and the promise that this therapeutic approach holds. Of course, there remain many questions about CBT for children and adolescents with ASD. Answering these questions will require considerably more research, novel methodological and analytic approaches, and collaboration among scientists and clinicians with different areas of expertise. Below we summarize what we see as some of the pivotal questions that will shape clinical research in this area and move the field forward.

1. Distillation and synthesis
   a. What are the common elements of effective treatment in CBT for people with ASD?
   b. Can we distill a set of *common features* to simplify clinical practice and reduce client–therapist confusion?
   c. Do the common features change over the course of development or are they different for individuals at different levels of developmental functioning?
   d. What levels of intensity are needed for clinically significant improvement to occur?
   e. What treatment settings or contexts promote generalizability?
2. Adaptation and fit
   a. In traditional CBT what, if anything, *must* be modified to make treatment effective for people with ASD?
   b. What kinds of assessments can we implement to determine whether an individual with ASD is prepared for and/or would benefit from CBT?
   c. Given the heterogeneity in ASD, to what degree does any

      treatment program need to be individually developed? Is it pos-
      sible that the utility of treatment manuals is different in this
      clinical population?
    d. Can treatments be modified to work with different levels of cog-
      nitive impairment or verbal ability?
    e. To what degree is parental involvement needed?
  3. Mechanisms and moderators of change with treatment
    a. Why/when does treatment work, and for whom is it most likely
      to be effective?
    b. Given high levels of comorbidity and clinical complexity in cli-
      ents with ASD, how do therapists determine treatment approach?
    c. To what degree can psychosocial treatment, such as CBT, effect
      change in neurobiological processes?
    d. How might CBT contribute to a positive prognosis?

The chapters in this edited volume have focused on promising CBT
interventions for specific problems often seen in higher-functioning youth
with ASD, namely, difficulties with anxiety and behavior problems, social
competence, and affection/sexuality. Clearly, these difficulties are interre-
lated and occur within a number of varied contexts, which can further add
to the complexity in treatment. Nonetheless, the interventions described
herein provide encouraging evidence for the benefit of CBT in improving
these problems that seriously impact the quality of life of individuals with
ASD. Future research in this field is therefore critical to further develop,
refine, and expand these initial CBT programs. We are excited to promote
this new era of scientific investigation in effective psychosocial treatment
approaches for young people with ASD.

REFERENCES

Attwood, T. (2004). *Exploring feelings: Cognitive-behavior therapy to manage anxiety.* Arlington, TX: Future Horizons.

Attwood, T., & Garnett, M. (2013). *From like to love within friendships and family: Cognitive behaviour therapy to understand and express affection.* London: Jessica Kingsley.

Bauminger, N. (2002). The facilitation of social-emotional understanding and social interaction in high functioning children with autism: Intervention outcomes. *Journal of Autism and Developmental Disorders, 32,* 283–298.

Bauminger, N. (2007). Group social-multimodal intervention for HFASD. *Journal of Autism and Developmental Disorders, 37,* 1605–1615.

Beaumont, R. (2009). *Secret Agent Society: Solving the mystery of social encounters—computer game.* Australia: The Social Skills Training Institute.

Beaumont, R. (2010). *Secret Agent Society. Solving the mystery of social encoun ters—facilitator manual.* Milton, Australia.

Beaumont, R., & Sofronoff, K. (2008). A multi-component social skills intervention for children with Asperger syndrome: The Junior Detective Training Program. *Journal of Child Psychology and Psychiatry, 49*(7), 743–753.

Chang, Y., Quan, J., & Wood, J. J. (2012). Effects of anxiety disorder severity on social functioning in children with autism spectrum disorders. *Journal of Developmental and Physical Disabilities, 24,* 235–245.

Chorpita, B. F., Becker, K. D., & Daleiden, E. L. (2007). Understanding the common elements of evidence-based practice: Misconceptions and clinical examples. *Journal of the American Academy of Child and Adolescent Psychiatry, 46*(5), 647–652.

Chorpita, B. F., Bernstein, A., & Daleiden, E. L. (2011). Empirically guided coordination of multiple evidence-based treatments: An illustration of relevance mapping in children's mental health services. *Journal of Consulting and Clinical Psychology, 79*(4), 470–480.

Garland, A. F., Hawley, K. M., Brookman-Frazee, L., & Hurlburt, M. S. (2012). Identifying common elements of evidence-based psychosocial treatments for children's disruptive behavior problems. *Journal of the American Academy of Child and Adolescent Psychiatry, 47*(5), 505–514.

Ghaziuddin, M., Ghaziuddin, N., & Greden, J. (2002). Depression in persons with autism: Implications for research and clinical care. *Journal of Autism and Developmental Disorders, 32*(4), 299–306.

Gresham, F. M., Sugai, G., & Horner, R. H. (2001). Interpreting outcomes of social skills training for students with high-incidence disabilities. *Teaching Exceptional Children, 67,* 331–344.

Hénault, I. (2006). *Asperger's syndrome and sexuality.* London: Jessica Kingsley.

Hénault, I., Forget, J., & Giroux, N. (2003). *Le développement d'habiletés sexuelles adaptatives chez des individus atteints d'autisme de haut niveau ou du syndrome d'Asperger [Developing adaptive sexual skills in individuals with high functioning autism or Asperger's syndrome].* Doctoral thesis, Department of Psychology, University of Québec, Montréal.

Kazdin, A. E. (2000). *Psychotherapy for children and adolescents: Directions for research and practice.* New York: Oxford University Press

Lickel, A., MacLean, W. E., Blakeley-Smith, A., & Hepburn, S. (2012). Assessment of the prerequisite skills for cognitive behavioral therapy in children with and without autism spectrum disorders. *Journal of Autism and Developmental Disorders, 42,* 992–1000.

Lopata, C., Thomeer, M. L., Volker, M. A., Toomey, J. A., Nida, R. E., Lee, G. K., et al. (2010). RCT of a manualized social treatment for high-functioning autism spectrum disorders. *Journal of Autism and Developmental Disorders, 40*(11), 1297–1310.

Lopata, C., Toomey, J. A., Dox, J. D., Volker, M. A., Chow, S. Y., Thomeer, M. L., et al. (2010). Anxiety and depression in children with HF ASDs: Symptom levels and source differences. *Journal of Abnormal Child Psychology, 38,* 765–776.

Lord, C., Wagner, A., Rogers, S., Szatmari, P., Aman, M., Charman, T., et al. (2005). Challenges in evaluating psychosocial interventions for autistic spectrum disorders. *Journal of Autism and Developmental Disorders, 35*(6), 695–708.

Mazefsky, C. A., & White, S. W. (in press). Adults with autism. In S. J. Rogers (Ed.), *Handbook of autism spectrum disorders* (4th ed.). Hoboken, NJ: Wiley.

McGinnis, E., & Goldstein, A. P. (1997). *Skillstreaming the elementary school child: New strategies and perspectives for teaching prosocial skills* (rev. ed.). Champaign, IL: Research Press.

Reaven, J., Blakeley-Smith, A., Nichols, S., & Hepburn, S. (2011). *Facing Your Fears: Group therapy for managing anxiety in children with high-functioning autism spectrum disorders* Baltimore: Brookes.

Rutter, M., & Sroufe, L. A. (2000). Developmental psychopathology: Concepts and challenges. *Development and Psychopathology, 12,* 265–296.

Scarpa, A., Wells, A. O., & Attwood, T. (2013). *Exploring feelings for young children with high-functioning autism or Asperger's disorder: The STAMP treatment manual.* London: Jessica Kingsley.

Silverman, W. K., Pina, A. A., & Viswesvaran, C. (2008). Evidence-based psychosocial treatments for phobic and anxiety disorders in children and adolescents. *Journal of Clinical and Adolescent Psychology, 37*(1), 105–130.

van Steensel, F. J. A., Bogels, S. M., & Perrin, S. (2011). Anxiety disorders in children and adolescents with autistic spectrum disorders: A meta-analysis. *Clinical Child and Family Psychology Review, 14*(3), 302–317.

White, S. W., Albano, A., Johnson, C., Kasari, C., Ollendick, T., Klin, A., et al. (2010). Development of a cognitive-behavioral intervention program to treat anxiety and social deficits in teens with high-functioning autism. *Clinical Child and Family Psychology Review, 13*(1), 77–90.

White, S. W., Oswald, D., Ollendick, T., & Scahill, L. (2009). Anxiety in children and adolescents with autism spectrum disorders. *Clinical Psychology Review, 29*(3),

Wood, J. J., Drahota, A., Sze, K., Har, K., Chiu, A., & Langer, D. A. (2009). Cognitive behavioral therapy for anxiety in children with autism spectrum disorders: A randomized, controlled trial. *Journal of Child Psychology and Psychiatry, 50*(3), 224–234.

Wood, J. J., & McLeod, B. D. (2008). *Child anxiety disorders: A family-based treatment manual for practitioners.* New York: Norton.

Index

Note. The letters *f*, *t*, or *n* following a page number indicate a figure, table, or note, respectively.

ABC model (Beck), 9
Aberrant Behavior Checklist, 59, 292
Abnormal behavior, as learned behavior, 8
ACTION program for depression, 17, 19–20
Activities, circumscribed, 201
Adaptive behavior, assessment of, 55, 56t
Adaptive Behavior Assessment, 2nd edition, 56t
Adaptive protection, FYF and, 111
Adaptive skills module, 85–86
Adolescents; *see also* MASSI
    affection and, 263–265
    anxiety disorders and, 127–128
    secondary psychiatric problems in, 123
    social skills interventions and, 126–127
Affection; *see also* CBT Affection Program; Expressing love and affection
    discomfort with expressing, 260–262
    health implications of, 267
    measures of, 268–269
    neurology of, 266–267
    to repair feelings, 265
    sensory sensitivity and, 266
    social conventions of, 260–261
Affection for Others Questionnaire, 269, 273–274

Affection for You Questionnaire, 269, 274
Affection Program; *see* CBT Affection Program
Affective education, 17, 28
    for anxiety disorders/ASD, 76–77
    in Exploring Feelings program, 152
Affective Matching Measure, 246
Aggression interventions, 20
Alexithymia, 35
Amygdalar pathology, emotional profile in ASD and, 266–267
Amygdalar volume, 75
Anger, SAS program and, 187
Anger management, 20
    future directions for, 165
    in STAMP, 158–159, 163
Anxiety
    about potential failure, 32–34
    versus ASD, 53–54
    with Asperger syndrome, 174–175
    assessment of, 58–59
    child's awareness of, 30
    exploring, in STAMP, 158–159
    exposures for, 83
    ranking levels of, 112
    SAS program and, 187
    social disability and, 125
    systematic desensitization and, 8

Anxiety disorders
  in adolescents, 127–128
  in HFASD, 150
  social disability and, 307
  social skills training and, 129–131
Anxiety Disorders Interview Schedule—
    IV, 52t
Anxiety Disorders Interview Schedule—
    Parent version, 110
Anxiety Disorders Inventory Schedule for
    Children—Parent Report, 115, 116
Anxiety disorders with ASD, 18, 74–75
  BIACA intervention in, 79–86
    case study of, 80–86
  CBT therapy for, 73–96
  cognitive modules in treatment of, 80–82
  contributing factors in, 99–104
    parental emotion and problem
        behaviors, 103–104
    parental mental health, 101–103
  developmental considerations in, 98–99
  impacts of, 98
  prevalence of, 97
  rates of, 73
  studies of treatments for, 129–130
  treatment of
    adaptive skills module in, 85–86
    behavioral/exposure modules in,
        83–85
    future directions for, 91–92
    limitations of, 91–92
    parental involvement in, 105–107
    stereotyped interests module in, 86
  in typically developing versus ASD
    youth, 73–75
Anxiety disorders with HFASD, 97–122
  treatment of
    future directions for, 116–117
    with group therapy, 109–114 (see
        also Facing Your Fears [FYF])
    parental involvement in, 107–109
    research on, 115–116
Arguments, avoiding, 193
Asperger, Hans, 173
Asperger syndrome; see also High-
    functioning ASD (HFASD)
  case example of, 61–63
  CBT for affection program and (see
    CBT Affection Program)

comorbid conditions of, 150
  development of interventions for,
      174–175
  and lack of sociosexual knowledge,
      279–280
  sexuality and, 278–279, 280 (see also
      Sexuality and Asperger syndrome)
  social skills training and (see Secret
      Agent Society [SAS]; Social skills
      training in Asperger syndrome)
Assessment, 45–69
  of anxiety and depression, 58–59
  of appropriateness of CBT, 50–51
  for ASD diagnosis, 47–50
  case example of, 60–63
  for comorbid psychiatric conditions,
      51–54
  of diagnostic changes, 54–55
  of general behavior problems, 59
  multiple-informant, 46–47
  purpose of, 47–59
  research needs in, 305
  of social skills and social cognition,
      56–58
Assessment measures
  age range and description, 49t
  choosing and administering, 46–47
  continuous, of symptom severity, 55,
      56t
  psychiatric interviews, 52t
  psychometric properties of, 46
  self-report, 46–47
Association for Behavioral and Cognitive
    Therapies (ABCT), guiding CBT
    principles of, 4–5
Attention-deficit/hyperactivity disorder
    (ADHD), ASD and, 30–32, 53
Australian Scale for Asperger's Syndrome,
    291–292
Autism, early interventions for, 173–174
Autism Comorbidity Interview, 52, 52t
Autism Diagnostic Interview—Revised,
    50
Autism Diagnostic Observation Schedule,
    50
Autism Mental Status Examination, 48
Autism Quotient, 49t
Autism Screening Questionnaire, 49t
Autism Social Skills Profile, 57

Autism-spectrum disorders (ASD); *see also* Asperger syndrome; High-functioning ASD (HFASD)
    ADHD and, 30–32, 53
    assessment of (*see* Assessment)
    cognitive profile in, 272
    deficits associated with, 28
    diagnosis of, 47–50
    early indicators of, 47
    heterogeneity of, 199–200
    interpersonal and social abilities in, 37–38
    language profile in, 36–37
    learning profile associated with, 29–36 (*see also* Learning profile)
    predictors of adult outcomes in, 226
    sensory profile in, 38–39
    sexuality and, 278–279
Awareness of Social Inference Test, 58

B

Bandura's model of self-efficacy, 9
Beck, Aaron, 9–11
Behavior Assessment System for Children—Second Edition, 48
Behavior modification techniques, 8
Behavior problems, general, assessment of, 59
Behavior therapy, early ASD applications of, 173–174
Behavioral aspects, in anxiety disorders/ASD, 77–78
Behavioral Assessment of Social Interactions in Young Children, 57
Behavioral Interventions for Anxiety in Children with Autism (BIACA), 74, 306; *see also* BIACA intervention
Behavioral management, in STAMP, 157
Behavioral monitoring, 11
Behavioral problems, CBT for, 306–308
Behavioral rehearsal, 12
Behavioral reinforcement system, in social skills summer program, 210–212
Behavioral techniques, for social interventions, 237–238
Behavior/exposure modules
    for anxiety/ASD, 83–85
    assignments in, 83–84

    developing hierarchy for, 83
    mentoring in, 85
    parent training in, 84
    playdates in, 84–85
    school involvement in, 85
    social coaching in, 85
Behaviors
    abnormal, as learned, 8
    adaptive, assessment of, 55, 56t
    circumscribed, 201
    linking with thoughts, 28
BIACA intervention, 79–86
    adaptive skills module in, 85–86
    behavioral/exposure modules in, 83–85
    cognitive modules in, 80–82
    research on, 86–87
    stereotyped interests module in, 86
    termination of, 86
Boredom, managing, 191
Breathing, diaphragmatic, 12
Building Confidence program, 109

C

CALM system, 84
C.A.T. Project for adolescents, 19
Cat-Kit program, 284
CBE interventions, 226–255, 309–310
    barriers to school assimilation of, 251
    components of, 242–245, 309–310
    conceptual basis for, 241–242
    future directions for, 250–251
    historical background and significance of, 226–227
    limitations of, 250
    and multidimensional social deficit in HFASD, 227 230
    and previous multifaceted procedures, 230–231, 232t–236t, 237–241
    research on, 245–250
        for dyadic intervention, 245–248
        for group intervention, 248–250
CBT Affection Program, 267–277, 311–312; *see also* Affection; Expressing love and affection
    aims of, 268
    cognitive profile of children with ASD and, 272
    future directions for, 275

CBT Affection Program (*continued*)
  group format for, 272–273
  historical background and significance
    of, 260–267
    in adolescence, 263–267
    in childhood, 260–262
  homework for, 272
  pilot programs for, 267–268
  practical considerations in, 268–270
  research on, 273–275
  sessions overview, 270–273
CBT interventions
  for anxiety disorders, 306–308
  for behavioral problems, 306–308
  client selection for, 306
  current knowledge about, 303–312
  future directions for, 312–313
  research on, 303
  theoretical grounding and
    conceptualization of, 304–306
CBT modifications, 27–44; *see also*
    Developmental modifications
  for interpersonal and social abilities,
    37–38
  research needs in, 305–306
CBT modifications for anxiety disorders,
    76–79
  in Asperger syndrome, 174–175
  emphasis on behavioral aspects, 77–
    78
  incorporating special interests, 78
  increased affective education, 76–77
  increased parental involvement, 78–79
  increased use of visual aids, 77
  targeting co-occurring difficulties, 79
CBT program
  assessment and (*see* Assessment)
  between-session projects in, 39–40
  components of, 39–41
  group participant selection in, 40
  post-session parent meetings and,
    40–41
Central coherence theory, weak, 262
Checklist for Autism Spectrum Disorder,
    48, 49t
Child and Adolescent Psychiatric
    Assessment, 51–52, 52t
Child Behavior Checklist, 48
Child Depression Inventory, 59

Childhood, affection in, 260–262
Childhood Autism Rating Scale, 50
Children's Automatic Thoughts Scale
    (CATS), 90
Children's Global Assessment Scale, 55
Chill-out zones, in SAS program, 193–
    194
Classical (respondent) conditioning, 7–8,
    12
Client–therapist collaboration, 4
Clinical Global Impressions Scale, 54–55,
    115
Cognitive ability, in very young children,
    18–19
Cognitive inflexibility, 32
Cognitive modules, for anxiety/ASD,
    80–82
Cognitive restructuring strategies, 10–11,
    28
  in Exploring Feelings program, 152
Cognitive revolution movement, 9
Cognitive techniques, for social
    interventions, 237
Cognitive therapy
  for depression, 11
  emergence of, 9–10
Cognitive-behavioral therapy (CBT); *see
    also* entries under CBT
  behavioral *versus* cognitive emphasis
    in, 7
  categories of, 10–11
  for children, research support for,
    12–13, 17–20
  definition and guiding principles of, 4–5
  description of, 3, 27
  determining appropriateness of, 50–51
  developmental modifications for,
    13–20 (*see also* Developmental
    modifications)
  disorders treated with, 27
  historical bases of, 7–10
  philosophical roots of, 5–7
  prevalence of, 10
  research support for, 21
  strategies used in, 10–12
  use with children, 3–4
Cognitive-behavioral-ecological
    intervention; *see* CBE interventions
Commercials, creating, 162

Communication; *see also* CBT Affection
  Program; Expressing love and
  affection
of affection, 260
nonverbal, 37–38
Communication deficits, 37–38
in HFASD, 202
Comorbid conditions, 51–54, 305
with anxiety disorders/ASD, 79
Comprehension deficits, in HFASD, 202
Comprehensive school-based
  interventions, need for, 220–221
Comprehensive treatment models
  (CTMs), focused interventions
  versus, 204–205
Computer game format, in Secret Agent
  Society, 177–178, 179f, 180, 180f,
  196
Conditioning; *see* Classical (respondent)
  conditioning; Instrumental (operant)
  conditioning
Consent, theory of mind and, 281
Consistency, desire for, 34
Constructivist epistemology, 5, 7
Contextual Assessment of Social Skills,
  57
Conversational skills, training in, 37
Cool Kids program, 90, 108
Cooperative skills
and CBE interventions, 247–248
developing, 244
Coping Cat program, 19
for anxiety/ASD, 78, 110
Coping skills strategies, 10–11

D

Decoding difficulties, in HFASD, 202
Depression, 103, 126, 127, 132, 186
ACTION program for, 17, 19–20
ASD and, 38, 53–54, 63
assessment of, 58–59
Beck's cognitive therapy of, 9–11
CBT and, 27, 308
SAS program and, 187, 195
social functioning and, 227, 240
Derogatis Sexual Functioning Inventory,
  292
Desensitization, systematic, 8, 12

Developmental, Dimensional, and
  Diagnostic Interview, 50
Developmental Disabilities Modification
  of CGAS, 55
Developmental modifications, 13–20, 21
affective education and, 17
for child's cognitive ability, 16
experiential learning and, 15
meeting frequency and, 14–15
motivation and, 13–14
play routines and, 16–17
relaxation strategies and, 16
in STAMP, 154
visual aids and, 15–16
Developmental Social Disorder content
  scale, 48
*Diagnostic and Statistical Manual of
  Mental Disorders,* autism diagnosis
  and, 173
Diagnostic changes, monitoring, 54–
  55
Diagnostic Interview Schedule for
  Children, 52t
Diaphragmatic breathing, 12
Drug therapy, review of, 31

E

Ellis, Albert, 9, 11
Emotion Inventory Measure, 246, 248
Emotion regulation
in ASD, 148–150
defined, 148
Emotion regulation skills, STAMP
  and, 147–148, 153–154, 163–164,
  308
Emotional competence, characteristics of,
  148
Emotional intelligence, AS and, 284
Emotional lability, 149
Emotional regulation intervention,
  significance of, 150–151
Emotional Toolbox, 152–153
appropriate and inappropriate tools in,
  161–162
for STAMP, 158–159
Emotional understanding and recognition
in CBE interventions, 243–244
deficits in, 228–229

Emotionality
   in ASD, 148–150
   negative, 149
Emotions
   complex, 228–229
      CBE interventions and, 247, 249
   converting to speech, 35–36
   education about, 77
   expression of, 38
   facial expressions for identifying, 284
   sexuality and AS and, 283–285
   simple, interventions for recognizing,
      239
Executive function, CBE interventions
   and, 248
Executive function deficits, 30–32
   ASD and, 30–32
   expression of affection and, 262
   MASSI program and, 135
Exploring Feelings program, 147–170,
   284; see also STAMP
   for children with HFASD, 151–154
   Emotional Toolbox of, 152–153,
      158–159, 161–162
   future directions for, 165–166
   historical background and significance
      of, 148–151
   research support for, 163–164
   stages of, 152
Exposure therapy, 12, 28; see also
   Behavior/exposure modules
Expressed emotion (EE), parental,
   103–104, 114
Expressing love and affection, 259–277;
   see also CBT program for affection
   current knowledge of, 311–312
   discomfort with, 260
   false assumptions about, 264–265
   frequency of, 265–266
   gender and, 261
   and learning about intimacy and
      sexuality, 284–285
   need for guidance in, 267
   social conventions regarding, 260–261
   theories about difficulties with, 262
Externalizing problems, in HFASD, 150,
   202
Extinction strategies, 12
Eysenck, Hans, 8

F

Face-emotion recognition
   deficits in, 35
   in summer program, 208, 209
Facial expression, for identifying
   emotions, 209, 284
Facing Your Fears (FYF), 109–114
   adolescent version of, 114
   components of, 110–111
   future directions for, 116–117
   parental involvement in, 111–117,
      307
   research on, 115–116
   session by session, 112–114
   treatment as usual (TAU) versus,
      115–116
Failure, fear of, 32–34
False-belief tasks, 58
Family involvement; see also Parental
      involvement; Parents
   in MASSI, 133–134
   treatment planning and, 13–14
Fear; see also Anxiety disorders; Social
      phobia
   ASD and, 75
   behavioral approach to, 8
   of failure, 32–34
   of speaking, 83
Feedback, in MASSI program, 134
Feelings; see also Expressing love and
      affection
   linking with thoughts, 28
   positive, exploring, 158
Focused interventions, versus
   comprehensive treatment models,
   204–205
Friendship Skills Observation Checklist,
   292
Friendships
   expressing affection and, 263–264
   sociosexual education program and,
      293–294
Functional behavioral assessment (FBA),
   for assessing comorbid disorders, 54

G

Games, incorporation of, 16–17
Gender, expressions of affection and, 261

General Affection Questionnaire, 269–271, 273
Generalized anxiety disorder, 74
  case example of, 61–63
Global Functioning Index, 56
Goals, 5
Ground rules, SAS, 190

H

Head trace activity, 161
Helper bugs, 112
High-functioning ASD (HFASD); *see also* Asperger syndrome
  adolescence and, 126–127
  anxiety disorders and, 97–122 (*see also* Anxiety disorders with HFASD)
  associated features of, 201–202
  circumscribed behaviors, interests, activities in, 201
  clinical and associated features of, 200–204
  defined, 109n2
  early indicators of, 47
  exploring feelings intervention in, 151–163 (*see also* STAMP)
  internalizing/externalizing problems in, 150
  intervention research on, 202–204
  practical considerations in, 204–206
  self-report and, 45
  social interaction impairments in, 200–201
  treatment as usual (TAU) and, 115–116

I

Individual daily note approach, 211–212
Instrumental (operant) conditioning, 8
Interests
  circumscribed, 201
  OCD and, 264
  special, 34–35, 78
  stereotyped, 86
Internalizing problems, in HFASD, 150, 202
Internet, sexuality on, 282–283
Interpersonal abilities, deficits in, 37–38

Interviews, psychiatric, 51–54, 52t
Intonation, insensitivity to, 36–37
IQ
  ASD and, 29
  MASSI program and, 132
  peer interaction outcomes and, 226–227

J

Junior Detective Training Program; *see* Secret Agent Society (SAS)

K

Kanner, Leo, 173
Keeping Your Cool program, 20
KICK plan, in cognitive module for anxiety/ASD, 81–82
Kiddie-Schedule for Affective Disorders and Schizophrenia, 52t

L

Language, nonliteral, 244
  skills groups for, 209
Language profile, 36–37
Learning, experiential, 15
Learning profile, 29–36, 304
  alexithymia in, 35
  consistency and certainty in, 34
  and conversion of thoughts and emotions to speech, 35–36
  fear of making mistakes and, 32–34
  one-track mind and, 32
  special interests and talents in, 34–35
Learning theory, CBT and, 4, 7
LEGO therapy, research on, 175–176
Logical thinking, 30
Loneliness Rating Scale, 246
Lovaas, Ivar, 173–174
Love and affection, expressing; *see* Expressing love and affection

M

Making Waves program, 285
Maladaptive thoughts, challenging, 11

Manualized interventions; *see* ACTION program for depression; Coping Cat program; Exploring Feelings program; Multimodal Anxiety and Social Skills Intervention (MASSI); Secret Agent Society (SAS); Social skills summer program; STAMP
Marcus Aurelius, 6
MASSI, 307
  case example of, 138–140
  CBT principles and, 129–131, 135–136
  content and delivery of, 131–133, 132*f*
  contraindications to, 132
  essential elements and unique components of, 133–136
  future directions for, 137–138
  IQ requirement for, 132
  parental involvement in, 129–131
  parent/family involvement in, 133–134
  research on, 136–137
  sessions overview, 131–136, 132*f*
Matson Evaluation of Social Skills with Youngsters, 57
Medications, review of, 31
Meltdowns in SAS, preventing/managing, 189–194, 189*t*
Memory, difficulties with, 30
Mentoring, in behavior/exposure module, 85
Mind Reading software, 284, 290, 295
Mindfulness, 6
Modified Checklist for Autism in Toddlers, 49*t*
Monitoring, 5
Mood and Feelings Questionnaire, 59
Motivation
  of child, 13–14
  cognitive factors in, 9
Multidimensional Anxiety Scale for Children, 59
Multifaceted social interventions, 230–241; *see also* CBE interventions
  agents and settings, 232*t*–236*t*, 237
  aims and targets of, 231, 232*t*–236*t*
  CBT techniques in, 232*t*–236*t*, 237–238
  outcomes of, 232*t*–236*t*, 238–241
  participants in, 231, 232*t*–236*t*, 237

Multimodal Anxiety and Social Skills Intervention (MASSI); *see* MASSI
Multimodal treatment for adolescents, 123–148; *see also* MASSI
  historical background and significance of, 124–128
Multimodality trauma treatment (MMTT), 20

N

National Institute of Mental Health (NIMH), research guidelines of, 213–214, 215*t*–217*t*, 218–220
Nonliteral language skills, 244
  in summer program, 209
Nonverbal communication, 37–38

O

Obsessive–compulsive disorder (OCD)
  in adolescents, 127
  versus ASD, 74
  response prevention strategies for, 12
  special interests and, 264
One-track mind, 32
Operant conditioning; *see* Instrumental (operant) conditioning

P

Parent Anxiety Management (PAM), 105–106
Parent training
  in adaptive skills module, 86
  in behavior/exposure module, 84
Parental involvement
  in anxiety interventions, 78–79, 306–307
  in Asperger interventions, 174
  in CBE-dyadic intervention, 243–244
  in Facing Your Fears, 111–117, 307
  in MASSI module, 130–131, 133–134
  research on, 163, 165
  in SAS program, 183–187
  in social interaction interventions, 240
  in social skills summer program, 212
  in STAMP, 155, 159–163, 308
  in treatment planning, 13–14

Parents
  CBT Affection Program and, 24–275
  exclusion of, 17–18
  expressed emotion and, 103–104, 114
  and expressions of affection, 261
  and fears about child's sexuality, 281–282
  Internet safety and, 283
  meetings with, 40–41
  Parent Anxiety Management program and, 105–106
  pathology of, 306–307
  sociosexual education program and, 295–296
  as treatment targets, 13
Pavlov, Ivan, 7
Pediatric Anxiety Rating Scale, 59
Peer aides, in CBE-dyadic intervention, 243–244
Peer interactions, IQ and, 226–227
Pervasive Developmental Disorder Behavior Inventory, 59
Phobia, classical conditioning of, 8
Play routines, incorporation of, 16–17
Playdates, in behavior/exposure module, 84–85
Positive feelings, exploring, 158
Positive reinforcement, 33–34
Pragmatics
  Exploring Feelings program and, 152
  problems with, 36–37
Preschool and Kindergarten Behavior Scale, 57
Problem solving, 28
  and CBE-dyadic interventions, 246–247
  social, 243–244
Problem Solving Measure, 246
Problem-solving therapy, 10–12
Programme d'Éducation Sexuelle, 288–289
Progressive muscle relaxation, 11
Protection
  adaptive versus excessive, FYF and, 111
  from Internet, 283
Psychiatric interviews, 51–54, 52t

Psychoanalytic approaches, challenges to, 8–9
Psychoeducation, 28
  in cognitive modules for SAD and social phobia, 80–82
  in MASSI program, 135
Psychometric properties, 46
Psychosocial interventions, NIMH research guidelines for, 213–214, 215t–217t, 218–220
Punishers, defined, 8
Puppet shows, as social tool, 160

Q

Questioning, Socratic method of, 6–7

R

Rational restructuring, systematic, 11
Rational-emotive behavior therapy, 9
Reciprocal determinism, Bandura's model of, 9
Reinforcers, defined, 8
Relationships, sexuality and AS and, 283–285
Relaxation gadgets, in SAS, 192–193
Relaxation strategies, 16, 28
  in STAMP, 158–160
Relaxation training, 11–12
Research support, 13, 17–20, 21
Resistance
  child, 193
  parental, 194–195
Response prevention, 12
Response–cost behavioral system, 210–211
Revised Child Manifest Anxiety Scale, 59
Revised Children's Manifest Anxiety Scale, 90
Reward system, in cognitive module for anxiety/ASD, 81
Ruler game, 158, 159

S

Sally Ann task, 58
Scales of Independent Behavior—Revised, 56t

School involvement
  in behavior/exposure module, 85
  in MASSI program, 137
  in SAS program, 185
School-based interventions; *see also* CBE
    interventions
  comprehensive, need for, 220–221,
    251
  outcomes for, 240–241
Screen for Child Anxiety Related
    Emotional Disorders (SCARED), 59,
    90, 115
Secret Agent Society (SAS), 173–198,
    176–177, 309, 310
  activity modifications for, 191–192
  caregiver characteristics and, 186–187
  characteristics of, 177
  child group meetings and resources in,
    181, 182*t*, 183, 183*f*
  child meltdowns and, 189–194, 189*t*
  clinic *versus* school delivery of,
    185–186
  cross-cultural trials of, 196–197
  emotional regulation and, 187
  future directions for, 196–197
  group composition and, 187–188
  overview of, 177–196
  parent group meetings and resources in,
    183–185
  parental resistance and, 194–195
  research on, 195–196
  school resources and support for,
    185
  selection criteria for, 186
  skills generalization and, 188–189
  structure and content of, 178, 179*f*,
    180, 180*f*
  synopsis of, 177–178
Secret Agent Society computer game,
    177–178, 179*f*, 180, 180*f*
  research on, 196
  website for viewing, 178
Self-control treatment, 11
Self-efficacy
  Bandura's model and, 9
  promotion of, 4–5
Self-instruction training (SIT), 11
Self-Perception Profile of Children, 246
Self-reflection, ASD and, 28

Self-report
  HFASD and, 45
  use of, 46–47
Sensory processing difficulties, SAS
    adaptations for, 192
Sensory profile, 38–39
Sensory sensitivity, expressions of
    affection and, 266
Separation anxiety disorder
  versus ASD, 51
  exposures for, 83
Set shifting, problem with, 32
Sex education programs; *see also*
    Sociosexual education program for
    AS
  critical elements of, 286–289
  interventions in, 286–287
  resources for, 287
Sex Information and Education Council
    of the United States, website for, 286
Sexual behaviors, inappropriate, 280–281
Sexual predators, vulnerability to,
    282–283
Sexual segregation, in Asperger syndrome,
    280
Sexuality and Asperger syndrome, 278–
    299; *see also* Sociosexual knowledge
  current knowledge of, 311–312
  environmental restrictions and, 280
  inappropriate behaviors and, 280–281
  Internet and, 282–283
  interpersonal relations, emotions, and,
    283–285
  intimacy and, 280
  relationships and, 278–299
  sexual segregation and, 280
  social skills and, 285
Sharing, difficulties with, 260–261
Singing activities, in STAMP, 158–159
Skills generalization, in SAS program,
    188–189
Skills modeling, in MASSI program,
    134–135
Social anxiety disorder, case example of,
    61–63
Social avoidance, potential causes of, 74
Social Circles exercise, 285
Social coaching, in behavior/exposure
    module, 85

Social cognition deficits, 228–229
  assessment of, 56–58
  CBE interventions and, 245–246, 248
Social Communication Questionnaire,
  49t
Social competence
  cognitive/behavioral composition of,
    310
  current knowledge about, 308–310
  defined, 125
Social constructs, in CBE interventions,
  243–244
Social context, treatment planning and,
  14
Social deficits, 229
  anxiety and, 125, 307
  ASD and, 124–125
  and CBE interventions, 247–250
  and co-occurring anxiety, 125
  current/potential intervention
    effectiveness, 310
  in HFASD, 200–201
  interventions for, 124–125
  multidimensional, 227–230
  multifaceted interventions and,
    239–240
Social functioning, defined, 226
Social initiations, teaching, 243–244
Social interventions, multifaceted; see
  Multifaceted social interventions
Social learning, in MASSI program,
  134
Social phobia
  in adolescents, 127–128
  versus ASD, 51
  exposures for, 83
Social problem solving, 243–244
Social reciprocity, training in, 37
Social Responsiveness Scale, 49t, 56–57
Social situations, high-challenge, 229
Social skills
  assessment of, 56–58
  deficits in, 37–38
  sociosexual education and, 285
Social Skills Rating System, 56
Social skills summer program, 199–225,
  309, 310
  behavioral reinforcement system and,
    210–212

face-emotion recognition groups in,
  208
fidelity monitoring in, 213
future directions for, 220–221
HFASD overview for, 200–204
historical background and significance
  of, 199–204
nonliteral language skills in, 209
overview of, 206–213
parent training in, 212
practical considerations for, 204–
  206
research on, 213–214, 215t–217t,
  218–220
  case study in, 214, 215t, 218
  manual development/pilot testing,
    218–219
  RCT in, 215t–217t, 219–220
social skills groups in, 207–208
staff training for, 212–213
summary of studies of, 215t–217t
therapeutic activities in, 209–210
Social skills training
  for adolescents, 126–127
  anxiety and, 79, 129–131
  effective techniques in, 203–
    204
  evidence supporting, 175
  focused versus comprehensive, 204
  for HFASD, 176
  research on, 202–203
  in sociosexual education for AS, 291,
    293–294
  in summer program, 207–208
Social skills training in Asperger
  syndrome, 173–198
  future directions for, 196–197
  group composition and physical space,
    187–188
  historical background and significance
    of, 173–177
  and optimizing skills generalization,
    188–189
  preventing/managing meltdowns in
    children's groups, 189–194
  preventing/managing resistance in
    parent groups, 194–195
  research on, 195–196
  selection criteria for, 186–187

Social skills training (*continued*)
  session overview, 177–186
    child group meetings and resources,
      181, 182*t*, 183
    clinic *versus* school delivery,
      185–186
    parent group meetings and
      resources, 183–185
    school resources and support, 185
    structure and content, 178–180
    synopsis, 177–178
Social tools, in STAMP, 160
Social understanding, interventions for,
  239
Social Use of Language Programme
  (SULP), research on, 175–176
Social Worries Questionnaire—Parent,
  89
Social-communicative reciprocity deficit,
  study of, 226
Social-emotional understanding,
  CBE intervention for; *see* CBE
  interventions
Socioemotional processing, difficulties
  with, 30
Sociosexual education program for AS,
  288–295, 311–312
  outcomes of, 293–294
  research on, 291–295
  social skills training and, 291
  structure of, 290–291, 294
  themes of, 288–291
  validation of, 290
Sociosexual Information Questionnaire,
  292
Sociosexual knowledge, lack of, 279–
  281
Socratic method, 5–7, 28
Software, for teaching emotional
  expression, 284
Speaking, fear of, 83–84
Special interest tools, in STAMP, 161
Special interests, 34–35
  incorporating, 78
    with anxiety disorders/ASD, 78
  in learning profile, 34–35
  OCD characteristics and, 264
Speech, converting thoughts/emotions to,
  35–36

Spence Child Anxiety Scale—Parent
  Version, 89
Staff training, for social skills summer
  program, 212
STAMP, 153–164, 307–308
  behavioral management in, 157
  CBT and, 153–154
  child eligibility for, 155
  Emotional Toolbox in, 152–153,
    158–159, 161–162
  exploring anxiety-anger in, 159–
    160
  exploring positive feelings in, 158–
    159
  future directions for, 164–166
  goal of, 153
  home projects for, 156
  overview of sessions, 158–163
  parental involvement in, 159, 161–162,
    308
  parental psychoeducation groups and,
    155
  relaxation tools in, 159–160
  research support for, 163–164
  room setup for, 155–156
  schedule for, 156
  therapist qualifications and number
    and, 154–155
  therapist training for, 154–155
  visual aids for, 156–157
Stereotyped interests module, 86
Stoicism, 5–6
Strengths and Difficulties Questionnaire,
  90
Stress, ASD and, 74–75
Stress and Anger Management Program
  (STAMP), 147–170; *see also*
  STAMP
Stress inoculation training, 11
Stress management, future directions for,
  165
Stress-o-meter, FYF and, 112–113
SULP approach; *see* Social Use of
  Language Programme (SULP)
Symptom severity, continuous measures
  of, 55, 56*t*
Systematic desensitization, 12
  for anxiety, 8
Systematic rational restructuring, 11

T

Tactile sensitivity, expressions of
 affection and, 266
Theory of mind
 assessment of, 58
 CBE interventions and, 248, 251
 Exploring Feelings program and,
  152
 interventions for, 237, 238–239
 notion of consent and, 281
 in STAMP, 160–161
Theory of Mind Inventory, 58
Thinking, inflexible, 32
Thinking tools, in STAMP, 160–161
Thoughts
 converting to speech, 35–36
 identifying, 160–161
 linking with feelings and behaviors,
  28
Time limits, 5
Token rewards, in SAS, 190–
  191

Transporters software, 284
Treatment targets, 208*t*
 derivation of, 205

V

Video, in anxiety treatment, 90
Vineland Adaptive Behavior Scales, 2nd
 edition, 56*t*
Visual aids, 15–16, 30
 for anxiety disorders/ASD, 77
 for STAMP, 156–157

W

Walk in the Forest measure, 270
Weak central coherence theory, 262
Wing, Lorna, 173
Workbooks, uses of, 39
Worry bugs, 112

Z

Zeno of Citium, 5–6